Basic Science Review
of
Anesthesiology

Basic Science Review
of
Anesthesiology

Guy L. Weinberg, M.D.

Editor

Assistant Professor of Anesthesiology
University of Illinois at Chicago College of Medicine
Staff Anesthesiologist
Veterans Administration West Side Medical Center
Chicago, Illinois

Associate Editors

Eric Moody, M.D.
David Stone, M.D.
Maria DeCastro, M.D.
Richard Berkowitz, M.D.
Charles Laurito, M.D.
Nancy Burk, M.D.
Timothy VadeBoncouer, M.D.
Guy Edelman, M.D.

McGRAW-HILL
Health Professions Division

New York   St. Louis   San Francisco   Auckland   Bogotá
Caracas   Lisbon   London   Madrid   Mexico City   Milan   Montreal
New Delhi   San Juan   Singapore   Sydney   Tokyo   Toronto

McGraw-Hill

A Division of The McGraw·Hill Companies

BASIC SCIENCE REVIEW OF ANESTHESIOLOGY

1234567890 MALMAL 9876

ISBN 0-07-069134-7

This book was set in Times Roman by Digitype, Inc.
The editors were Martin Wonsiewicz and Pamela Touboul;
the production supervisor was Anna Lieggi;
the cover designer was Marsha Cohen.
Malloy was printer and binder.

This book is printed on acid-free paper.

Library of Congress Cataloging-in-Publication Data

Basic science review of anesthesiology / editor, Guy L. Weinberg
     p.   cm.
   Includes bibliographical references and index.
   ISBN 0-07-069134-7
   1. Anesthesiology—Outlines, syllabi, etc.   2. Anesthesiology—
Examinations, questions, etc.   I. Weinberg, Guy.
   [DNLM: 1. Anesthetics—pharmacology—outlines.   2. Anesthetics—
pharmacology—examination questions.   3. Physiology—outlines.
4. Physiology—examination questions.   5. Anatomy, Regional—
outlines.   6. Anatomy, Regional—examination questions.   QV 18.2
B311 1997]
RD82.4.B37   1997
618.9′6′076—dc20
DNLM/DLC
for Library of Congress

This book is dedicated to
my wife and children,
the residents and staff of the Department of Anesthesiology at
the University of Illinois at Chicago College of Medicine,
and to the memory of
Dr. Harold Carron.

Contents

Contributors*

Associate Editors

Richard A. Berkowitz, MD [17]
Assistant Professor of Anesthesiology and Pediatrics
Director, Division of Pediatric Anesthesiology
University of Illinois at Chicago College of Medicine
Chicago, IL

Nancy S. Burk, MD [12, 13, 14, 16]
Assistant Professor of Anesthesiology
University of Illinois at Chicago College of Medicine
Chicago, IL

Maria A. DeCastro, MD [6, 10, 22]
Assistant Professor of Anesthesiology
University of Illinois at Chicago College of Medicine
Chicago, IL

Guy Edelman, MD [15]
Assistant Professor of Anesthesiology
University of Illinois at Chicago College of Medicine and
Staff Anesthesiologist
Veterans Administration West Side Medical Center
Chicago, IL

Charles Laurito, MD [4, 5, 19]
Associate Professor of Anesthesiology
Director, Pain Management Program
University of Illinois at Chicago College of Medicine
Chicago, IL

Eric Moody, MD [1, 2, 3]
Assistant Professor
Department of Anesthesiology and Critical Care Medicine
The Johns Hopkins Hospital
Baltimore, MD

David Stone, MD [21]
Assistant Professor of Anesthesia
Director of Neurosurgical Anesthesiology
University of Virginia
Charlottesville, VA

Timothy VadeBoncouer, MD [7, 8, 20]
Assistant Professor of Anesthesiology
University of Illinois at Chicago College of Medicine and
Staff Anesthesiologist
Veterans Administration West Side Medical Center
Chicago, IL

Theodore Alston, MD, PhD [1]
Associate Professor of Anesthesia
Harvard Medical School
Boston, MA

Juan Chediak, MD [15]
Associate Professor of Medicine
Rush Presbyterian St. Luke's Medical Center
Chicago, IL
Director of Thrombosis and Hemostasis Laboratory
Illinois Masonic Medical Center

Andrew Chenelle, MD [21]
Chief Resident, Neurological Surgery
University of Virginia Health Sciences Center
Medical Center, Box 395
Charlottesville, VA

Robin Chorn, BSc, MBChB, FRCP(C) [24]
Assistant Professor of Anesthesiology
University of Southern California
Los Angeles, California

*The numbers in brackets following the contributor name refer
to chapter(s) authored or coauthored by contributor.

James Christon, MD [9]
Fellow, Respiratory and Critical Care Medicine
University of Illinois at Chicago College of Medicine
Chicago, IL

Steven Donatello, MD [13]
Fellow, Memorial Sloan-Kettering Cancer Center
Cornell University Medical Center
NY, NY

Phillip Factor, DO [9]
Associate Director of Intensive Care
Pulmonary and Critical Care Medicine
Michael Reese Hospital
Assistant Professor of Medicine
University of Illinois at Chicago College of Medicine
Chicago, IL

Jeffrey E. Fletcher, PhD [8]
Professor of Anesthesiology and Biochemistry
Medical College of Pennsylvania and Hahnemann University
School of Medicine
Philadelphia, PA

Benjamin Gruber, MD, PhD, FACS [23]
Assistant Professor of Otolaryngology
University of Illinois at Chicago College of Medicine
Attending Physician, Department of Head Neck Surgery
Michael Reese Hospital
Chicago, IL

Bradford Harris, MD [2]
Neuroscience Fellow
Laboratory of Neuroscience
National Institute of Diabetes, Digestive and Kidney
Disorders
National Institute of Health
Bethesda, MD

Hugh C. Hemmings, Jr, MD, PhD [3]
Associate Professor of Anesthesiology and Pharmacology
Director of Research in Anesthesiology
Cornell University Medical College
NY, NY

J. Michael Jaeger, MD, PhD [11]
Assistant Professor of Anesthesiology and Neurological
Surgery
University of Virginia Health Sciences Center
Charlottesville, VA

Bruce James, MD [7]
Staff Anesthesiologist
Iowa Methodist Medical Center
University of Iowa College of Medicine
Des Moines, IO

James R. Laidler, MD [5]
Director of Pain Management
Providence Alaska Medical Center
Anchorage, Alaska

James P. Lash, MD [14]
Assistant Professor of Medicine
University of Illinois at Chicago College of Medicine
Chicago, IL

Barry S. Levin, MD [12]
Assistant Professor of Anesthesia and Critical Care Medicine
Northwestern University Medical Center
Chicago, IL

Timothy McDonald, MD [17]
Assistant Professor of Pediatrics and Anesthesiology
University of Illinois at Chicago College of Medicine
Director of Anesthesia Services, Eye and Ear Infirmary
University of Illinois at Chicago College of Medicine
Chicago, IL

Janet R. Newman, MD [18]
Assistant Professor of Anesthesiology
University of Illinois at Chicago College of Medicine and
Staff Anesthesiologist
Veterans Administration West Side Medical Center
Chicago, IL

Christopher Shaffrey, MD [21]
Assistant Professor of Neurological Surgery
University of Virginia Health Sciences Center
Charlottesville, VA

Mark Shaffrey, MD [21]
Assistant Professor of Neurological Surgery
University of Virginia Health Sciences Center
Charlottesville, VA

Sabet M. Siddiqui, MD [15]
Fellow, Hematology and Oncology
Rush Presbyterian St. Luke's Medical Center
Chicago, IL

Timothy P. Staudacher, MD [14]
Assistant Professor of Anesthesiology
University of Illinois at Chicago College of Medicine
Chicago, IL

Paul E. Stensrud, MD [10]
Instructor of Anesthesiology
Mayo Graduate School of Medicine
Mayo Medical School
Rochester, MN

Jaye J. Stricker, MD [4]
Staff Anesthesiologist and Pain Management Specialist
Marshfield Clinic, Inverventional Pain Management Clinic
Marshfield, WI

Guy L. Weinberg, MD [8, 10]
Assistant Professor of Anesthesiology
University of Illinois at Chicago College of Medicine and
Staff Anesthesiologist
Veterans Administration West Side Medical Center
Chicago, IL

David Young, MD [16]
Attending Physician
Department of Anesthesiology
Lutheran General Hospital
Park Ridge, IL

Preface

Basic Science Review of Anesthesiology is designed to serve two purposes. First, it is a general survey of the basic scientific principles on which anesthesia practice is based, and, second, it is an aid to preparing for in-training and board examination. The term *basic science* is used here to specify the disciplines, among those typically addressed in the first 2 years of medical school, possessing the greatest relevance to anesthesiology. As anesthesiologists, we are fortunate to practice a medical discipline that is firmly moored to scientific principle. This fact does not diminish the art required in clinical anesthesia practice but certainly strengthens the logic and reasoning behind our therapeutic decisions.

What topics are most germane to the stated goal of this book? With a bit of effort and imagination, one can easily justify including disciplines at the extremes of a macroscopic-microscopic scientific spectrum. Population genetics, for instance, explains the observed frequency of pseudocholinesterase deficiency and the corresponding sensitivity to succinylcholine. Bioenergetics clarifies molecular dynamics at an end point of the oxygen stream that our specialty is dedicated to maintaining. However, clinical anesthesiology is rooted somewhere between these extremes. Our primary purpose is to stay pain and shepherd patients through the stress of an operation. Thus, ours is a humanistic specialty in both temperament and scale. It is also, at heart, rather simple. We administer drugs, establish vascular and airway access, perform nerve blocks, and monitor and maintain physiologic homeostasis. The scientific disciplines that correspond to these activities are pharmacology, physiology, and anatomy. Together, they reflect a perspective quite specific to the anesthesiologist. This is consistent with the old saw describing the anesthesiologist as the internist in the operating room. The surgeon has a structural take on the treatment of disease, while the internist uses a medicinal approach, and both rely on physiology to inform the pathway from clinical diagnosis to treatment. The anesthesiologist blends these viewpoints and obtains a distinct vantage point based essentially on an equal mix of pharmacology, physiology, and anatomy. Recognizing that we practice hands-on medicine in the best and truest sense of the term, I have chosen to cover the topics with the most palpable character and practical scale. They also happen to be those I believe are most important to the anesthesiologist.

Although not entirely separable into these categories, the chapters are generally divided into sections corresponding to the three topics just described: pharmacology, physiology, and anatomy. The first eight chapters develop practical pharmacology from principles of pharmacokinetics and drug-receptor interaction to the specific pharmacologies of inhaled and intravenous anesthetics, local anesthetics, opioids, muscle relaxants, and cardiotonic agents; the latter chapter also provides an opportunity to address anatomy and physiology of the autonomic nervous system. The final chapter in this section, "Pharmacogenetic Disease," is limited to covering the mendelian traits that confer nonimmunologic hypersensitivity to anesthetic agents.

Chapters 9 through 19 comprise the physiology section. Chapters 9 through 15 bring a modern outlook to classical organ-system-based physiology. They cover lung, heart, nerve, liver, the endocrine organs, renal and acid-base physiology, and coagulation. Chapters 16 through 19 take on the special cases of maternofetal physiology, the extremes of age, and our current understanding of the phenomenon of pain. Chapter 19 also provides an opportunity to revisit the pharmacology of pain management.

Chapters 20 through 23 cover the anatomy topics most relevant to anesthesia practice. "Peripheral Neuroanatomy" provides a basis for performing nerve blocks. "Central Neuroanatomy" emphasizes the surgical considerations that inform neuroanesthesia perioperative care. The next chapters review cardiac anatomy as the anesthesiologist sees it, via transesophageal echocardiography, and airway anatomy, innervation, and embryology. Chapter 24 surveys the principles of basic physics as they pertain to the anesthesiologist.

Obviously, a book of this scope requires the efforts of a large number of dedicated individuals. First, I must acknowledge my family, without whose love, support, and incredible patience I would never have completed this undertaking. The colleagues who agreed to assist in editing the 24 chapters herein deserve recognition and credit for their wisdom, persistence, and energy. I must also thank the many faculty members at the University of Illinois Hospital, Michael Reese Hospital, and the Veterans Administration West Side Medical Center whose efforts provided me the time and space required to finish this book. I thank Richard Berlin, MD for his assistance and contribution to sections in Chapter 8. Special recognition is due my editors, Michael Houston, Jamie Kircher, and Pamela Touboul, who directed me through the most difficult parts of this journey; Kate Nolan, the project manager, who got things done; Diane Raeke, the medical illustrator, whose drawings bring many difficult concepts into focus; and the secretarial staff in the several affiliated Departments of Anesthesiology, particularly Robin Saunders, Jeannine Drish, and Denise Marshall.

Introduction

One Anesthesiologist's View of Studying the Basic Sciences

Anesthesiology is a bastion of the generalist. This statement runs contrary to popularly held depictions of the specialty, but an anesthesiologist has more in common with a family practitioner than with practitioners of many narrowly defined clinical disciplines. Simply put, every organ system is subject to substantial alterations in the perioperative period, and, obversely, a pathologic condition of any organ system has a probable or potential effect on the course and conduct of the anesthesia care plan. The anesthesiologist's role differs from that of the medical generalist, not so much by the type of problem or organ system derangement, but rather by the differences in approach to diagnosing and managing such problems. The different settings demand different strategies. Whereas the medical clinic allows for reflective deliberation in caring for problems through chronic, iterative management, the operating room environment requires analytic solutions to most clinical issues. The time frame for such action is also significantly compressed in the operating suite compared to the clinic setting.

Therefore, the anesthesiologist must often rapidly integrate extensive information about several organ systems to choose an appropriate therapeutic course. Commonly, the clinical situation further requires the anesthesiologist to institute treatment while the diagnostic process is ongoing. Successfully applying a knowledge base to interpret a complex clinical data base, particularly under time pressure, requires a deeper understanding of how the systems in question work than is entailed by the ability merely to recall facts and figures. Some clinicians might call the necessary, distinguishing ingredient judgment. Judgment comes in part from experience, but it is also an outlook. It is derived from a way of seeing the big picture.

This book serves as both an adjunct to clinical practice and a study aid. It will serve both purposes more effectively if the reader approaches the material with the more subtle and challenging goal of finding the deeper meanings among the facts and figures. As described in the Preface, anesthesiology is uniquely based on a blend of three scientific disciplines: pharmacology, physiology, and anatomy. I propose a method of study and a way of thinking about these fields, each potentially daunting in their scope. This approach is based on three general principles of study plus three specific recommendations one can apply to any given subject. Finding the logical framework underlying this material allows one to build a coherent foundation on which to base further study and practice.

☐ THREE GENERAL PRINCIPLES OF STUDY

HEURISTIC TRIANGULATION

The concept of heuristic triangulation is based on the thesis that one achieves a better understanding of a concept by finding several ways of thinking about it or defining it. This is a bit like the parable of the blind men, each of whom sees an elephant differently in his mind's eye as he touches different parts of it. Imagine that they are normally sighted but blindfolded, and imagine further their amazement at removing the blindfolds. Suddenly, each of the different viewpoints is integrated into an entirely different, more comprehensive, and accurate image. The term *heuristic triangulation* is based on the analogy of navigating or positioning by triangulation. One gets a better fix on the meaning of a topic after viewing it from several angles. Further, one attains a deeper appreciation of any concept when one sees, as the unblinded viewers in the first allegory, that each of several definitions represents a different but equivalent way of describing the same thing.

Dead space, for instance encompasses several concepts, including 1) anatomic dead space, the volume of conducting, non-gas-exchanging airways, measured as the inflection point of the single-breath washout curve; 2) alveolar dead space, contributed by the alveoli which excrete gas with a carbon dioxide composition closer to that of inhaled gas than of arterial blood; 3) physiologic dead space, the sum of anatomic and alveolar dead space, or the difference between minute ventilation and alveolar ventilation; 4) the Bohr relationship, a measure of V_D/V_T, the ratio of dead space to tidal volume, or the wasted fraction of each tidal volume, given by the difference of arterial and mixed exhaled carbon dioxide tensions normalized to arterial carbon dioxide tension; 5) the ventilation-perfusion (V/Q) mismatch obverse to shunting, that is, ventilation in excess of perfusion and causing arterial hypercarbia, as opposed to arterial oxygen desaturation; 6) lung zone 1, that is, nondependent lung where alveolar pressure exceeds pulmonary capillary hydrostatic pressure; 7) the portion of a circle breathing system to the patient's side of the "Y" in the corrugated tubing; 8) the portion of any circuit, with or without valves, where end-tidal gases reside at end-exhalation, implying the risk of rebreathing alveolar gas; and so on. A similar litany of equivalent definitions can be surmised for virtually any important concept.

SEARCH FOR RECURRING THEMES

The search for commonalities, or recurring patterns and relationships where they are not immediately apparent, will reveal deeper meanings and understanding that make the additional effort worthwhile. One example of a recurring theme is provided by the frequent use of volume (V) and pressure (P) measurements in describing physiological relationships that are important to the anesthesiologist. Taking V as a function of P renders a curve whose slope is defined as compliance. Compliance curves are seen throughout a typical anesthesia text, particularly in chapters covering pulmonary physiology. The inverse function of compliance, P as a function of V, yields elastance. This curve is typically seen in descriptions of the cardiac cycle. The product of P and V, given by integration of the area under an elastance curve, provides an estimate, in certain systems, of work performed.

Another, but less obvious, recurring theme is given by the "elbow-in-the-curve" phenomenon, which describes the precipitous fall in function of a parenchymal organ only after a large portion of its physiologic reserve is spent. These organs comprise a large number repeating functional units, and the elbow is shown in curves graphing the fraction of remaining functional units versus some measure of organ performance. Examples of such organs, with the functional

unit, or horizontal axis, and measure of organ performance, or vertical axis, given respectively in parentheses, include lung (alveoli, arterial carbon dioxide tension), kidney (nephron, creatinine), liver (lobule or acinus, prothrombin time or serum albumin concentration), skeletal muscle (neuromuscular junction, twitch height). Thus, the elbow pattern recurs in many organs and is useful when thinking about the means to avoid aggravating functional deterioration in a patient at or near such an elbow.

SEARCH FOR THE PARADOX

Paradoxes abound in science, but usually at a relatively superficial level of understanding. Once the origin of a paradox is revealed, as made possible by a deeper understanding of underlying principles, the paradox generally evaporates. A typical paradox is given by asking whether the Starling curve is a measure of compliance or elastance, as defined above. This is related to the common description of how, of necessity, our typical means of measuring left ventricular preload—that is, the pulmonary artery occlusion pressure—is indirect at best. The vertical axis of the Starling curve one typically uses in the operating room is given by some volume or flow-related measure of cardiac performance, such as stroke volume or cardiac output. Meanwhile, the horizontal axis is given by an indirect measure of preload, say, the wedge pressure. However, the original Starling curve describes contractility as a function of myocardial presystolic stretch, or ventricular dimension. The paradox, then, is that, while the Starling curve we usually draw in the operating room is a compliance curve, the proper Starling relationship is actually given by the inverse function, an elastance curve.

☐ THREE SPECIFIC PRINCIPLES OF STUDY

METAPHOR AS MEANING

Virtually every obscure, arcane concept will yield some aspect of its meaning to the appropriate metaphor. Since the best metaphor to explain an idea often differs from person to person, the challenge to the reader is to find the one that best explains, for him/her, a specific difficult idea. The concept of tension, for instance, as given by the law of LaPlace, is relatively clear: it increases in a sphere as the radius increases. But what does this mean, and what is tension? The metaphor of a soap bubble makes the idea transparent for me. Blow a bubble, and you watch the radius and tension increase. What happens then? At some point the bubble bursts. After blowing many bubbles, it will occur to one that tension is the force vector within the bubble wall that has a direction tangential to the bubble surface in such a manner as to pull the bubble surface apart, causing it to explode. Now it is easy to see why the diameter of an aortic aneurysm is so important. The intramural tension, that is, the force causing it to rupture, is directly related to the aneurysm diameter.

Another conundrum is the relationship of cardiac work to myocardial oxygen consumption. Returning to the elastance curves described above, it is clear that the area within the cardiac cycle gives a measure of left ventricular work. I find it difficult to reconcile that this value, when normalized to a single contraction and the patient's body size (left ventricular stroke work index) does not correspond to myocardial oxygen consumption. However, if one returns to elastance, that is, pressure, or force, as a function of volume and thinks of a rubber band, elastance can be thought of as "snappiness." A lax rubber band (relaxed state) has no capacity to do work, but if one stretches a rubber band until it is taut (stretched state 1), further increases in diameter (to stretch state 2) provide energy that can be expended as the rubber band contracts, or "snaps," when returning to stretch state 1. Now visualize the rubber band as a left ventricle in the short-axis view on a transesophageal echocardiogram. The oscillation between two positions in a stretched state corresponds to the cardiac cycle: stretch state 1 is end systole, and stretch state 2 is end diastole. If one measures only the work done in each cycle, an important component of the total energy of the entire system is neglected: that required to move from the relaxed state to stretch state 1. Thus, an intrinsic part of the energy required for cardiac performance is that needed to stretch the heart into the dimensions where it can do useful work. The sum of energy expended in this manner, the potential energy, and that spent pumping blood, doing the external work of the cardiac cycle, accurately depicts myocardial oxygen consumption (Suga, 1990).

SEEK THE ORIGINAL SOURCES

Scientific assertions long separated from their original sources and often expressed as fact are passed from one generation of physicians to the next by practice, word of mouth, and text books. Propagation in this manner tends to fossilize material into dogma. Although blithly repeated and rarely questioned, such "facts" are often obsolete or incorrect, and the same can be said of the clinicians basing their practice on such data. Conversely, attaching an idea to its origins can enliven and strengthen it in the reader's mind, like putting a building onto its foundation. In the same way that I recommended viewing a topic from many directions, it is extremely revealing to review a pertinent literature base at various times during its development, looking forward and back. Reading the most recent articles on a topic is the obvious way to stay current. Understanding an idea, however, is also enhanced by reviewing its scientific origins and development. Taking a closer look, as it were, at the giants on whose shoulders our contemporary academicians are standing is al-

ways an interesting and valuable exercise, well worth the time.

Extending the example of dead space used above to illustrate this principle, one can trace the original measurement of anatomic dead space to Zuntz, who took postmortem casts of the tracheobronchial tree (Zuntz, 1882). The concept was later expanded by Bohr in his calculations of dead space (Bohr, 1891). Fowler pioneered the washout method of determining anatomic dead space (Fowler, 1948), and the concept of dead space has been subsequently refined many times (Fletcher, 1984).

SEARCH FOR CLINICAL IMPLICATIONS

Obviously, aside from the academic rewards, such intellectual exertions as described above gain substance only when they can be translated into better care of patients. The contemplation must have a practical application. Continuing the example of dead space, it is a valuable exercise to consider the clinical relevance of many of the several definitions given earlier. Consider that when a patient is hypotensive, the lung zone 1 is expanded due to pulmonary hypoperfusion. This is essentially an increase in dead space and so obtains in any situation where lung perfusion is dramatically reduced, as in pulmonary embolus (e.g., a clot, fat, or amniotic fluid) or overdose with a vasodilator (e.g., an inadvertently administered bolus of nitroprusside). In these situations, the event can be detected by a sharp reduction of end-tidal carbon dioxide and an increase in the arterial-end tidal P_{CO_2} difference. The latter quantity is a rough equivalent of the Bohr relationship measure of dead space, which is properly given by the difference between the arterial and the *mixed* exhaled P_{CO_2}. Since the capnograph is the only simple measure we have of organ perfusion in the operating room, a normal trace is comforting in patients whose other monitors are for some reason obscured. Obversely, an abrupt, severe drop in exhaled carbon dioxide reflects a corresponding increase in dead space and indicates a serious problem. Consider also that virtually all circuits, with and without valves, are designed to minimize the rebreathing of end-tidal gases, in other words, to reduce dead space. The efficiency of every Mapelson circuit is given by a diagram that shows the relative position of the mask, corrugated tubing, reservoir bag, pop-off valve, and fresh gas flow. This indicates the path of end-tidal gases between end exhalation and inhalation and therefore yields a measure of the effective dead space created by the circuit for any given ratio of fresh gas inflow and minute ventilation.

Applying all of these several techniques of study will require more thought, time, and effort than simply committing the fine details to memory. However, this approach will also provide a better understanding of the scientific principles on which our practice is based. It offers the possibility of speeding the acquisition of that aforementioned trait we all seek: judgment.

BIBLIOGRAPHY

Bohr C: Über die Lungenathmung. *Skand Arch Physiol* 2:236, 1891.

Fletcher R: Airway dead space, end-tidal CO_2 and Christian Bohr. *Acta Anaesthesiol Scand* 28:408, 1984.

Fowler WS: Lung function studies: Part 2, The respiratory dead space. *Am J Physiol* 154:405, 1948.

Suga H: Cardiac mechanics and energetics: from E_{max} to PVA. *Front Med Biol Eng* 2:3, 1990.

Zuntz N: Physiologie der Blutgase und des respiratorischen Gaswechsels. *Hermann's Handb Physiol* 4:1, 1882.

Basic Science Review
of
Anesthesiology

Pharmacokinetics and Drug-Receptor Interactions

Theodore A. Alston

Pharmacology is often divided conceptually into kinetics and dynamics. Pharmacokinetics has been aptly called "what the body does to the drug," while pharmacodynamics is "what the drug does to the body." Pharmacokinetics, then, deals with the absorption, distribution, and elimination of drugs. Most often, pharmacokinetic parameters relate those processes to the plasma concentration of a drug.

☐ ONE-COMPARTMENT MODEL AND FIRST-ORDER KINETICS

First-order reactions are those in which the velocity is directly proportional to the concentration of the reactant. At high concentrations of the reactant, an enzyme or transport protein required to degrade or eliminate the reactant may become saturated so that an additional increase in reactant concentration cannot increase reaction velocity. Under saturating conditions, reaction velocity is independent of reactant concentration and said to be of zero order. Zero-order kinetics are unusual in pharmacology, but ethanol, aspirin and barbiturates at very high doses, are often cited as examples of drugs that sometimes saturate their metabolizing enzymes. The rate at which halothane is oxidized by the liver probably also achieves saturation velocity under some clinical circumstances.

Absorption, distribution, and elimination tend to be first-order exponential processes. The rate of a first-order process is directly proportional to the concentration of the reactant. For instance, consider the slow rate of absorption of a hypothetical drug from a subcutaneous depot. Suppose that, once absorbed, the drug rapidly and reversibly distributes throughout the tissues of the body to which there is access. Kinetically, then, the body can be regarded as comprising a single compartment for the drug. For further simplicity, suppose that the rate of elimination is negligible. Figure 1–1 shows the expected plot of plasma concentration versus time. The plasma concentration rises at an initial rate, which halves as the size of the drug depot halves. The first-order process can be completely described by its half-time and its final value.

The half-time is the time during which the amount of drug in the depot, and its rate of absorption decreases by 50%. A short half-time indicates rapid absorption, while a long half-time indicates that a long time is required for absorption to approach completion. A first-order process is essentially complete after four or five half-times. That is, four half-times are required for the process to become 93.75% complete (50% + 25% + 12.5% + 6.25%). Strictly speaking, a first-order process can closely approach but never actually reach completion.

Half-times ($t_{1/2}$) are interchangeable with first-order rate constants (k). The relationship is given in Eq. 1, where the natural logarithm of 2 is approximately 0.693:

$$t_{1/2} = (\ln 2)/k \qquad (1)$$

Since the parameters are reciprocally related, a high rate constant indicates that the process approaches completion quickly. Rate constants have dimensions of reciprocal time. Suppose, for instance, that a process has a half-time of 69.3 min. The rate constant for the process, then, is 0.01 min^{-1}, and the process reaches almost 1.0% of completion during the first minute.

The use of rate constants stems from the calculus of first-order exponentials. If D_0 is the initial size of a depot from which drug is absorbed via first-order kinetics, then $D = D_0 e^{-kt}$ and $dD/dt = -k$. Since $D = D_0/2$ when $t = t_{1/2}$, then $1/2 = e^{-k(t_{1/2})}$. Taking logarithms of the terms of the last equation provides Eq. 1.

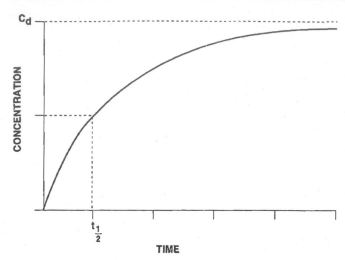

Figure 1–1 First-order absorption of a hypothetical drug exhibiting a relatively negligible rate of elimination. The absorption is 94% complete after four half-times.

As mentioned, the plot in Fig. 1–1 needs two parameters for complete description. In addition to a parameter for the rate at which absorption approaches completion, a parameter providing the extent of distribution is required. In the hypothetical case of Fig. 1–1 (rapid distribution, negligible rate of elimination), the plasma concentration that is approached with time is the concentration achieved when the entire dose of the drug is completely distributed throughout the phases of the body to which there is access. This concentration, C_d, is directly proportional to the dose of the drug. That is, doubling the dose under the conditions of Fig. 1–1 will double the concentration that the drug approaches. The proportionality constant may be viewed as a dose-independent parameter. Consequently, the extent of distribution of a drug is usually expressed in terms of this parameter, V_d, the volume of distribution:

$$\text{Systemic dose} = V_d C_d \qquad (2)$$

V_d is an imaginary volume into which a drug would apparently distribute if its tissue concentrations at equilibrium were equal to that of the plasma. The higher the V_d (which can exceed the volume of the body), the greater the extent of distribution from the plasma to other sites. V_d values are somewhat predictable on the basis of molecular structure. For instance, highly charged water-soluble drugs (e.g., pancuronium) typically exhibit V_d values approximating the size of the extracellular fluid volume (about 0.3 L/kg), whereas lipid-soluble drugs (e.g., propofol) exhibit large V_d values. Dose and V_d are usually normalized to body mass, in which case V_d is given in units of liters per kilogram. Alternatively, the V_d may be normalized with respect to body surface area and given in units of liters per square meter.

The V_d is calculated from the amount of drug that reaches the systemic circulation. That quantity may be less than the total dose of the drug. For instance, only part of an enterally administered drug may prove to be absorbed into the portal bloodstream. Furthermore, a large fraction of the drug that reaches the portal bloodstream may prove to be eliminated by the liver and so not reach the systemic circulation. The ability of the liver to block enterally absorbed drugs from reaching the systemic circulation is termed the first-pass effect.

Drug absorption adds drug to the conceptual volume of distribution, while elimination removes drug from that volume. However, both processes can often be described by means of first-order rate constants. The progress curve of Fig. 1–2 exhibits an absorption phase and an elimination phase, for which k_{abs} and k_{elim} can be respectively assigned. Again, when distribution is rapid with respect to absorption and elimination, then the rate of distribution of the drug from the plasma to the various tissues of the body is not kinetically significant, and the body can be viewed as constituting one compartment for the drug. The size of the imaginary single compartment is given by the V_d value, which can be defined and determined in various ways. When, as in the case of Fig. 1–2, more than one exponential term is involved in the calculation of the V_d, one approach is to calculate $V_{d\,(area)}$ from the area under the concentration versus time curve (AUC):

$$V_{d\,(area)} = (\text{systemic dose})\text{AUC}^{-1}k_{elim}^{-1} \qquad (3)$$

Elimination kinetics are often discussed in terms of a parameter termed clearance:

$$\text{Clearance} - V_d k_{elim} \qquad (4)$$

For a drug that is carried by the plasma (rather than by the blood cells), clearance is the flow of plasma (generally normalized per kilogram of body mass) from which the drug must be completely removed to account for the rate of elimination of a thoroughly distributed drug. For instance, if a parenterally administered drug is eliminated from the plasma

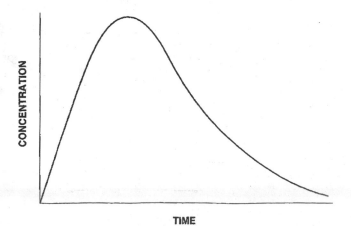

Figure 1–2 Biphasic profile of a drug which is detectably eliminated during the sampling period. Rate constants can be assigned to the absorption phase and to the elimination phase.

exclusively by the liver, then the clearance of the drug would be less than or equal to the rate of hepatic plasma flow. Similarly, a drug that is eliminated exclusively by the kidneys exhibits a clearance that is less than or equal to the renal plasma flow. A clearance value exceeding the cardiac output of plasma would imply that a drug is eliminated in the bloodstream, for instance, by a circulating esterase.

Equations 3 and 4 can be combined to afford Eq. 5:

$$\text{Total clearance} = (\text{systemic dose})\text{AUC}^{-1} \qquad (5)$$

Equation 5 is analogous to the Stewart-Hamilton equation, used to calculate cardiac output from thermodilution data. A small AUC indicates high clearance of drug or high flow of indicator.

Clearance can be calculated from the rate of disappearance of drug from the blood or from the rate of appearance of voided drug. For instance, urinary clearance of drugs can be calculated according to Eq. 6, also used to calculate the creatinine clearance ability of the kidneys:

$$\text{Urinary clearance} = (\text{urine flow})\,C_{\text{plasma}}C_{\text{urine}}^{-1} \qquad (6)$$

Clearance depends upon two types of processes: excretion and biotransformation. Excretion refers to the removal of intact drug molecules from the body via the bile, urine, or exhaled breath. Biotransformation refers to the covalent destruction of drug molecules. Biotransformation is generally mediated by enzymes, although atracurium is an example of a drug that can undergo nonenzymatic destruction in the plasma.

☐ TWO-COMPARTMENT MODEL

The kinetics of drug distribution cannot always be neglected. Many drugs administered as an intravenous bolus achieve an initial plasma concentration that declines in a biphasic manner. The two phases are particularly apparent from semilogarithmic plots exemplified by Fig. 1–3. An initial rapid phase of drug decline can be ascribed largely to distribution of the drug from the plasma to extravascular sites. After distribution nears completion, a slower phase of drug decline becomes evident and can be ascribed primarily to drug elimination. Rate constants for the distribution and elimination phases are usually designated α and β, respectively. The y-intercept of the alpha phase of Fig. 1–3 can be used to calculate the volume of the so-called central compartment and provides a measure of the peak plasma concentration expected from a rapid intravenous bolus of drug. The volume of distribution can be variously defined but is often calculated according to Eq. 3, taking β to be k_{elim}.

A two-compartment model is sometimes inadequate to describe the rate at which C_{plasma} declines following an intravenous injection. When a triphasic progress curve is obtained, the first phase is ascribed mainly to distribution of drug into richly perfused tissues. The second phase is caused mainly by distribution of drug into less-perfused tissues. The final phase is again ascribed largely to elimination.

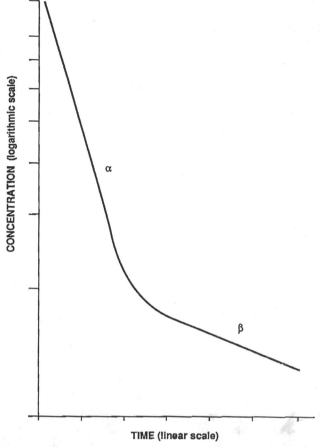

Figure 1–3 Semilogarithmic profile of an intravenously injected drug exhibiting kinetically detectable distribution and relatively slow elimination.

☐ STEADY STATE

It is often desirable to maintain a nearly constant plasma concentration of a drug. In the case of intravenously administered drugs that can be described by means of a one-compartment model, the V_d value permits calculation of the size of the loading dose required for the targeted concentration (Eq. 2). The maintenance dose is then given by the product of the loading dose and k_{elim}. The maintenance dose can be provided as continuous infusion or by periodic boluses of the drug. In the latter case, the steadiness of the plasma concentration will, or course, depend on the frequency of the maintenance doses. For instance, the plasma level will fall by more than 50% between doses if the maintenance doses are spaced apart by intervals longer than $0.693/k_{\text{elim}}$ (Eq. 1).

Intravenous infusion at a given rate will ultimately achieve the same steady-state plasma concentration of drug whether or not a loading dose is provided (Fig. 1–4). In the case of a drug described by a one-compartment model, the concentration of drug at plateau provides a V_d value according to Eq. 7, and the V_d so measured is termed the volume of distribution at steady state:

$$\text{Infusion rate} = V_{d(ss)}C_{ss}k_{\text{elim}} \qquad (7)$$

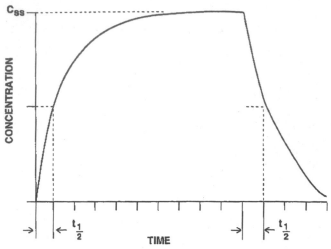

Figure 1–4 Achievement of a steady plasma concentration of drug by means of intravenous infusion at a constant rate. In case of a drug described by a one-compartment model, the concentration rises in a first-order process described by a rate constant equal to that for the fall in concentration upon termination of the infusion.

The time required for the infusion to nearly achieve the steady-state plasma level of drug depends on the elimination rate constant. The plasma concentration will reach 50% of the steady-state value after one elimination $t_{1/2}$ and will reach 93.75% of C_{ss} value after four times the elimination $t_{1/2}$ value. Loading doses, then, are generally required for drugs that exhibit slow elimination rate constants (long elimination half-times).

☐ REDISTRIBUTION

Pharmacokinetic measurements of drug concentration generally involve blood sampling because of the availability of blood specimens. However, drug concentrations in various tissues may not be related to plasma levels in a simple manner. For instance, an intravenous bolus of thiopental will rapidly achieve its peak tissue levels in the brain and other richly perfused tissues. The peak tissue level in muscle tissue occurs several minutes after that in the brain, and the peak tissue level in poorly perfused adipose tissue may not occur until over an hour after the injection (see Chap. 3). This phenomenon of drug transfer into richly perfused tissue and then out to less well-perfused tissues is termed redistribution. Alterations in redistribution caused, for instance, by hypo-volemia can significantly potentiate the actions of a given dose of thiopental. In case of hypovolemia, blood flow to the brain and heart tends to be preserved at the expense of blood flow to other tissues, and the rate of drug redistribution is thereby slowed.

Despite rich perfusion of the central nervous system, the blood-brain diffusion barrier may prevent brain levels of a drug from equilibrating with the plasma levels. For instance, morphine is more polar than fentanyl and is less able to diffuse through the barrier in either direction. Consequently, following intravenous injections, the peak action of morphine

on the brain occurs later than that of fentanyl. In a more extreme example, the tertiary amine physostigmine exhibits anticholinesterase activity in the brain, while the quaternary amine neostigmine does not reach the central nervous system.

☐ RECEPTORS

Absorption and distribution generally bring a given drug to the site of pharmaceutical action, while further distribution (redistribution) and elimination remove the drug from its site of action. In most cases, the pharmaceutical effect is caused by interaction of the drug molecule with a discrete macromolecular structure termed the receptor. Pharmacodynamics deals, first, with the interaction of a drug with its receptor and, second, with the ensuing biological response.

Macromolecular receptors for drugs are usually proteins or protein-containing structures. As outlined in Table 1–1, examples include enzymes (acetylcholinesterase for neostigmine), voltage-gated ion channels (axonal sodium channels for local anesthetics), and chemically gated ion channels (nicotinic receptors). In many cases, the receptor for an exogenous drug ordinarily functions as a receptor for some neurotransmitter, hormone, or other endogenous regulatory molecule. Classically, the concept of receptors for drugs evolved concomitantly with the concept of receptors for neurotransmitters. In particular, acetylcholine receptors were among the first entities to be appreciated as receptors for bioactive molecules. A key element leading to the concept of discrete receptors was the availability of blocking compounds (antagonists) that could bind to the receptors and so prevent stimulants (agonists) from binding and eliciting responses. For instance, atropine blocked the stimulant effect of pilocarpine on salivation, and curare blocked the ability of nicotine to contract skeletal muscle.

Quantification of drug-receptor interactions is facilitated by concentration-response curves (or, similarly, dose-response curves) such as those in Fig. 1–5. At low levels of the drug, the strength of the response increases as the concentration of the drug increases. Increasing the drug concentration eventually achieves a level at which essentially all of the drug-binding sites are occupied by drug. At full occupancy (saturation) of the receptors, the response is maximal; further increases in drug concentration will not increase the strength of the response. In the simplest of cases, the concentration-response curve has the shape of a hyperbola (Fig. 5a). In practice, most curves prove to have a sigmoid shape (Fig. 5b) and thus resemble the Bohr curve of hemoglobin (saturation versus P_{O_2}). A sigmoid curve suggests that the receptor is polymeric (e.g., hemoglobin, a tetramer) and that the subunits exhibit cooperativity. A hyperbola can be completely described by two parameters, usually the maximal response and the drug concentration, termed EC_{50}, at which response is half-maximal. Sigmoid curves require an additional parameter for complete description, and the Hill coefficient, originally applied to hemoglobin, is one such descrip-

Table 1–1
SELECTED EXAMPLES OF SOME COMMONLY RECOGNIZED CLASSES OF RECEPTORS

ENZYMES

Acetylcholinesterase is directly inhibited by neostigmine.
Phosphodiesterase is inhibited by amrinone.
Many antibiotics are inhibitors of microbial enzymes.
Vitamin K-dependent enzymes are inhibited by dicumarol.
Heparin facilitates inactivation of thrombin.
Guanylate cyclase is activated by nitroprusside.

ION PUMPS

The gastric proton pump is inhibited by omeprazole.
Na,K-ATPase is inhibited by digoxin.

VOLTAGE-GATED ION CHANNELS

Verapamil blocks calcium channels.
Lidocaine blocks axonal sodium channels.

LIGAND-GATED ION CHANNELS

Striated muscle nicotinic sodium channels are activated (and then
   desensitized) by succinylcholine or blocked by pancuronium.
GABA-gated chloride channels are positively modulated by
   diazepam in a manner blocked by flumazenil.

G PROTEIN-COUPLED RECEPTORS

β-Adrenergic receptors are activated by isoproterenol or blocked by
   propranolol and are coupled via G proteins to adenylate cyclase.
Opioid receptors are activated by fentanyl or blocked by naloxone
   and are coupled via G proteins to adenylate cyclase.
α_1-Adrenergic receptors are activated by phenylephrine or blocked
   by phentolamine and are coupled via G proteins to transducers
   other than adenylate cyclase.

MEMBRANE-SPANNING PROTEIN KINASE

The insulin receptor binds extracellular hormone, with resultant
   stimulation of the tyrosine-specific protein kinase activity of its
   cytosolic domain.

LIGAND-ACTIVATED TRANSCRIPTION FACTORS

The steroid hormones and drugs activate these cytoplasmic and
   nuclear proteins.

---

tion of the sigmoidicity of a concentration-response curve. Sigmoidicity (caused by cooperativity of receptors) increases the steepness of part of a concentration-response curve so that, at drug concentrations near the EC_{50}, there is increased response to a small change in drug concentration.

Two of the parameters used to describe an agonist, then, are the maximal magnitude of its response and the EC_{50} value, the concentration at which the response is half-maximal. The former parameter is a measure of the efficacy (or power or strength) of the agonist, and the latter parameter is a measure of the potency of the agonist. For instance, drug C of Fig. 1–5 is more efficacious than drug B, but drug B is more potent than drug C.

Agonist drugs bind to a receptor, and, upon binding, cause a conformational change in the receptor that produces the response. Congeners (mechanistically similar drugs sharing a receptor) can vary in ability to bind to the receptor and thus vary in EC_{50} values. Congeners can also vary in ability to cause the receptor to elicit the response. Thus, when compared to drug C, drug B of Fig. 1–5 may be termed a partial agonist. One example of a partial agonist in anesthesia is the analgesic pentazocine, which is less efficacious than morphine at opioid receptors.

Other drugs, termed antagonists, bind to a given receptor but are virtually unable to cause the receptor to elicit the response. Antagonists can thus block the effects of agonists. A variety of receptor-blocking drugs are commonly administered during anesthetic care, including naloxone, atropine, pancuronium, propranolol, flumazenil, and diphenhydramine, to name a few. Furthermore, through competition for the receptor, a drug of low efficacy can partially block the effect of a drug of high efficacy, and the partial agonist pentazocine is therefore sometimes termed an agonist-antagonist.

Attachment of a drug to its binding site on a receptor involves complementarity of surfaces and is often likened to the fitting of a key in a lock. All sorts of chemical bonds can be involved: ionic bonds, ion-dipole and dipole-dipole interactions, van der Waals forces, hydrophobic interactions, charge-transfer complexation, and aromatic stacking. In some cases, even covalent bonds are involved. For instance, the α-adrenergic blocking agent phenoxybenzamine is long-acting because it covalently attaches to its receptor. Covalent attachment of drugs to receptors is common in the case of receptors that are enzymes. For instance, long-acting monoamine oxidase (MAO) inhibitors become covalently bound to MAO, neostigmine transiently attaches to acetylcholinesterase, and penicillin reacts covalently with bacterial cell-wall enzymes.

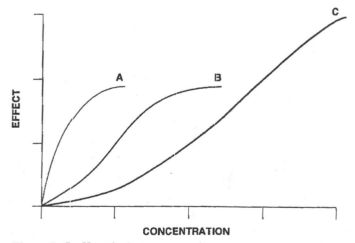

Figure 1–5 Hypothetical concentration—response curves. Curve A is hyperbolic while curves B and C are sigmoid. A hyperbolic curve is expected when receptors function independently, while a sigmoid curve indicates cooperativity among interactive receptor molecules. Drug B is more potent than drug C, but drug C is more efficacious than drug B.

In many cases of drugs with well-defined receptors, it is possible to appreciate the structural similarity of the drugs to endogenous agonists. For instance, all of the commonly used neuromuscular blocking agents resemble acetylcholine in structure.

☐ SIGNAL TRANSDUCTION

The binding of an agonist to its receptor has to be transduced into a response. Attractive forces between the drug and the receptor change the shape of the receptor, and this conformational change sets off other biochemical events that culminate in the response. The series of biochemical events can be complex and is ill-defined in most cases. The complexity is well-illustrated by the β-adrenergic receptor, activated by isoproterenol and blocked by propranolol.

As outlined in Table 1–2, one β-adrenergic effect of isoproterenol is to stimulate glycogen breakdown in skeletal muscle and the liver. This intracellular response is triggered by extracellular isoproterenol. The drug binds to β-receptors on the cell surface. The receptor then changes conformation, and this event triggers conformational changes in other proteins in contact with the receptor. These proteins are called G proteins because their function requires the guanine nucleotides GTP and GDP. The activated G proteins contact and activate adenylate cyclase, an enzyme present on the inner aspect of the cell membrane. The activated enzyme then converts cytoplasmic ATP into cyclic AMP (cAMP), which is then said to function as a second messenger for the isopro-

Table 1–2
STEPS IN THE STIMULATION OF GLYCOGENOLYSIS BY ISOPROTERENOL

1. Isoproterenol binds to a complementary cleft in the adrenergic receptor protein on the cell surface.
2. A conformational change in the receptor permits the receptor to bind to and perturb a membrane-bound G protein complex (composed of three subunits).
3. The G protein subunit on the inner aspect of the membrane releases bound GDP in exchange for cytosolic GTP.
4. Binding of the GTP causes dissociation of the G protein trimer.
5. The G protein subunit bearing the GTP then binds to and activates adenylate cyclase on the cytosolic aspect of the cell membrane.
6. The activated cyclase converts cytosolic ATP to cAMP.
7. The cAMP diffuses through the cytosol and binds to regulatory subunits of soluble protein kinase.
8. The regulatory subunits dissociate from protein kinase and thereby activate the kinase.
9. Protein kinase uses ATP to phosphorylate other enzymes.
10. Phosphorylation of glycogen synthetase turns that enzyme off, while the enzyme that breaks down glycogen is turned on by phosphorylation.
11. Negative regulation is provided by the hydrolytic cleavage of phosphate ester linkages in the GTP, the cAMP, and/or the phosphoproteins.

terenol. The cAMP diffuses through the cytoplasm and binds to a regulatory site on an enzyme, protein kinase. The protein kinase is inactive in the absence of bound cAMP. Upon activation, the kinase covalently modifies other enzymes by transferring phosphate groups from ATP to the enzymes. In this case, the enzyme that generates glycogen is turned off by phosphorylation, and the enzyme that breaks down glycogen is turned on by phosphorylation.

There are many variations on Table 1–2. Many surface receptors are linked to G protein transducers, but these transducers can be coupled to a number of effector systems. For instance, α_2-adrenergic receptors activate alternative G proteins, which, in turn, inhibit adenylate cyclase instead of activating the enzyme. In other cases, G proteins can control ion channels and/or control enzymes other than adenylate cyclase. In addition to cAMP, then, second messengers include cyclic GMP and inositol phosphates. Furthermore, various protein kinases differ in their regulatory properties and substrate preferences.

In another large group of receptors, signals are transduced through membranes without G proteins as intermediaries. Many drug receptors are ion channels that necessarily span the cell membrane and bind drugs in various ways. Examples include chemically gated channels, voltage-gated channels, and ion pumps. Since chemically gated channels are opened by neurotransmitters, they can be activated or blocked by structural analogs of the respective neurotransmitter. For instance, the nicotinic receptors of skeletal muscle are acetylcholine-gated sodium channels, which can be activated (and then desensitized) by succinylcholine or blocked by pancuronium. The opening of the sodium channel of the nicotinic receptor by acetylcholine has recently been imaged by means of electron microscopy. The ion channel or pore of that protein is lined by five α-helical segments, which tend to come together as a gate in the absence of acetylcholine. Binding of acetylcholine to two of the segments results in transient rotation of the subunits and opening of the pore.

Other drugs bind to regulatory sites on chemically gated channels. For instance, the γ-aminobutyric acid ($GABA_A$) receptors of the central nervous system are chloride channels opened upon binding of synaptically transmitted GABA. Many anesthetic drugs significantly perturb that receptor at regulatory sites. Thus, diazepam potentiates the effect of GABA on chloride conductance, and flumazenil blocks the diazepam effect. Voltage-gated ion channels also possess regulatory sites that can bind drugs. For example, diltiazem blocks certain calcium channels. Other drugs, such as digoxin or omeprazole, block the ability of ion pumps to utilize ATP.

The vast majority of drugs, then, bind to structurally complementary receptors that are proteins, and the binding ultimately leads to either the activation or inhibition of an enzyme or an ion channel. However, the coupling of the drug-binding site to the enzyme or channel can be direct or else quite tortuous. *Whether volatile anesthetics act in this fashion is a topic of debate and is discussed in the next chapter.*

BIBLIOGRAPHY

Abeles RH, Frey PA, Jencks WP: *Biochemistry.* Boston, Jones and Bartlett, 1992.

Higashida H, Yoshioka T, Mikoshiba K: *Molecular Basis of Ion Channels and Receptors Involved in Nerve Excitation, Synaptic Transmission and Muscle Contraction.* New York, New York Academy of Science, 1993.

Hughes MA, Glass PSA, Jacobs JR: Context-sensitive half-time in multicompartment pharmacokinetic models for intravenous anesthetic drugs. *Anesthesiology* 76:334–341, 1992.

Jencks WP: Catalysis in Chemistry and Enzymology. New York, Dover, 1987.

Shafer SL, Varvel JR: Pharmacokinetics, pharmacodynamics, and rational opioid selection. *Anesthesiology* 74:53–63, 1991.

Silverman RB: *The Organic Chemistry of Drug Design and Drug Action.* San Diego, Academic Press, 1992.

Unwin N: Acetylcholine receptor channel imaged in the open state. *Nature* 373:37–43, 1995.

Walsh C: *Enzymatic Reaction Mechanisms.* New York, Freeman, 1979.

2 Inhalational Anesthetics

Bradford Harris and Eric Moody

Volatile anesthetics have been the mainstay of clinical anesthesia for nearly 150 years. While these agents remain the backbone of clinical anesthesia, they are frequently used in combination with other drugs, such as barbiturates, benzodiazepines, and opiates, as well as with regional anesthesia. These balanced and combined techniques exploit the desirable characteristics of various agents by limiting the doses of each. This chapter discusses the kinetics and pharmacology of inhalation anesthetics and their various organ system effects.

PHYSICAL CHARACTERISTICS

Inhalational anesthetics differ from most other drugs in that they are volatile liquids that are administered as gas. Thus, special equipment is needed to administer them and monitor their concentrations. By administering these agents via the lungs, various kinetic factors become an issue. The structures of commonly used volatile agents are shown in Fig. 2–1, and the physical characteristics of several anesthetics are summarized in Table 2–1.

The relative lack of safety of volatile anesthetics is an important feature of these drugs. These agents possess low therapeutic indices compared to most other classes of drugs. The therapeutic index is the ratio of the LD_{50} to the ED_{50}. The therapeutic index of volatile anesthetics is about 2 to 4 as compared to 300 to 1000 for potent opiates such as sufentanil. This narrow therapeutic index results from significant toxic effects on organs such as the heart.

Since volatile anesthetics are therapeutic at high micromolar to low millimolar concentrations, the agents are much less potent than many other commonly used drugs. For example, benzodiazepines act in the low nanomolar range and are

about 10,000 times more potent than volatile anesthetics. This low potency of volatile anesthetics may contribute to the prevalence of side effects, since high concentrations of the anesthetics are found in all tissues.

PHARMACOKINETICS OF VOLATILE ANESTHETICS

When volatile anesthetics are administered to a patient, there exist a number of gradients between the source of the anesthetic and the target site in the body. Since the desired effect—anesthesia—depends on the anesthetic concentration in the central nervous system (CNS), an understanding of these pharmacokinetic parameters is of considerable importance. During the induction of anesthesia the highest concentration of volatile anesthetic is found in the anesthesia machine output, with correspondingly lower concentrations in the inspired gas, the alveoli, the arterial blood, and various tissues. The rate of equilibration of each of these sites is determined by the solubility of the drug, the concentration gradient, and the delivery of anesthetic. When the volatile anesthetic is at equilibrium, the partial pressures are identical in the brain, systemic arterial blood, pulmonary capillary bed, and alveoli; thus, alveolar anesthetic tension indicates brain anesthetic tension. Thus, at equilibrium, end-tidal anesthetic pressures will reflect brain anesthetic partial pressures. Note that while the *partial pressures* (tensions) are the same in various tissues, the *content* is not the same, since volatile anesthetics have high lipid solubilities and are present at higher concentrations in tissues with more lipid.

The relationship between the inspired and alveolar concentrations is frequently referred to as the F_A/F_I ratio. A more rapid rise in the F_A/F_I ratio indicates a more rapid equilibration

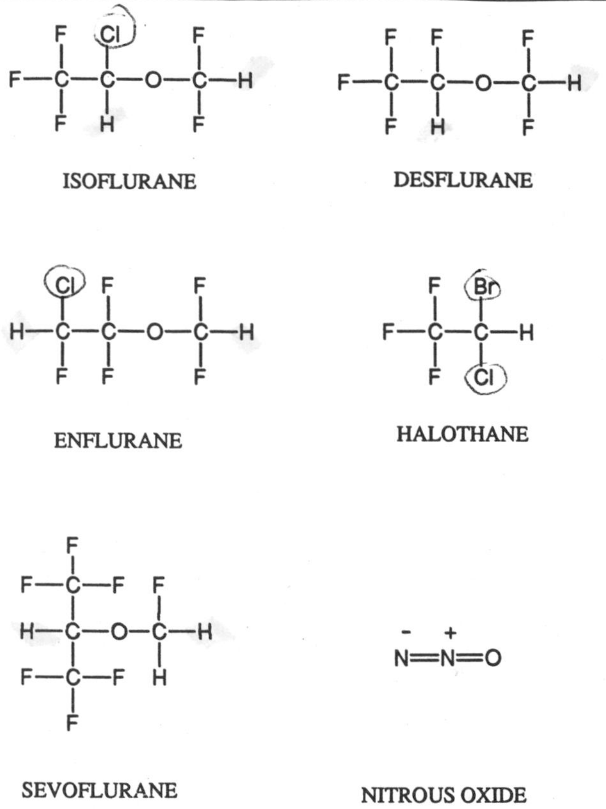

Figure 2–1   Structure of commonly used volatile anesthetics.

Alveolar anesthetic concentration reflects the counterpoise of the anesthetic delivery and the uptake from the alveoli. Therefore, agents that have large apparent volumes of distribution have a slower rate of rise of F_A/F_I ratio due to the uptake and redistribution of gas into tissue reservoirs. Conversely, agents that are less soluble in the body as a whole have more rapid equilibration of the F_A/F_I ratio. Thus, poorly soluble agents, such as nitrous oxide, have more rapid equilibration than the more soluble anesthetics, such as halothane. In other words, a higher tissue-blood solubility coefficient results in lower induction and slower equilibration between the inspired and alveolar tensions. Figure 2–2 demonstrates the effect of solubility on the rate of equilibration of an inhaled anesthetic. The rank order of speed of equilibration for volatile agents is roughly desflurane > sevoflurane > isoflurane > enflurane > halothane.

The distribution of anesthetic from the blood into other tissues is determined by the solubility, as mentioned above, and the blood flow to that tissue. Tissues with a higher relative blood flow will equilibrate sooner and contribute to a much faster rise in the F_A/F_I ratio than tissues with less blood flow. The tissues with a high blood flow to mass ratio, sometimes termed the vessel-rich group, include the brain, heart, kidneys, and liver. Muscle represents a major body compartment that has intermediate blood flow. Fat has a relatively low blood flow but a high capacity for volatile anesthetics. Thus, it is very slow to equilibrate and does not contribute significantly to uptake from blood until the more highly perfused areas have equilibrated. A final compartment of the body—bone, cartilage, and the like—has very little blood flow and does not contribute significantly to the body uptake of anesthetic. Thus, during the initial phases of anesthesia induction with a volatile agent, the uptake of anesthetic into the highly perfused areas accounts for most of the body uptake. As that compartment equilibrates, the less well perfused organs account for a greater proportion of the uptake. The fat takes a very long time to equilibrate and continues to

between the two values. A number of factors affect the gradient between the inspired and alveolar concentrations, including the uptake of anesthetic gas from the alveoli and the rate of delivery of the anesthetic to the alveoli. The rate of delivery, in turn, is the product of the inspired concentration and the alveolar ventilation. Therefore, increasing the alveolar ventilation will increase the rate of rise of F_A/F_I and result in a more rapid induction. This effect is less pronounced with a drug such as nitrous oxide, which equilibrates rapidly.

Table 2–1
PHYSICAL PROPERTIES OF CLINICALLY USED INHALATION ANESTHETICS

Physical Property	Halothane	Isoflurane	Desflurane	Sevoflurane	Enflurane	Nitrous Oxide
EC_{50} (% atmosphere)	0.77	1.15	6	2	1.7	110
Blood: gas	2.5	1.43	0.42	0.60	1.82	0.47
Specific gravity	1.87	1.50	1.47	1.50	1.52	NA
Boiling point (°C)	50	48.5	22.8	58.5	56.5	−88.5
Vapor pressure (mmHg, 20°C)	243	238	669	120	175	Gas
Molecular weight	197.4	184.5	168	200	184.5	44.0
Metabolism	++	−	−	−	+	−
Specific toxicity	Hepatitis	−	−	−	Seizures	Bone marrow depression, neuropathy
Degrades in soda lime	−	−	−	++	−	−
Reacts with metal	+	−	−	−	−	−
Photodegradation	+	−	−	−	−	−
Releases fluoride	−	+	−	+	++	−

+, presence of effect
−, no effect

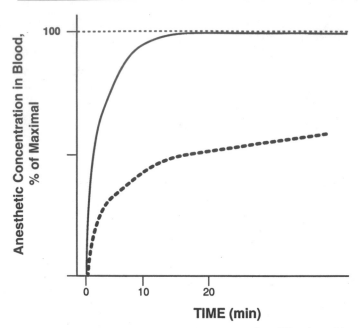

Figure 2–2 Effect of agent solubility on rate of equilibration with blood. Agents which are poorly soluble in blood achieve their steady state concentrations in blood more rapidly than more soluble agents. The maximal achievable level in blood will be at equilibrium when the partial pressure of the anesthetic in the alveolus equals the inspired partial pressure. This is indicated by the dashed line at the top of the graph. The solid line indicates the rate of equilibration of a relatively insoluble agent such as nitrous oxide or desflurane. The dotted line represents the blood concentrations of more soluble agents such as halothane. During recovery from anesthesia, reciprocal changes will occur.

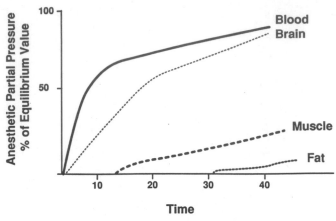

Figure 2–3 Uptake of volatile anesthetics into tissue. Equilibration of volatile anesthetics in tissue is determined by the relative blood flow to that tissue as well as the solubility of drug in the tissue. The solid line represents the uptake of anesthetic into blood for a representative volatile anesthetic [See Figure 2-1]. The brain partial pressure [dotted line] will lag slightly behind the blood partial pressure but will follow it closely. Tissue with less relative blood flow than the brain [dashed line] will take proportionally longer to achieve levels comparable to those in the blood. Tissues such as fat (circles) have relatively low blood flow but considerable capacity for soluble anesthetics. The rate of washout of anesthetics during the recovery from anesthesia will be the reverse of the uptake curves. Thus, concentrations will fall very slowly from the poorly perfused groups.

absorb anesthetic after the other tissues have equilibrated (Fig. 2–3).

The rate of anesthetic uptake from the alveoli is also influenced by the cardiac output. Increased blood flow through the lung increases rates of anesthetic uptake and tissue distribution, resulting in a *less* rapid rise in the F_A/F_I ratio and a slower anesthetic induction. By the same token, a decrease in cardiac output results in a more rapid F_A/F_I rise. It is important to note that increased uptake of volatile anesthetic is usually inversely related to the speed of induction.

The uptake of volatile anesthetic is also slowed in patients who have significant ventilation-perfusion mismatch in their lungs. The F_A/F_I ratio rises more slowly in the presence of pulmonary shunting. With increased pulmonary dead space, the F_A/F_I is also slowed as a greater proportion of the minute ventilation does not perfuse alveoli. If minute ventilation is increased to maintain the alveolar ventilation, then an increase in pulmonary dead space should have little effect on the rate of anesthetic uptake. A similar slowing in uptake of volatile agent into blood is seen in patients with intracardiac shunting. Patients with a *right-to-left shunt* will have a slower rise in anesthetic blood concentration because of admixture to the arterial circulation of blood from the right side of the heart, which is unexposed to alveolar anesthetic concentrations. The presence of the more common *left-to-right shunt* may speed the rate of rise of alveolar anesthetic concentrations but will decrease tissue delivery because of the

lower systemic cardiac output. However, if systemic cardiac output is maintained, the shunt will have no effect on the speed of inhalation induction, since the shunted blood has already been exposed to the anesthetic and does not absorb any more on its subsequent passage through the lungs. Table 2–2 summarizes factors that alter the rate of rise in the F_A/F_I ratio.

Two special cases of the uptake require mention due to the attention that they have received. These are the *concentration* and the *second gas effects*. The concentration effect states that the higher the inspired concentration of volatile agent, the more rapid the equilibration between the alveolar and the inspired concentrations of that gas. As anesthetic is absorbed from the alveoli its concentration falls, but the incremental decrease is less pronounced at higher concentrations since there is bulk flow of inspired gas, which replaces the lost volume with higher anesthetic concentrations. Thus, higher inspired concentrations lead to more rapid rise in F_A/F_I. The contribution of the concentration effect on anesthetic uptake is significant only for anesthetics such as nitrous oxide, which are taken up in relatively large volumes.

Table 2–2
FACTORS THAT SLOW THE RISE OF F_A/F_I RATIO

High cardiac output
Cardiac shunting
Decreased alveolar ventilation
Highly soluble agents

The second gas effect states that coadministration of an anesthetic with a gas that is rapidly absorbed (e.g., nitrous oxide) leads to a more rapid equilibration between inspired and alveolar anesthetic concentrations. Thus, when there is significant volume loss in the alveoli due to gas absorption, the concentration of the anesthetic (i.e., the second gas) is increased. Replacement of the absorbed first gas by bulk flow of inspired gas will also result in a concentration of alveolar anesthetic (second gas) that is higher than the inspired concentration. Both the concentration and second gas effects speed the equilibration of anesthetic between alveoli and blood and result in a more rapid induction.

☐ ANESTHETIC EFFECTS ON ORGAN SYSTEMS
See also Table 2–3.

RESPIRATORY SYSTEM

Volatile agents generally decrease the responsiveness of the airways and decrease bronchospasm. These effects are more profound with halothane. The pungency and odor of these drugs can cause significant coughing in the unanesthetized patient during induction. Thus, desflurane has a significant risk of laryngeal spasm during induction, which may be due to the relatively high concentrations needed. Both halothane and sevoflurane are well tolerated and result in smooth inhalation inductions.

Volatile anesthetics inhibit hypoxic pulmonary vasoconstriction when used in high concentrations but have relatively little effect at lower concentrations.

Volatile anesthetics cause a dose-dependent suppression of respiration with a concomitant increase in Pa_{CO2}. Tidal volume is decreased and respiratory rate is increased.

CARDIOVASCULAR SYSTEM

All of the volatile anesthetics cause dose-dependent decreases in blood pressure due to both a decrease in vascular tone and depression of cardiac contractility. The agents differ in their relative effects on vascular tone and cardiac contractility. At similar planes of anesthesia, halothane predominantly lowers blood pressure via depression of myocardial function, while isoflurane and desflurane predominantly affect vascular tone. Enflurane has intermediate effects. The effects on cardiac depression are probably due to alterations in calcium sequestration in cardiac sarcoplasmic reticulum. Isoflurane and desflurane can significantly increase the heart rate, especially with rapid increases in concentration, while bradycardia may be a presentation of anesthetic overdose.

Halothane can cause ventricular arrhythmias and may sensitize the heart to the arrhythmogenic effects of epinephrine. The other volatile anesthetics are much less likely to do this. Isoflurane, presumably because of its vasodilating properties, has been shown experimentally to cause coronary *steal*. Thus, its vasodilation may shunt blood away from areas at risk for ischemia. However, this is not a significant clinical problem.

Table 2–3
PROPERTIES OF INHALATION ANESTHETICS

HALOTHANE

Causes significant myocardial suppression
Significantly metabolized
Associated with very rare hepatic toxicity (adults only)
Sensitizes the heart to arrhythmogenic effects of β-agonists
Suppresses airway reflexes well and is useful for inhalation inductions
Slower recovery relative to other agents, possibly resulting from pharmacokinetics
Very inexpensive

ISOFLURANE

Not significantly metabolized
Decreases blood pressure predominately via decreased vascular tone
Results in isoelectric EEG at very high concentrations
Much more expensive than halothane

ENFLURANE

Significant release of fluoride ion with prolonged use and high doses
May cause seizures with high doses and hypocarbia (rare)
Less probability of arrhythmias than with isoflurane and halothane
Can be used for inhalation inductions but less ideal than halothane
Similar in price to isoflurane

DESFLURANE

Rapid equilibration between inspired concentration and body, resulting in rapid awakening and changes in depth
Not significantly metabolized
Not indicated for inhalation induction due to risk of laryngeal spasm
Special delivery system, which meters it as a gas, dictated by low boiling point
Cost higher than isoflurane under similar conditions

SEVOFLURANE

Clinical experience relatively limited
Some fluoride ion release with high doses
Desirable pharmacokinetics for rapid changes in blood levels
Very satisfactory for inhalation inductions
Has reactive byproduct of undetermined toxicity, which may accumulate at low flow rates
Cost is similar to desflurane

NITROUS OXIDE

Low potency (> 1 atm)
Very rapid changes in blood concentrations due to solubility, which is similar to sevoflurane and desflurane
Useful only in combination with other agents due to potency
Little cardiovascular depression relative to volatile agents
May be associated with postoperative nausea and vomiting
Suppresses airway reflexes and is very useful for inhalation inductions
Will expand volume of gas pockets within the body (e.g., pneumothorax)
Inhibits activity of vitamin B_{12}, which may result in anemia and neuropathy from chronic use in patients at risk
Supports combustion
Inexpensive

NEUROMUSCULAR SYSTEM

Volatile anesthetics potentiate the neuromuscular blocking effects of nondepolarizing muscle relaxants. Isoflurane, desflurane, and enflurane exhibit the most profound potentiation and are roughly three times more active in this regard than halothane at equal planes of anesthesia.

RENAL SYSTEM

Volatile anesthetics significantly decrease renal blood flow and urine output. However, if cardiac output and blood pressure are maintained, these effects should revert to normal. Fluoride ion is released with the metabolism of some anesthetics (e.g., enflurane and sevoflurane) and can impair the concentrating ability of the kidneys (see below).

CENTRAL NERVOUS SYSTEM

Volatile anesthetics cause unconsciousness and alter the electroencephalogram (EEG). Generally, they cause slowing and decreased frequency at therapeutic concentrations. At low concentrations, inhalational agents cause an increase in frequency and voltage, reflecting an excitatory stage of anesthesia. At concentrations of about 2 times the anesthetic EC_{50}, isoflurane, as well as desflurane, can cause an isoelectric EEG. Enflurane can cause seizure activity, especially in the presence of low Pa_{CO_2}. Brain blood flow is increased by volatile anesthetics, but this effect is suppressed by hyperventilation. The agents also inhibit autoregulation of brain blood flow, especially at high concentrations.

EFFECTS ON OTHER ORGAN SYSTEMS

Blood sugar levels may be increased as insulin secretion and action are suppressed. Volatile anesthetics suppress uterine contraction by inhibiting smooth muscle action. This may cause increased bleeding during uterine surgery and may inhibit labor contractions.

Nitrous oxide has some considerably different properties from the other inhalational anesthetics. It is considerably less potent than the other clinically used inhalational agents. Because the concentration needed for anesthesia is greater than 1 atm, it is used to supplement other inhalational agents, thereby lowering the requirement for the respective inhalational agent (e.g., halothane). The anesthetic effects of nitrous oxide are additive to the other agents, suggesting that they have a common mechanism of anesthetic action. In addition to its anesthetic effects, nitrous oxide has analgesic effects that are naloxone reversible, indicating that it interacts with the opiate system. Long-term toxicity is notable for bone marrow depression and neuropathy.

An additional concern in the use of nitrous oxide is based on the physical characteristics of the gas. Relatively large volumes of nitrous oxide gas are absorbed during anesthesia, and this gas will equilibrate throughout the body. Thus, it will increase the volume of any gas spaces in the body, such as bowel gas, pneumothorax, and air emboli. Typically, nitrous oxide is avoided when these conditions may exist. Nitrous oxide also supports combustion and should be replaced by a nonflammable gas when the risk of airway fires is present.

☐ TOXICITY

Volatile anesthetics are largely excreted via the lungs unchanged. Relative to most other drugs, only small portions are metabolized. The proportion of agent metabolized depends on the concentration of administration and may be zero order under some circumstances (see Chap. 1). The relative metabolism of the commonly used volatile agents is halothane > sevoflurane > enflurane > isoflurane > desflurane. Note that isoflurane and desflurane are minimally metabolized. The other three drugs have significant degrees of metabolism. The metabolism of these drugs can lead to significant accumulations of fluoride and bromide. Enflurane particularly can result in serum fluoride concentrations of up to ~20 μm. Levels above 50 μm can cause loss of concentrating ability of the kidney. Fluoride toxicity is unusual with enflurane but occurs occasionally with methoxyflurane, which is used only in veterinary practices in this country. Sevoflurane metabolism releases fluoride, but the magnitude and clinical consequences of this have not been documented. Drugs that induce the P450 system in the liver can result in increased metabolism of volatile agents. These substances include isoniazid, phenobarbital, chlorpromazine, and insecticides.

Chronic exposure to low levels of volatile anesthetics is possibly associated with a number of health risks, including an increased risk of spontaneous abortions in operating room personnel, though this is a point of considerable controversy. Currently, with effective scavenging techniques, exposure of operating room personnel should be much lower than the mandated air limits of 2 ppm for volatile agents and 50 ppm for nitrous oxide.

All of the volatile anesthetics (but not nitrous oxide) can trigger malignant hyperthemia. This hypermetabolic state is characterized by high temperature and sustained contractions of skeletal muscles. Volatile anesthetic interactions with the skeletal muscle ryanodine receptor is implicated in some families with this disease. This is discussed in detail in Chap. 8.

Halothane is unique among the volatile agents in that it has been associated with a rare form of liver failure, halothane hepatitis (incidence about 1 in 35,000). This is felt to be immunologically mediated and related to the byproducts of metabolism. It is seen more frequently after repeated exposures to the drug. The primary metabolites of halothane are trifluoroacetic acid and bromide. Antibodies against the liver have been detected in patients with halothane hepatitis. Hepatitis is not seen with the less extensively metabolized volatile agents.

Sevoflurane reacts with the CO_2 absorbent soda lime to produce a number of reactive products, including one called substance A. The clinical significance of these products is unclear at present. Sevoflurane has been in clinical use in Japan for a number of years without significant side effects and was recently approved for use in the United States. Current studies indicate that there is not significant accumulation of substance A if fresh gas flows are kept at 2 L/min or higher.

There is a recent report implicating desflurane in the generation of carbon monoxide because of an interaction with soda lime. If confirmed, the conditions under which this reaction takes place will need to be studied thoroughly.

Prolonged exposure to nitrous oxide is associated with bone marrow depression (megaloblastic anemia and agranulocytosis) and peripheral neuropathy, which is probably secondary to inactivation of the vitamin B_{12} methionine synthase.

☐ ANESTHETIC POTENCY

The measurement of anesthetic potency presents some problems relative to intravenous drugs because of the pharmacokinetics issues described above. Notably, a significant gradient may exist between the inspired concentration and the concentration at the site of action. Thus, measurements are typically performed at equilibrium when the partial pressure of anesthetic in the blood is stable. Minimum alveolar concentration (MAC) is a measure of anesthetic potency and can be used to compare the effects of different agents. It is defined as the concentration of anesthetic, at one atmosphere, needed to suppress reaction to a painful stimulus in 50% of the population. MAC is an EC_{50} measurement under a defined set of circumstances. It should be noted that other paradigms are also used to study anesthetic phenomena and yield EC_{50} values that differ from MAC. Thus, other stimuli (tail clamp, surgical incision, or supine positioning) and different endpoints (loss of righting reflex versus gross movement versus blood pressure changes) result in different values of anesthetic potency. The abolition of movement seems to require higher anesthetic concentrations than does unconsciousness. While all inhalational anesthetics are low in potency (~0.2–0.8 mM), the rank order potency of clinically used agents is halothane > isoflurane > enflurane > sevoflurane > desflurane > nitrous oxide.

The experimental measurement of MAC is primarily a measure of a motor (movement) response to a painful stimuli. The recent reports that MAC is unchanged in rats after lesions separating the brain from the spinal cord are intriguing, and they suggest that MAC is a spinal reflex. If these findings are confirmed, they support the notion that MAC may be measuring effects that parallel the unconsciousness that results in anesthesia. These findings also suggest that other "sites" of anesthetic actions will be found that mediate other components of anesthesia. Further experimental studies on the mechanism of action of anesthetics should help clarify these issues (see below).

Table 2–4
FACTORS THAT INFLUENCE APPARENT ANESTHETIC POTENCY

DECREASE
Hypernatremia
Hyperthyroidism
Excitatory states
Hyperthermia
Tolerance to CNS depressants

INCREASE
Hypothermia
Hyponatremia
Acute ethanol intoxication
Concurrent use of CNS depressants (e.g., benzodiazepines, barbiturates, opiates, etc.)
Old age
Hypothyroidism

MAC has been studied under a variety of conditions to determine which physiological states are associated with alterations in anesthetic requirement. Studies have demonstrated that the coadministration of CNS depressants increases the apparent anesthetic potency. Conversely, physiological states associated with excitation (e.g., hyperthermia and hypernatremia) lead to a decrease in anesthetic potency (i.e., a greater anesthetic requirement). Likewise, individuals tolerant of CNS depressants may require larger doses of anesthetics. Two disease states may also lead to increased anesthetic potency. Diabetes involves biochemical alteration, including acylation, of many brain enzymes and in animals is associated with an increase in anesthetic potency. Hepatic failure is associated with increases in endogenous benzodiazepine-receptor agonists, and ammonia, which are both CNS depressants and are likely to be associated with increased sensitivity to anesthetics, although this remains to be confirmed clinically. Table 2–4 summarizes states that are associated with alterations in anesthetic requirement.

☐ MECHANISM OF ACTION

Despite their clinical use for almost 150 years, the mechanism by which anesthetics induce anesthesia remains unknown. At the turn of the century the Meyer-Overton hypothesis correlated the lipid solubility of an anesthetic and its clinical potency. This suggested that lipids may be a primary locus of anesthetic action. While the Meyer-Overton hypothesis accounts for an enormous array of chemical structures from anesthetics that have simple structure, such as xenon, to complex compounds like alphaxalone, multiple mechanisms of action may exist for different classes of anesthetics. Any valid explanation of anesthesia must account for the fact that these compounds of varied structure all result in anesthesia. Thus, it has been difficult to imagine a single site of action that would accommodate all of these compounds. Moreover, the anesthetic state is a complex one comprising, at least, unconsciousness, amnesia, analgesia, and lack of movement. These multiple facets of anesthesia also suggest that there may be different mechanisms for the various components—a view supported by the fact that drugs vary in their potencies in producing various measures of anesthesia. Thus, some anesthetics suppress movement more than others, while certain drugs (e.g., barbiturates) lack any significant analgesic component. These various components, measures, and definitions of anesthesia make it important to specify what is meant by anesthesia. For the purposes here, anesthesia is referred to in the clinical sense as measured by MAC, while it is recognized that, scientifically, unconsciousness is perhaps the most interesting component.

These multiple components of anesthesia, as well as the diversity of compounds, has led to the hypothesis that there are multiple sites of anesthetic action. This concept is in contrast to a unitary hypothesis, which maintains that there is a common mechanism of anesthesia. A receptor complex with multiple binding sites for different compounds might account for the diversity of structure among anesthetic drugs. A target, such as lipid, which would have less stringent structural requirements for an interaction than a protein site, might also be a candidate.

Lipid theories of action include increased permeability, fluidity, and membrane expansion as well as general disordering of the lipid environment. Under experimental conditions, high pressures have been known to reverse some of the effects of anesthetics. This finding has been interpreted as support for volume expansion theories of anesthesia, since hyperbaric pressure may reverse the expansion of a lipid. It is unclear whether this reversal is a direct pharmacologic antagonism or the result of a complex physiologic response, such as the generalized excitation seen in the high-pressure neurologic syndrome. The observation that volatile anesthetics can modulate the activity of the bacterial enzyme luciferase in a lipid-free state, however, is strong evidence that these anesthetics can directly affect proteins. This observation has led to the further observation that volatile anesthetics can modulate a variety of receptor sites. These findings have, however, failed to resolve the question of whether the primary anesthetic action is perturbation of the phospholipid bilayer or discrete interactions with specific protein sequences.

Anesthetics affect many enzymes and other proteins, including ion channels for potassium, calcium, and sodium. Several ligand-gated ion channels have been extensively studied and are modulated by inhalational anesthetics, including nicotinic acetylcholine, n-methyl-D-aspartate (NMDA), and γ-aminobutyric acid$_A$ (GABA$_A$) receptor complexes. A significant problem in the interpretation of volatile anesthetic effects is determining which of the myriad interactions are actually pharmacologically relevant to the anesthetic process and which either mediate side effects or have no relevance. The careful correlation between behavioral, in vivo studies and the observed in vitro effects will be helpful in evaluating hypothetical sites of anesthetic action.

The recent availability of the stereoisomers of volatile anesthetics may be useful as well. Stereoisomers are mirror-image compounds with similar physical and chemical properties. The presence of stereoselectivity is considered to be strong evidence of protein-receptor-mediated events, since it indicates that the receptor is able to distinguish subtle conformational differences between the two mirror-image compounds. "Nonspecific" sites would be unlikely to exhibit stereoselectivity, since their requirements of interaction are less stringent. Stereoisomers have been useful in defining the receptor sites of action of other compounds, such as opiates and benzodiazepines. Preliminary studies with the stereoisomers of isoflurane indicate that they exhibit modest stereoselectivity in some in vivo models as well as stereoselectively modulating a number of sites on the GABA$_A$ receptor complex. Moreover, these compounds lack stereoselective effects at a number of other receptors. If these findings are confirmed, the use of these compounds may represent a way of distinguishing relevant sites for anesthesia from nonanesthetic effects.

It is possible, indeed, some say likely, that anesthesia results from modulation of various receptors at the same time. For example, anesthesia might result, not from a single receptor interaction, but from inhibition of excitatory synapses in combination with augmentation of inhibitory neurotransmitter systems as well as effects elsewhere. This proposal might explain the effects of anesthetics at a wide variety of receptor systems. It would also account for the difficulties in any single site fulfilling the requirements of anesthetic action. If multiple sites are involved in anesthetic action, a clear, testable hypothesis will need to be developed in order to accumulate supporting data.

The GABA$_A$ receptor complex has recently attracted considerable attention as a possible site at which many nonvolatile anesthetics have actions (see Chap. 3). GABA is the primary inhibitory neurotransmitter in the brain, and it is possible that augmentation of the inhibitory tone in the brain would result in significant CNS depression. GABA-induced inhibitory postsynaptic potentiation (IPSP) is a measure of GABA activity, and volatile anesthetics augment this activity. It has been hypothesized that this augmentation of GABA-IPSP may be a common property whereby many anesthetics are also effectors at GABA$_A$ receptors, including barbiturates, propofol, etomidate, and anesthetic steroids. If those actions at the GABA$_A$ receptor result in their anesthetic effects, it is likely that some volatile anesthetic effects can be attributed to this site as well, since volatile and nonvolatile agents share many properties. The use of purified receptors, genetically altered animals, site-directed mutagenesis and other strategies common to molecular biology holds promise in answering some of these questions.

BIBLIOGRAPHY

Eger EI II: *Anesthetic Uptake and Action.* Baltimore, Williams & Wilkins, 1974.

Felman SA, Paton W, Scurr C: *Mechanisms of Drugs in Anaesthesia.* London, Edward Arnold, 1993.

Franks NP, Lieb WR: Molecular and cellular mechanisms of general anaesthesia. *Nature* 367;607–614, 1994.

Tanelain DL, Kosek P, Mody I, MacIver MB: The role of the GABA$_A$ receptor chloride channel complex in anesthesia. *Anesthesiology* 78:757–776.

Pharmacology of Nonopioid Intravenous Anesthetics

Hugh C. Hemmings, Jr.

Induction of general anesthesia by the administration of intravenous agents is a safe and effective technique that is preferred for its rapid onset and patient acceptability. Intravenous induction is usually employed regardless of the technique used for maintenance of anesthesia; it can be combined with inhalation anesthesia, opioid anesthesia, balanced anesthesia, or total intravenous anesthesia. This chapter reviews the intravenous anesthetic agents that are most frequently utilized for the induction of general anesthesia. Appropriate use of these agents requires an understanding of their pharmacokinetic and pharmacodynamic properties (Chap. 1). Pharmacokinetic concepts that are particularly relevant to intravenous anesthetics include the half-time ($t_{1/2}$), volume of distribution (V_d), and clearance. The volume of distribution of a drug varies with such properties as its pK_a, degree of protein binding, partition coefficient into fat (lipophilicity), and so on, and can also vary with patient age, gender, body composition (% fat), and disease state. Some drugs, including many intravenous anesthetics, have very large apparent volumes of distribution at steady state ($V_{dss} > 100$ L) due to high tissue-plasma partition coefficients or to protein binding, both of which are reflected in a large apparent compartment volume. A useful concept of the relationships among half-time, clearance (CL), and volume of distribution is provided by

$$t_{1/2} \cong 0.693 \, V_d/CL$$

The half-time, a useful clinical parameter, is directly proportional to the volume of distribution and inversely proportional to the clearance.

☐ BARBITURATES

CHEMISTRY AND FORMULATION

The barbiturates (Table 3–1) include a number of derivatives of barbituric acid that are weak acids and are poorly soluble in water. The commonly used barbiturates, which include thiopental, thiamylal, and methohexital (Fig. 3–1), are formulated as racemic mixtures of their water-soluble sodium salts. Sodium carbonate is included to maintain an alkaline pH of 10 to 11, which prevents precipitation of the free acids due to acidification by atmospheric CO_2. The alkalinity of these solutions can result in severe tissue damage if injected extravascularly or intraarterially and will induce precipitation of many weak bases, such as pancuronium, vecuronium, lidocaine, and morphine sulfate. As acidic lipophilic compounds, most barbiturates bind to plasma albumin.

The barbiturates are broadly classified as thiobarbiturates (sulfur at C2; thiopental, thiamylal) and oxybarbiturates (oxygen at C2; methohexital). Substitution of sulfur for oxygen at C2 increases lipophilicity, which results in increased potency, a more rapid onset, and a shorter duration of action (e.g., pentobarbital versus thiopental, its thio-analog). Alkylation of N1 also increases lipophilicity and thereby speeds onset but increases excitatory side effects, such as spontaneous involuntary movements (e.g., methohexital, a methylated oxybarbiturate). The anesthetic potency of the L isomers of thiopental and thiamylal are more than twice that of the D isomers.

Table 3-1
PROPERTIES OF INTRAVENOUS BARBITURATES

Property	Thiopental	Methohexital
Water solubility	Yes (sodium salt)	Yes (sodium salt)
pK_a	7.6	7.9
Initial $t_{1/2}$ (min)	8.5	5.6
Intermediate $t_{1/2}$ (min)	62	58
Terminal $t_{1/2}$ (h)	12	3.9
V_{dss} (L/kg)	2.4	2.4
Clearance (mL/kg/h)	3.4	11
Protein binding (%)	85	85
Induction dose (mg/kg IV)	2.5-4.5 adult 5-6 children 7-8 infants	1-1.5

SOURCE: Data adapted with permission from Hull, 1989. Pharmacokinetic data are derived from a three-compartment model.

PHARMACOKINETICS

The short duration of action of thiopental, thiamylal, and methohexital can be explained by their pharmacokinetic behavior. Following rapid bolus intravenous administration, these agents distribute rapidly within the intravascular space and to the highly perfused (vessel-rich) tissues, such as the brain (Fig. 3-2), resulting in induction of anesthesia within one arm-brain circulation time, or about 60 s, depending on the cardiac output. Data for thiopental and methohexital indicate that the central volumes of distribution (equivalent to the central compartment) exceed the intravascular volume, which is consistent with their rapid distribution to brain and other highly perfused tissues. The action of a single bolus injection of these drugs is terminated primarily by redistribution to the much larger V_{dss}, which includes lean, vessel-rich tissues, such as muscle. Since the short duration of a single bolus dose of these drugs depends on redistribution to lean tissues, the appropriate induction dose should be calculated based on lean body mass; this explains the apparent increased sensitivity to barbiturates among women and the aged. The high fat-plasma partition coefficient of the lipophilic barbiturates has little effect on their initial distribution, since adipose tissue, although providing a large reservoir for delayed drug uptake, is very poorly perfused.

The pharmacokinetic properties of barbiturates also help explain the mechanism of delayed recovery observed from large or repeated doses or after prolonged infusions of these agents. Their short duration depends on a redistribution mechanism that is limited by the mass of lean tissue and is easily overwhelmed by a large cumulative dose, which saturates this reservoir. At this point, the duration of action is no longer related to the initial redistribution half-time ($t_{1/2}\alpha$), but to the terminal elimination half-time ($t_{1/2}\beta$), which is relatively slow given the high V_{dss} and low CL of, for example, thiopental (Table 3-1). Under these conditions, methohexital is eliminated more quickly than thiopental due to its higher CL (despite a similar V_{dss}). The ultimate elimination of the barbiturates is very slow relative to drug uptake by lean tissue; it is due primarily to hepatic extraction and metabolism and makes little contribution to terminating the effect.

MECHANISM OF ACTION

The mode of action of general anesthetics remains controversial. Synaptic transmission is more sensitive to the effects of general anesthetics than is axonal conduction. A consensus is building that the principal targets of general anesthetics in the central nervous system are ion channel proteins, particularly ligand-gated channels, although voltage-gated channels may also be affected. Electrophysiological evidence suggests that the anesthetic barbiturates inhibit excitatory synaptic transmission, possibly by blocking presynaptic Ca^{2+} influx

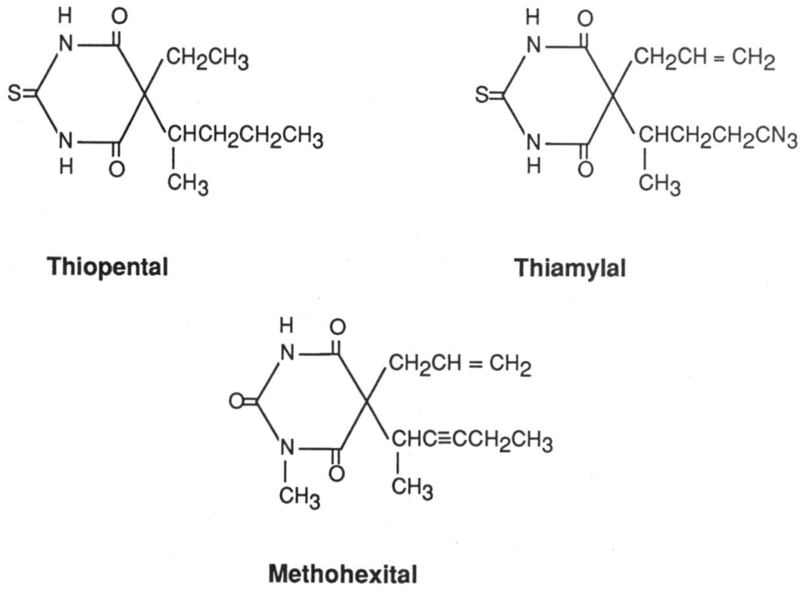

Figure 3-1   Chemical structures of intravenous barbiturates. The sodium salts are formed by association of Na^+ with one of the deprotonated ring nitrogens.

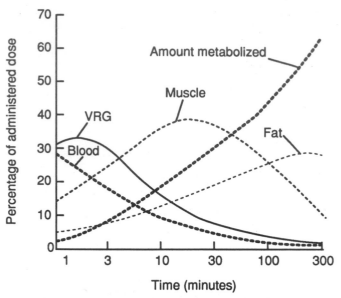

Figure 3–2 The uptake and redistribution of an intravenous bolus of thiopental. The amount of thiopental in the blood rapidly decreases as drug moves from blood to body tissues. Time to peak tissue levels is a direct function of tissue capacity for barbiturate relative to blood flow. Thus, a larger capacity or smaller blood flow is related to a longer time to a peak tissue level. Initially, most thiopental is taken up by the VRG (vessel-rich group) tissues because of their high blood flow. Subsequently, thiopental is redistributed to muscle and, to a lesser extent, to fat. Throughout this period, small but substantial amounts of thiopental are removed by the liver and metabolized. Unlike removal by the tissues, this removal is cumulative. The rate of metabolism equals the early rate of removal by fat. The sum of this early removal by fat and metabolism is the same as the removal by muscle. (Modified with permission from Saidman LJ: Uptake, distribution and elimination of barbiturates, in Eger EJ (ed): *Anesthetic Uptake and Action.* Baltimore, Williams & Wilkins, pp 264–284, 1974.)

through voltage-dependent Ca^{2+} channels and inhibiting neurotransmitter release. They also facilitate inhibitory synaptic transmission by both enhancing and mimicking GABA-mediated Cl^- influx at the $GABA_A$ receptor. A variety of pharmacologic evidence indicates that effects at the $GABA_A$ receptor are primarily responsible for the anesthetic effects of barbiturates.

CLINICAL USE

Until recently, the barbiturates were the most popular anesthetic induction agents, a role that is being challenged by propofol, especially in ambulatory anesthesia. Thiopental, thiamylal, and methohexital induce anesthesia rapidly and effectively within one arm-brain circulation time (peak effect in ~60 s) following intravenous injection, with a duration of about 4 to 8 min. The usual induction dose of thiopental in healthy patients is 2.5 to 4.5 mg/kg for adults, 5 to 6 mg/kg for children, and 7 to 8 mg/kg for infants, based on lean body mass. Dose requirements are reduced by opioid or benzodiazepine premedication, acute ethanol intoxication, anemia, malnutrition, uremia, shock, or severe systemic disease. Reduced cardiac output prolongs induction and decreases the

dose requirement, due to higher peak blood drug levels. Thiamylal is equipotent with thiopental; methohexital is about 2.7 times as potent as thiopental.

Barbiturates are occasionally used by anesthesiologists as anticonvulsants in acute situations; for brain protection during neurosurgery, cardiac valvular surgery or circulatory arrest; and for reduction of intracranial pressure in patients with intracranial hypertension. The cerebroprotective effects of the barbiturates may be due to a reduction in cerebral metabolism of oxygen (CMR_{O_2}; normal value 3 to 6 mL O_2/min/100 g brain tissue) as a result of a dose-related reduction in neuronal activity. This is reflected in a depression of the electroencephalogram (EEG), which progresses through high-amplitude and low-frequency delta and theta activity to burst suppression and then to complete silence (at a thiopental dose of about 4 mg/kg/h), at which point there is a maximal decrease in CMR_{O_2} of 55%. There is a parallel reduction in cerebral blood flow and intracranial pressure, preserving cerebral perfusion pressure despite reduction in mean arterial pressure. The normal coupling between cerebral blood flow and CMR_{O_2} (autoregulation) is not affected. Barbiturates are useful in reducing focal or regional cerebral ischemia by suppressing oxygen consumption in the ischemic zones. Another salutary effect of barbiturates on cerebral ischemia is the so-called inverse steal, or increased perfusion of ischemic zones due to vasoconstriction in nonischemic areas secondary to decreased CMR_{O_2}. These properties make the barbiturates particularly useful in neurosurgical procedures. Barbiturates are not effective in the treatment of global cerebral ischemia.

Continuous infusion of barbiturates for maintenance of anesthesia has been largely supplanted by propofol, which allows more rapid recovery; however, the barbiturates are occasionally used as infusions to treat intracranial hypertension. Continuous infusion or repeated doses of barbiturates lead to drug accumulation as the lean tissue reservoir for redistribution becomes saturated. Drug elimination from plasma then depends on hepatic metabolism, which can also be saturated at high plasma concentrations. Methohexital, with a terminal elimination half-time of about 4 h, is the most suitable barbiturate for continuous infusion. This contrasts with thiopental, which has a terminal elimination half-time of almost 12 h due to its 30% lower clearance.

Methohexital is occasionally used per rectum (at a dose of 30 mg/kg) as a premedication for longer surgical procedures in children less than 20 kg. However, benzodiazepines have replaced barbiturates as premedications in most cases.

CARDIOVASCULAR EFFECTS

The principal hemodynamic effects of the barbiturates administered by bolus intravenous injection for induction of anesthesia in healthy, normovolemic patients are transient reductions in systemic arterial pressure and cardiac output and an increase in heart rate, with no change or an increase in systemic vascular resistance. The hypotension results from marked venodilation with peripheral pooling of blood and decreased cardiac filling pressures, which reduces cardiac output and arterial pressure. Usual doses of thiopental produce minimal myocardial depression, although higher doses reduce contractility. The increased heart rate, which is more marked with methohexital than with thiopental, results from baroreceptor reflex sympathetic stimulation of the heart and may partially mask the negative inotropic effects. Thiopental and thiamylal, but not methohexital, can induce histamine release, which will worsen hypotension.

The hypotensive effects of the barbiturates are more pronounced in treated or untreated hypertensive patients and in conditions such as hypovolemia, valvular or ischemic heart disease, or shock, where compensatory mechanisms are impaired. The hemodynamic effects of the barbiturates are particularly deleterious in conditions worsened by reduced preload or tachycardia, such as myocardial ischemia, congestive heart failure, pericardial tamponade, and valvular heart disease. The barbiturates are not arrhythmogenic and do not sensitize the heart to catecholamines.

RESPIRATORY EFFECTS

The intravenous barbiturates are potent central respiratory depressants. They produce dose-dependent decreases in both minute volume and tidal volume. Respiratory rate may increase slightly at lower doses but is reduced by higher doses that lead ultimately to apnea. The medullary center ventilatory responses to both hypercarbia and hypoxia are depressed by barbiturates. Laryngeal and tracheal reflexes are not depressed by the usual doses of barbiturates, so laryngospasm and, rarely, bronchospasm can occur with barbiturate induction of anesthesia. Upper airway stimulation by secretions, artificial airway, or laryngoscopy enhance this response. Cough and hiccough are not uncommon, especially with methohexital.

OTHER EFFECTS

Pain on intravenous injection is rare with thiopental but more common with methohexital. Venous thrombosis and phlebitis may occur up to several days postoperatively. Intraarterial or subcutaneous injection can cause tissue irritation or necrosis, depending on the amount and site of injection.

The barbiturates do not acutely affect gastrointestinal or hepatic function with induction of anesthesia. There is a low incidence of postoperative nausea and vomiting due to barbiturates. Chronic administration can lead to hepatic enzyme induction, resulting in accelerated metabolism of the barbiturates as well as of other drugs. Stimulation by barbiturates of the mitochondrial enzyme δ-aminolevulinic acid reductase, the rate-limiting enzyme in porphyrin biosynthesis, can exacerbate acute intermittent porphyria in susceptible patients; barbiturates are therefore contraindicated in porphyria.

Barbiturates can contribute to intraoperative oliguria by reducing renal blood flow and glomerular filtration; this is effectively prevented by treating hypotension and providing adequate intravenous fluid. In contrast to etomidate, barbiturates do not suppress adrenocortical stimulation.

Thiopental is safe for anesthetic induction for cesarean section; however, doses greater than 8 mg/kg may cause neonatal depression due to placental transfer. This effect can be minimized by delivery of the baby within 10 min of induction. Thiopental has little effect on uterine contractions.

Undesirable central nervous system effects observed with barbiturates include paradoxical excitement with small doses (possibly due to central disinhibition, especially in the presence of pain) and involuntary skeletal muscle movements (a central excitatory effect seen with methohexital, which can also precipitate seizures in susceptible patients). Prolonged neurobehavioral effects can be observed for several hours after induction with large or repeated doses. Significant effects on neuromuscular transmission or skeletal muscle function do not occur with barbiturates.

☐ PROPOFOL

CHEMISTRY AND FORMULATION

Propofol (2,6-diisopropyl phenol) is a lipophilic alkylated phenol (Fig. 3–3) that exists as an oil at room temperature and is insoluble in water (Table 3–2). It is a very weak acid ($pK_a = 11$), and is essentially fully unionized at physiological pH. Because of its poor aqueous solubility, propofol is formulated at 1% in an oil-water emulsion containing 10% soy bean oil, 1.2% egg lecithin, and 2.25% glycerol (as an osmotic agent) with a pH of 6 to 8.5. A previous formulation, in Cremophor EL (Blagden, UK), was withdrawn due to anaphylactic reactions. The oil-water emulsion is an excellent medium for microbial growth; care must be taken to avoid contamination and to minimize the time between withdrawal from the ampule and administration. Propofol is extensively bound to plasma albumin.

PHARMACOKINETICS

Like the intravenous barbiturates, propofol is a rapidly acting intravenous anesthetic that will induce anesthesia within one arm-brain circulation time following intravenous injection. Following bolus intravenous injection, plasma concentration decreases rapidly due to the combined effect of redistribution and elimination. When plasma concentrations are fitted to a two-compartment pharmacokinetic model, the initial redistribution half-time ($t_{1/2}\alpha$) is 2 min, and the terminal half-time ($t_{1/2}\beta$) is approximately 5 h. The initial and steady-state volumes of distribution are extremely large (40 and 320 L, respectively) compared to that of thiopental (26 and 170 L, respectively). In contrast to thiopental, the clearance of

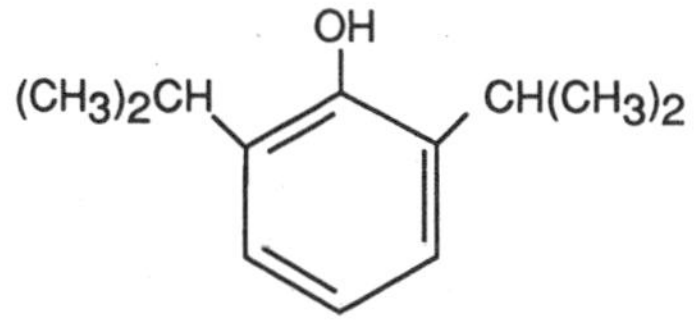

Figure 3–3   Chemical structure of propofol (1,6-diisopropylphenol).

Table 3–2
PROPERTIES OF PROPOFOL, ETOMIDATE, AND KETAMINE

Property	Propofol	Etomidate	Ketamine
Water solubility	No	No	Yes
pK_a	11	4.2	7.5
Initial $t_{1/2}$ (min)	2	1	16
Intermediate $t_{1/2}$ (min)	50	12	———
Terminal $t_{1/2}$ (h)	4.8	5.4	3.0
V_{dss} (L/kg)	4.6	5.4	3.0
Clearance (mL/kg/h)	25	18	19
Protein binding (%)	98	75	12
Induction dose (mg/kg IV)	1–2.5	0.2–0.6	0.5–2 (5–10 IM)
Active metabolites	No	No	Yes (minimally)

SOURCE: Modified with permission from Hull, 1989. Pharmacokinetic data for propofol and etomidate are derived from a three-compartment model, and for ketamine from a two compartment model.

propofol is also extremely high (25–31 mL/min/kg for propofol versus 4 mL/min/kg for thiopental) and exceeds hepatic blood flow, which suggests extrahepatic metabolism. Propofol is rapidly and completely metabolized by the liver to inactive compounds that are eliminated by the kidney. Despite its hepatic metabolism, the clearance of propofol is not impaired in patients with cirrhosis. Clearance is also unaffected by renal failure. The high lipophilicity of propofol contributes to its rapid uptake into the brain; redistribution and a high clearance result in a short duration of action.

MECHANISM OF ACTION

The mechanism of action of propofol, as of other general anesthetics, is not fully understood. As is the case with a number of other anesthetics, propofol potentiates inhibitory synaptic transmission by interacting with $GABA_A$ receptors at both spinal and supraspinal synapses. In contrast to other anesthetics, propofol appears to have marked subcortical effects that may be involved in mediating some of its atypical actions (see below).

CLINICAL USES

Use of propofol as an intravenous induction agent has supplanted the use of other agents in many situations since its introduction in the United States in 1988. Rapid redistribution and elimination, which result in a rapid return to consciousness with minimal residual effects, and a low incidence of nausea and vomiting make propofol particularly useful for short procedures and outpatient surgery. The average induction dose of propofol in healthy patients under 60 years is 2 mg/kg (range 1.5 to 2.5 mg/kg). This dose should be reduced in elderly or premedicated patients.

The rapid clearance of propofol makes it useful for maintenance of anesthesia by continuous infusion without significant cumulative effects; plasma concentrations decrease rapidly when the infusion is terminated. Continuous infusion of propofol can also be combined with infusions of other short-acting drugs, such as alfentanil, sufentanil, and mivacurium, for balanced intravenous anesthesia. Continuous infusion of propofol has also found widespread use as a sedative technique in monitored anesthesia care, as an adjunct to regional anesthesia and in the intensive care unit. Subhypnotic doses of propofol do not cause an increased sensitivity to somatic pain and may even provide analgesia, in contrast to thiopental, which has been reported to cause hyperalgesia.

Propofol has recently been found to possess a number of unique characteristics, including antiemetic, antipruritic, and anxiolytic properties, which may be due to effects at subcortical sites. Propofol may also have anticonvulsant properties, and can be used for treating refractory epilepsy.

CARDIOVASCULAR EFFECTS

An intravenous injection of propofol (2 mg/kg) in healthy patients decreases arterial blood pressure 15 to 40%; reductions in blood pressure are generally greater with propofol than with comparable doses of thiopental. Propofol produces significant reductions in systemic vascular resistance and myocardial contractility. The effect of propofol on heart rate is variable, but in general it produces less tachycardia than thiopental. Propofol resets baroreceptor reflex control of heart rate, resulting in an unchanged heart rate despite lower levels of blood pressure compared to controls; this mechanism has been used to explain the greater hypotensive effect of propofol compared to thiopental. The pressor response to tracheal intubation is less marked with propofol compared to the barbiturates. Plasma levels of histamine are not affected by intravenous propofol injection.

The hemodynamic effects of propofol may be magnified in hypovolemic or elderly patients and in patients with impaired left ventricular function. These patients benefit from a reduced dose of propofol in conjunction with an intravenous opioid or benzodiazepine to reduce the propofol requirement and minimize cardiovascular effects. Propofol is not arrhythmogenic and does not sensitize the heart to catecholamines.

RESPIRATORY EFFECTS

Propofol is a potent respiratory depressant and often produces an apneic period of 30 to 60 seconds following a normal induction dose. Hiccough, cough, and laryngospasm are less common than with the barbiturates; this may be due to a greater depression of laryngeal reflexes.

OTHER EFFECTS

Pain on injection remains a significant problem with intravenous propofol, although the incidence is somewhat lower than with the previous Cremophor (Blagden, UK) formulation. Pain on intravenous injection can be minimized by using larger veins with a rapid carrier infusion rate, injecting lidocaine before or with the propofol emulsion, or injecting a synthetic opioid before the propofol emulsion. The incidence of venous thrombosis and phlebitis following propofol injection is quite low.

Propofol does not have adverse gastrointestinal or hepatic effects. Even high doses produce no significant changes in hepatic transaminases, alkaline phosphatase, or bilirubin. Coagulation and fibrinolytic activities are also unaffected. Propofol has significant antiemetic activity, even at subanesthetic doses (10 mg IV). Propofol is also an effective antipruritic and can be used to relieve pruritus associated with neuraxial opioids.

Propofol has no significant direct effects on renal function and does not interfere with cortisol secretion. Propofol has not been reported to trigger malignant hyperthermia or to exacerbate acute intermittent porphyria.

Excitatory phenomena such as tremor, hypertonus, and spontaneous or dystonic movements can occur rarely with induction or emergence from anesthesia induced by propofol. Proconvulsant effects of propofol have not been clearly demonstrated; the majority of apparent propofol-induced "seizures" are likely due to spontaneous excitatory movements secondary to selective disinhibition of subcortical centers by subadequate doses. Cerebral blood flow, CMR_{O_2}, and intracranial pressure are all reduced by propofol; these properties, together with its rapid recovery and antiemetic effect, make propofol a useful drug in neuroanesthesia. Propofol has no direct effect on neuromuscular transmission, nor are there significant interactions between propofol and neuromuscular blocking agents.

☐ ETOMIDATE

CHEMISTRY AND FORMULATION

Etomidate is a carboxylated imidazole derivative that is chemically unrelated to other general anesthetics (Fig. 3–4 and Table 3–2). It is a weak base that is poorly water soluble and is therefore formulated as a solution in 35% propylene glycol. Etomidate is about 75% bound to albumin in plasma.

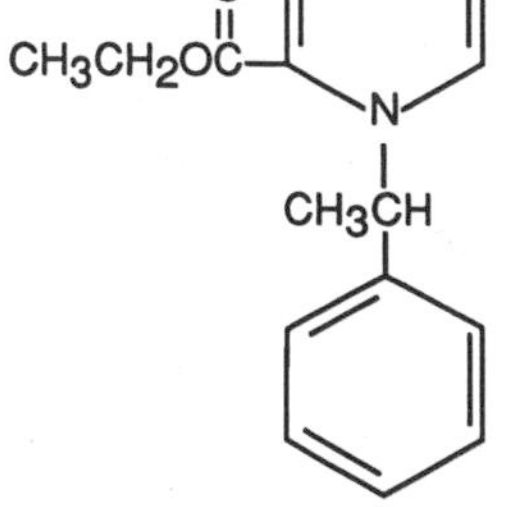

Figure 3–4   Chemical structure of etomidate.

PHARMACOKINETICS

The onset of unconsciousness following intravenous injection of etomidate occurs in one arm-brain circulation time. This rapidity is due to its lipophilicity, which facilitates penetration of the blood-brain barrier. Duration is dose-dependent and is usually 3 to 5 min with an average dose (0.3 mg/kg). Awakening following a single injection of etomidate is rapid due to its rapid and extensive redistribution to peripheral tissue. This is reflected in a large but variable V_{dss} (~5.4 L/kg). Pharmacokinetic investigations of plasma etomidate concentrations following rapid bolus intravenous injection reveal its rapid distribution ($t_{1/2}\alpha = 1$ min) and slower terminal elimination ($t_{1/2}\beta = 5.4$ h). Etomidate is rapidly and essentially completely metabolized in plasma and liver by ester hydrolysis to the inactive etomidate carboxylic acid. Etomidate clearance is relatively high (18 to 24 mL/min/kg), similar to propofol clearance. The larger terminal elimination half-time of etomidate compared to propofol is due primarily to the larger V_{dss} of etomidate. Although etomidate has been used by continuous infusion without evidence of cumulation, large doses will result in cumulative effects due to the terminal $t_{1/2}$ of 5 h. Limited pharmacokinetic data suggest that in hepatic cirrhosis the V_{dss} and terminal $t_{1/2}$ are approximately twice normal.

MECHANISM OF ACTION

Considerable evidence suggests that the general anesthetic properties of etomidate are due to facilitation of inhibitory synaptic transmission at GABAergic synapses through potentiation of $GABA_A$ receptor function. The (+)-isomer of etomidate, which is more potent as an anesthetic than the (−)-isomer, stereoselectively mimics the action of GABA in a number of neuronal preparations in vitro.

CLINICAL USES

Despite its rapid onset and short duration of action, a number of troublesome side effects limit the routine use of etomidate as an intravenous induction agent. Etomidate (0.2 to 0.6 mg/kg; average dose 0.3 mg/kg) has found a niche as an induction agent when less cardiovascular and respiratory depressant actions are tolerated than with thiopental. It is therefore particularly useful in the induction of general anesthesia in patients with impaired ventricular function, cardiac tamponade, or hypovolemia. A short duration of action makes it useful as a sole anesthetic agent in short, painless procedures such as electroconvulsive therapy or cardioversion for patients with ventricular dysfunction or hypovolemia.

Etomidate has effects on the central nervous system similar to those of the barbiturate anesthetics. Dose-dependent changes in the EEG culminating in burst suppression result from doses greater than 0.3 mg/kg. Etomidate also decreases CMR_{O_2} (by about 45%) and cerebral blood flow (by about 35%) similarly to thiopental but without reducing arterial blood pressure or cerebral perfusion pressure. This produces an increase in the cerebral oxygen supply-demand ratio. These properties make it attractive for neurosurgical procedures, where its short duration is also advantageous. Although etomidate has anticonvulsant activity, it can also activate seizure foci in patients with focal seizure disorders; although this property limits its use in these patients, it may facilitate the identification of seizure foci in patients undergoing the resection of epileptogenic tissue. Etomidate, unlike most other anesthetic agents, also enhances somatosensory evoked potential amplitude; this makes it a useful agent in procedures that employ this monitor.

CARDIOVASCULAR EFFECTS

Etomidate is remarkable for its relative lack of effects on the cardiovascular system. In normal patients or patients with mild cardiovascular disease, etomidate (0.15 to 0.3 mg/kg) has minimal effects on heart rate, stroke volume, cardiac output, and ventricular filling pressures; arterial blood pressure is also minimally affected at doses less than 0.3 mg/kg, although decreases of up to 20% can occur in patients with valvular heart disease. The hemodynamic stability of etomidate is related to its lack of effects on the sympathetic nervous system and baroreceptor reflex responses. Etomidate produces a smaller change than thiopental or ketamine in the balance of myocardial oxygen supply and demand and has a two-fold lower negative inotropic effect than equianesthetic doses of thiopental. (Studies in vitro suggest that the minor negative inotropic effect of etomidate may be due to the propylene glycol vehicle and not to etomidate itself.) Etomidate does not evoke histamine release and has a low incidence of allergic reactions.

RESPIRATORY EFFECTS

Etomidate causes less respiratory depression than the barbiturates, which makes it a useful induction agent for cases in which maintenance of spontaneous ventilation is desirable. Transient apnea may occur, especially in geriatric patients. Etomidate does depress the sensitivity of the medullary respiratory center to CO_2, but ventilation is usually greater at a given Pa_{CO_2} than with barbiturates. In most patients, minute ventilation and tidal volume are decreased, while respiratory rate is increased.

OTHER EFFECTS

Pain on injection and myoclonus are the most frequent undesirable side effects of etomidate. Pain on injection occurs in up to 80% of patients, but its incidence varies with the size and location of the vein used, the vehicle, the speed of injection, and premedication. The incidence is higher with small veins, particularly those in the hand. Use of large veins, a rapid carrier infusion, or opioid premedication decreases the incidence.

Induction of anesthesia with etomidate is accompanied by a high incidence of excitatory phenomena, including spontaneous muscle movement, hypertonus, and myoclonus. Although these effects may resemble seizure activity, they are not associated with epileptiform EEG activity. They appear, as with propofol, to result from disinhibition of subcortical extrapyramidal pathways. The incidence of myoclonus associated with etomidate is reduced by the prior administration of opioids or benzodiazepines.

Etomidate administered by both single injection or by continuous infusion directly suppresses adrenal cortical function. Although the clinical significance of this effect following single injections is unclear, increased mortality is observed in critically ill patients receiving long-term etomidate infusions. Etomidate reversibly inhibits 11-β-hydroxylase activity, an effect that persists 6 to 8 h after an induction dose and is unresponsive to ACTH.

Etomidate has no significant effects on hepatic and renal function; in contrast to other intravenous anesthetics and volatile anesthetics, there is no reduction in renal blood flow.

Nausea and vomiting are more common following induction of anesthesia with etomidate than with other induction agents. Etomidate is potentially porphyrinogenic and should be avoided in patients with porphyria. Etomidate is an inhibitor of plasma cholinesterase and may prolong the action of succinylcholine in patients with plasma cholinesterase deficiency and may also potentiate the action of nondepolarizing neuromuscular blockers.

There is insufficient data to support the use of etomidate in pregnancy and obstetrics.

☐ BENZODIAZEPINES

CHEMISTRY AND FORMULATION

The benzodiazepines include a large number of structurally related compounds with similar pharmacodynamic effects that differ primarily in their pharmacokinetic properties. The benzodiazepine receptor agonists routinely used in clinical anesthesia are diazepam, lorazepam, and midazolam (Fig. 3–5 and Table 3–3). All contain a benzene ring fused with the characteristic seven-membered 1,4-diazepine ring and are lipid-soluble at physiologic pH. Due to their insolubility in water, diazepam is formulated in propylene glycol/ethanol and lorazepam is formulated in polyethylene glycol 400/propylene glycol for intravenous use. Midazolam is unique in being the only water-soluble benzodiazepine available for intravenous use. This property is due to a reversible pH-dependent reaction that opens the diazepine ring of midazolam at pH < 4 and converts it to a water soluble prodrug (Fig. 3–6). Midazolam is formulated as a solution buffered to pH 3.5, which maintains the open ring and water solubility; at physiological pH following intravenous injection, cyclization occurs, converting midazolam to a highly lipid soluble active compound.

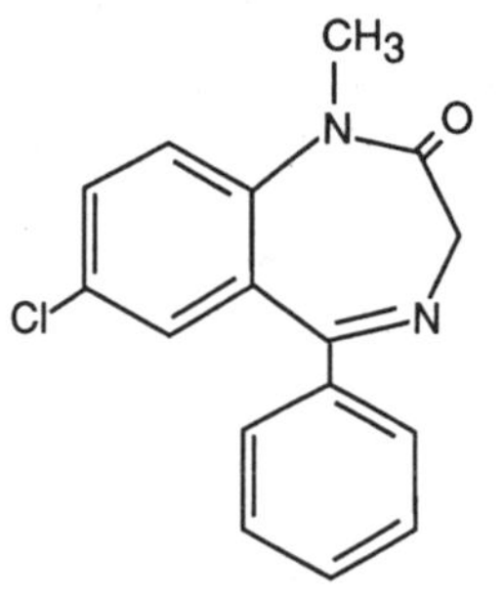

Diazepam 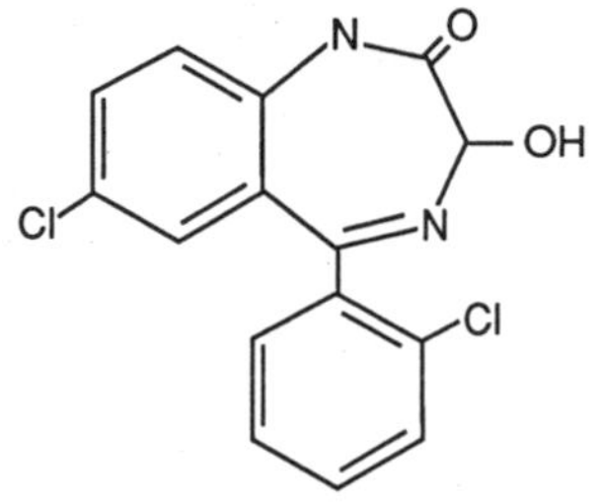   **Lorazepam** 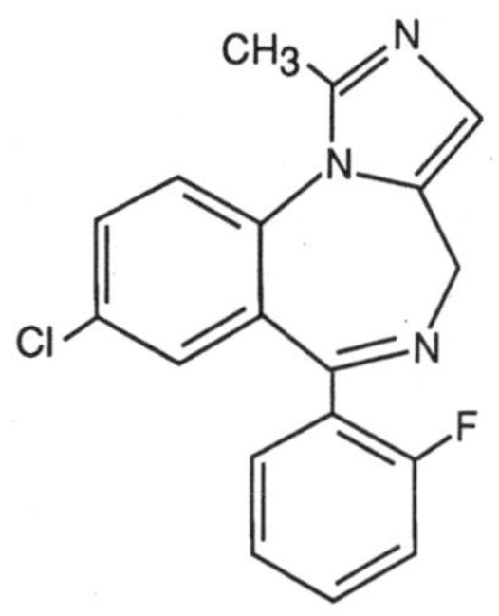   **Midazolam**

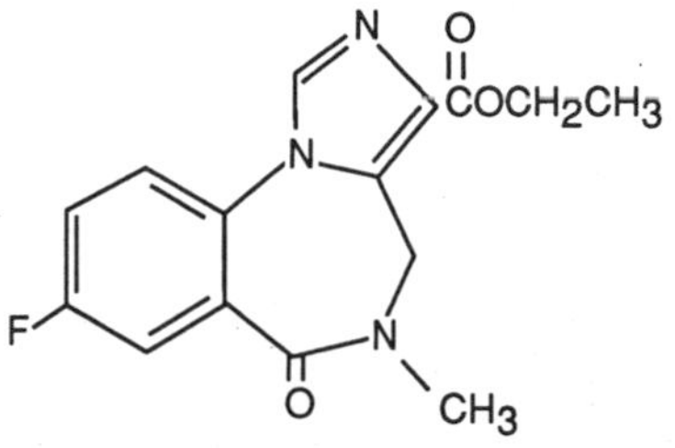

Flumazenil

Figure 3-5   Chemical structures of intravenous benzodiazepines and the antagonist flumazenil.

PHARMACOKINETICS

The high lipophilicity of the benzodiazepines (midazolam $\cong$ diazepam > lorazepam) accounts for the rapid onset of their central nervous system effects. The lipophilic benzodiazepines are also highly protein bound (96 to 99%), which may account for their moderate volumes of distribution despite their high lipophilicity (V_{dss} = 0.7 to 1.7 L/kg for diazepam). They are rapidly taken up into the brain and subsequently redistributed to peripheral tissues, including fat;

Table 3-3
PROPERTIES OF INTRAVENOUS BENZODIAZEPINES

Property	Diazepam	Lorazepam	Midazolam
Water solubility	No	No	Yes (pH-dependent)
pK_a	3.3	11.5	6.2
$t_{1/2}\alpha$ (min)	30–66	3–10	6–15
$t_{1/2}\beta$(h)	24–57	11–22	1.7–2.6
V_{dss} (L/kg)	0.7–1.7	0.8–1.3	1.1–1.7
Clearance (mL/kg/min)	0.2–0.5	1–2	6–11
Protein binding (%)	96–99	86–93	97
Induction dose (mg/kg IV)	0.3–0.5	0.05–0.1	0.1–0.3
Active metabolites	Yes	No	No

SOURCE: Modified with permission from Reves et al., 1994, and Reves and Berkowitz, 1993.

this redistribution to adipose tissue is used to explain the large V_{dss} in women, elderly, and obese patients. The termination of action of the benzodiazepines following a single small dose is primarily due to redistribution; after continuous infusion or large bolus doses, drug clearance becomes the dominant mechanism. Based on their differences in clearance, the benzodiazepines are classified as short- (midazolam; 6 to 11 mL/kg/min), intermediate- (lorazepam; 0.8 to 1.8 mL/kg/min), or long-acting (diazepam; 0.2 to 0.5 mL/kg/min). The clearance of diazepam is reduced in older patients, while the clearance of lorazepam and midazolam is less sensitive to age.

The benzodiazepines are metabolized in the liver by hepatic microsomal oxidation (phase I) and glucuronide conjugation (phase II). Both diazepam and midazolam undergo phase I oxidation reactions, which are depressed under certain conditions including old age, hepatic cirrhosis, and coadministration of certain drugs (i.e., cimetidine). Lorazepam, which is metabolized primarily by phase II conjugation reactions, is less sensitive to these factors.

The metabolism of the benzodiazepines is important, since many of their metabolites have pharmacologic activity. Diazepam is metabolized primarily by N-demethylation to desmethyldiazepam, which is only slightly less potent than its parent diazepam. Diazepam is metabolized more slowly to oxazepam, which is also active. Both of these metabolites contribute to the prolonged effects of diazepam. The elimination half-time ($t_{1/2}\beta$) of diazepam is 24 to 57 h in healthy volunteers (prolonged by liver disease, old age, and obesity), and that of desmethyldiazepam is extremely long at 48 to 96 h. Prolonged pharmacologic effects are common, particu-

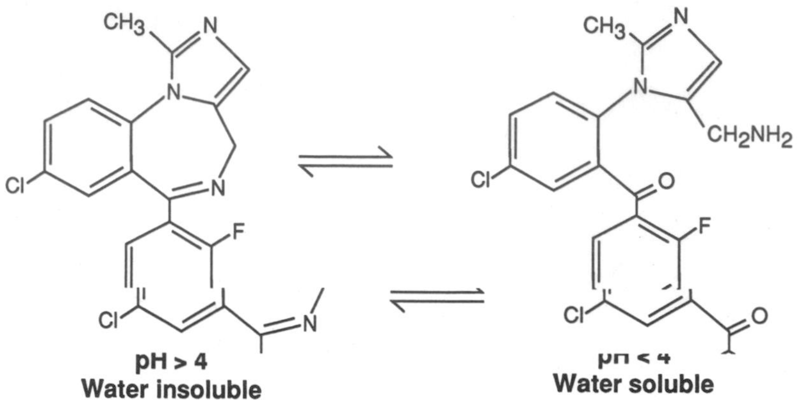

Figure 3–6 Reversible ring opening of midazolam above and below a pH of 4. The ring closes at pH >4, converting midazolam from a water-soluble to a lipid-soluble drug.

larly with chronic use in elderly patients. Midazolam undergoes hydroxylation to 1-hydroxymidazolam (major) and 4-hydroxymidazolam (minor), which have minimal pharmacologic activity; its elimination half-time is 1.7 to 2.6 h, which can double in elderly patients. Lorazepam is metabolized principally by glucuronidation to inactive metabolites; its elimination half-time is 11 to 22 h. Given the similarities in their volumes of distribution, the different elimination half-times of these drugs can be accounted for by their different rates of hepatic clearance.

MECHANISM OF ACTION

Compared to other intravenous anesthetics, the mechanism of action of the benzodiazepines is reasonably well understood. The amnesic, anxiolytic, anticonvulsant, and hypnotic effects of the benzodiazepines all appear to result from interactions with the benzodiazepine binding site of the $GABA_A$ receptor. Benzodiazepines modulate $GABA_A$ receptor function by facilitating GABA binding. $GABA_A$ receptor activation leads to the opening of an integral Cl^- channel, which stabilizes membrane potential near the Cl^- equilibrium potential (-70 mV) and inhibits neuronal excitation.

CLINICAL USE

The important applications of the benzodiazepines in clinical anesthesia include preoperative medication, intravenous sedation, induction and maintenance of general anesthesia, and anticonvulsant therapy. Preoperative medication to provide an anxiolytic and amnesic effect is usually accomplished by oral administration of diazepam (0.1 to 0.2 mg/kg) or lorazepam (0.05 mg/kg), or by intramuscular injection of midazolam (0.1 mg/kg). Midazolam has also been used by the oral or nasal route as a premedicant in children. The most widespread use of benzodiazepines in anesthesia currently is for intravenous sedation. Midazolam is particularly effective for this application, especially during short procedures under local or regional anesthesia, due to its more rapid onset and shorter elimination half-time. The anticonvulsant effect of the benzodiazepines also protects against the central nervous system toxicity of local anesthetics during regional anesthetic techniques.

The principal advantage of the benzodiazepines in the induction of general anesthesia is their hemodynamic stability. Midazolam has essentially supplanted diazepam and lorazepam in this role due to its more rapid onset, shorter duration of action, and lack of venous irritation. Induction of anesthesia with midazolam is accomplished by the intravenous injection of 0.1 to 0.2 mg/kg. Onset of anesthesia, identified by unresponsiveness and loss of the eyelash reflex, is slower than with thiopental and can be unpredictable, especially in younger patients. The induction dose is lower in premedicated, elderly, or chronically ill patients. Synergistic interactions are observed when midazolam is combined with opioids and other anesthetics. This allows reduced doses of each agent, when used in combination, to achieve anesthetic induction with minimal side effects and rapid recovery (coinduction). The barbiturates, propofol, and etomidate, as well as the volatile anesthetics, augment benzodiazepine binding to the $GABA_A$ receptor, which may be the mechanism underlying these synergistic interactions.

Emergence following induction of anesthesia with benzodiazepines occurs primarily due to drug redistribution. In general, the emergence time from anesthesia induced with midazolam is somewhat longer than it is with thiopental or propofol, although discharge from the recovery room is not delayed. Use of supplemental benzodiazepines may reduce volatile anesthetic requirements during balanced anesthesia and may reduce nausea, vomiting, and excitement during emergence.

CARDIOVASCULAR EFFECTS

The hemodynamic effects of the benzodiazepines used alone for anesthetic induction are minimal. The predominant effect is a slight reduction in arterial blood pressure due to a decrease in systemic vascular resistance. Filling pressures and cardiac output are usually unchanged; there are variable but small changes in heart rate. Myocardial contractility is unaffected by diazepam, which may also reduce left ventricular end-diastolic pressure while preserving coronary blood flow and cardiac output in patients with coronary artery disease. Midazolam causes slightly more hypotension than diazepam or lorazepam, possibly due to a direct negative inotropic effect. Generally, this effect is clinically negligible; however, the hypotensive effects of the benzodiazepines are magnified in the presence of hypovolemia and by combination with intravenous opioids, probably due to a reduction in sympathetic tone. Benzodiazepines alone do not block the hemodynamic responses to endotracheal intubation or surgery; this requires the use of adjuvant anesthetics, principally opioids. The hemodynamic stability provided by the benzodiazepines (maintenance of blood pressure and cardiac output) makes these agents useful for the induction of anesthesia in unstable patients.

RESPIRATORY EFFECTS

Benzodiazepines produce dose-related central respiratory depression, consisting of a decrease in tidal volume and minute ventilation. The slopes of the ventilatory response curves to CO_2 are decreased but are not shifted to the right, as with opioids. Chronic obstructive pulmonary disease, severe chronic disease, old age, and concurrent respiratory depressant drugs all increase the degree of respiratory depression and incidence of transient apnea observed with the benzodiazepines.

OTHER EFFECTS

The benzodiazepines have no appreciable adverse effects on renal or hepatic function. They do not suppress adrenal function or release histamine. The major side effects of diazepam and lorazepam are venous irritation and thrombophlebitis due to their formulation in organic solvents; these complications are minimized by injection into large veins with a rapid carrier flow rate.

Benzodiazepines produce a centrally mediated muscle relaxant effect; they do not affect neuromuscular transmission or influence requirements for neuromuscular blockers.

☐ FLUMAZENIL

The benzodiazepines are unique among the nonnarcotic intravenous anesthetic induction agents in having a specific antagonist available for clinical use. Flumazenil is a competitive benzodiazepine receptor antagonist with minimal intrinsic agonist activity or side effects. Although flumazenil has a high affinity for benzodiazepine binding sites, it has a short half-time due to rapid clearance. This creates the potential for resedation in cases where flumazenil is used to reverse the effects of high doses or prolonged infusions of benzodiazepines. The usefulness of flumazenil is limited in routine anesthetic practice; its principal roles are in the diagnosis of suspected benzodiazepine overdose (in increments of 0.5 mg/min given intravenously up to 3 to 5 mg) and in cases of accidental overdose or hypersensitivity to benzodiazepines following intravenous sedation or general anesthesia (0.2 mg/min intravenously up to 1 mg). Flumazenil is free of cardiovascular effects. It may induce severe withdrawal

reactions in patients who use benzodiazepines chronically. Administration of flumazenil can precipitate seizures in patients taking benzodiazepines as anticonvulsants, in the presence of other proconvulsant drugs (e.g., toxic levels of cyclic antidepressants), or in patients who are benzodiazepine-dependent.

☐ KETAMINE

CHEMISTRY AND FORMULATION

Ketamine is a partially water-soluble phencyclidine derivative with a pK_a of 7.5 (Fig. 3–7; Table 3–2). It is formulated as a racemic mixture of two optical isomers in aqueous solution with sodium chloride. The S(+) enantiomer is 2 to 4 times as potent as the R(−) enantiomer in producing anesthesia.

PHARMACOKINETICS

Following an intravenous injection of an induction dose of ketamine, its plasma concentration shows rapid distribution ($t_{1/2}\alpha$ = 16 min) and elimination ($t_{1/2}\beta$ = 3 h). Ketamine is extremely lipophilic (5 to 10 times more lipid-soluble than thiopental) with a moderate volume of distribution (V_{dss} = 3 L/kg). As a result of its high lipophilicity and pK_a near physiologic pH, it is rapidly taken up into the brain and has a fast onset of action. The rapid elimination of ketamine is a result of its high clearance (19 mL/kg/min), which is roughly equal to hepatic blood flow. Ketamine is metabolized by hepatic microsomal enzymes by N-demethylation and hydroxylation to derivatives that are glucuronidated and excreted in the urine. The metabolites of ketamine have significantly less pharmacologic activity than the parent compound and are not clinically significant. Ketamine is not significantly bound to plasma proteins.

Redistribution from highly perfused tissues to lean tissue is responsible for ketamine's short duration of action, which is unaffected by hepatic or renal dysfunction following a single dose. With repeated doses or continuous infusion, cumulative drug effects can occur, since ketamine is ultimately dependent on hepatic metabolism for clearance. Chronic administration of ketamine can result in induction of the hepatic enzymes involved in its metabolism. Tolerance to ketamine on repeated exposures may be due in part to this mechanism, although pharmacodynamic tolerance is also thought to occur.

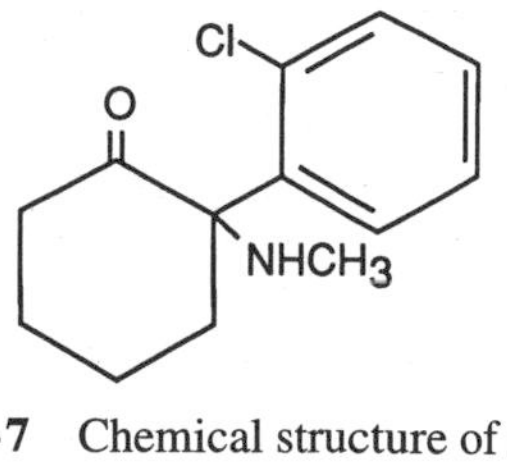

Figure 3–7   Chemical structure of ketamine.

MECHANISM OF ACTION

Considerable evidence suggests that the general anesthetic effects of ketamine are due to inhibition of excitatory synaptic transmission by antagonism of the N-methyl-D-aspartate (NMDA) receptor, an ionotropic (or ion-channel coupled) glutamate receptor subtype (i.e., a glutamate-gated excitatory cation channel). Ketamine is relatively selective for inhibition of NMDA receptors, and its stereoselectivity in producing anesthesia is also observed in its effects at the NMDA receptor, which suggests this as a site of action. Ketamine may be unique among general anesthetics in not producing its effects primarily through interactions with the $GABA_A$ receptor, although it also affects this receptor. The anesthetic effects of ketamine are also clinically distinguishable from other agents. It is described as producing "dissociative anesthesia" because of electroencephalographic evidence of dissociation between the thalamocortical and limbic systems. Dissociative anesthesia is characterized by intense analgesia, amnesia, and a cataleptic-like state of unresponsiveness and occasional purposeful movements. The analgesic effects of ketamine, which occur at subanesthetic doses, may be related in part to effects of the S(+) enantiomer at μ opioid receptors.

CLINICAL USE

Ketamine possesses a number of properties that limit its routine clinical use, although some can be advantageous in specific situations. The psychotomimetic effects of ketamine are therapeutically undesirable as well as a source of its abuse potential. Emergence reactions occur most frequently during the first hour of recovery from anesthesia and include excitement, confusion, euphoria, fear, vivid dreaming, and hallucinations. The incidence of emergence reactions (10 to 30%) in adult patients is lower in children and the elderly, and can be reduced by coadministration of a benzodiazepine with a lower dose of ketamine.

The sympathomimetic properties of ketamine give it an important role in the induction of anesthesia under specific conditions (0.5 to 2 mg/kg). Specifically, ketamine is useful in the rapid induction of anesthesia in hemodynamically unstable patients with acute hypovolemia, hypotension, cardiomyopathy, constrictive pericarditis, cardiac tamponade, congenital heart disease (with the potential for right-to-left shunting), or bronchospastic disease. Indeed, ketamine may be the agent of choice for induction of anesthesia in the patient with acute asthma. Ketamine is also effective by intramuscular injection and can be used for the induction of anesthesia in children and uncooperative adult patients without intravenous access (usual dose 4 to 6 mg/kg intramuscularly).

Subanesthetic doses of ketamine by intermittent bolus (0.2 to 0.5 mg/kg IV) or by continuous infusion (10 to 20 μg/kg/min) can provide intravenous sedation and intense analgesia. These properties are beneficial in short, painful procedures (e.g., debridement, dressing changes, skin graft-ing, closed reduction of bone fractures, biopsies, etc.) and as a supplement to regional anesthesia, both during placement of painful blocks and for inadequate or resolving blocks. Ketamine is also useful for sedation of pediatric patients for procedures outside the operating room (e.g., cardiac catheterization, dressing changes, radiation therapy, diagnostic radiology, etc.).

CARDIOVASCULAR EFFECTS

The cardiovascular effects of ketamine result primarily from direct central stimulation of the sympathetic nervous system. Ketamine also has a direct myocardial depressant effect that is usually masked by its sympathomimetic effect, except in patients with depletion of catecholamine stores or exhausted sympathetic nervous system compensatory mechanisms. Thus, it may cause significant hypotension in critically ill patients or patients in shock. Ketamine also inhibits catecholamine reuptake by neuronal and extraneuronal sites; whether this mechanism potentiates its direct excitation of the sympathetic nervous system is unclear.

The stimulatory effects of ketamine on the cardiovascular system include increases in systemic and pulmonary arterial blood pressure, heart rate, cardiac output, myocardial oxygen consumption (MV_{O_2}), coronary blood flow, and cardiac work. These effects contrast with the effects of other anesthetic drugs, which usually produce no change or cause hypotension and myocardial depression. The S(+) enantiomer is equipotent with the racemic mixture in its hemodynamic effects but is 2 to 4 times more potent than the R(−) enantiomer in its anesthetic potency. Equianesthetic doses of the S(+) enantiomer may allow for decreased cardiovascular side effects as well as a quicker recovery (due to the reduced dose). The hemodynamic effects of ketamine are not dose-related and are usually less pronounced following a second dose. The cardiac stimulation produced by ketamine can be blocked by a number of pharmacologic methods, including α- and β-receptor antagonists, clonidine, benzodiazepines, and volatile anesthetics. Ketamine is relatively contraindicated in patients with coronary artery disease (due to the increase in myocardial work and MV_{O_2}) or pulmonary hypertension (due to a potential further increase in pulmonary vascular resistance).

RESPIRATORY EFFECTS

Ketamine does not appreciably depress the ventilatory response to CO_2. Respiratory rate may decrease transiently immediately following induction of anesthesia, and, rarely, apnea occurs following rapid administration. Upper airway reflexes and muscle tone are maintained, which is beneficial during deep sedation. However, ketamine stimulates salivary and tracheobronchial secretions, which can lead to cough, airway obstruction, and laryngospasm. For this reason, an antisialagogue is recommended in conjunction with ketamine; glycopyrrolate is preferred to atropine or scopolamine due to its lack of central nervous system effects.

The bronchodilatory effect of ketamine makes it extremely useful in patients with reactive airway disease or active bronchospasm. Ketamine can improve pulmonary compliance in these patients by its sympathomimetic effect and by a direct smooth muscle relaxant effect.

OTHER EFFECTS

Ketamine is a potent cerebral vasodilator that increases cerebral blood flow, CMR_{O_2}, and intracranial pressure; it is therefore contraindicated in patients with intracranial hypertension. The increase in intracranial pressure can be attenuated by hypocapnia or prior administration of barbiturates or benzodiazepines. Ketamine also produces mydriasis, nystagmus, and excitatory central nervous system effects, evident in the development of theta activity on EEG. However, ketamine does not appear to decrease the seizure threshold in patients with seizure disorders. Ketamine enhances the amplitude of somatosensory-evoked potentials but suppresses the amplitudes of auditory and visual evoked potentials.

Ketamine does not impair hepatic or renal function. It does not evoke histamine release; allergic reactions are rare, although a transient erythematous rash is not uncommon. Ketamine enhances the action of nondepolarizing neuromuscular blockers by an undefined mechanism. In contrast to phencyclidine, it does not significantly prolong the action of succinylcholine by inhibition of plasma cholinesterase. Ketamine does not trigger malignant hyperthermia.

OTHER AGENTS

A number of other compounds with general anesthetic properties have been used as induction agents but are not currently available for clinical use. Of these, the steroid anesthetics are of particular interest. Althesin, a mixture of alphaxalone (the active anesthetic) and alphadolone, is poorly soluble in water. A formulation in Cremophor EL was withdrawn due to the high incidence of hypersensitivity reactions. Minaxolone was developed as a water-soluble steroid anesthetic but was associated with a high incidence of excitatory phenomena. Pregnanalone (Eltanolone) is currently under development as an intravenous induction agent. It is water-soluble and is formulated in a lipid emulsion. Advantages of this agent include minimal hemodynamic side effects, a short duration of action, and a low incidence of venous irritation; however, excitatory phenomena are occasionally a problem. The mechanism of action of the steroid anesthetics appears to be through effects at the $GABA_A$ receptor.

☐ CONCLUSION

There is no ideal intravenous anesthetic agent for all patients. A variety of drugs are available with differing pharmacologic profiles and hemodynamic side effects. The astute clinician selects and administers the appropriate drugs based on the anesthetic goals for each individual patient, which are dictated by the procedure to be performed and the pathophysiological state of the patient.

BIBLIOGRAPHY

Borgeat A, Wilder-Smith OHG, Suter PM: The nonhypnotic therapeutic applications of propofol. *Anesthesiology* 80:642–656, 1994.

Bowdle TA, Horita A, Kharasch ED: *The Pharmacologic Basis of Anesthesiology.* New York, Churchill Livingstone, 1994.

Franks NP, Lieb WR: Molecular and cellular mechanisms of general anaesthesia. *Nature* 367:607–614, 1994.

Fragen RJ, Avram M: Barbiturates, in Miller RD (ed): *Anesthesia,* 4th ed. New York, Churchill Livingstone, pp 229–246, 1994.

Hull CJ: Pharmacokinetics and pharmacodynamics, with particular reference to intravenous anesthetic agents, in Nunn JF, Utting JE, Brown BR Jr (eds): *General Anaesthesia,* 5th ed. London, Butterworth, pp 96–114, 1989.

Olsen RW: Barbiturates. *Int Anesthesiol Clin* 26:254–261, 1988.

Reves JG, Berkowitz DE: Pharmacology of intravenous anesthetic drugs, in Kaplan J (ed): *Cardiac Anesthesia,* 3d ed. Philadelphia, Saunders, pp 512–534, 1993.

Reves JG, Glass PSA, Lubansky DA: Nonbarbiturate intravenous anesthetics, in Miller RD (ed): *Anesthesia,* 4th ed. New York, Churchill Livingstone, pp 247–290, 1994.

Stoelting RK: *Pharmacology and Physiology in Anesthetic Practice,* 2d ed. Philadelphia, Lippincott, 1991.

Tanelian DL, Kosek P, Mody I, MacIver MB: The role of the $GABA_A$ receptor/chloride channel complex in anesthesia. *Anesthesiology* 78:757–776, 1993.

Opioid Pharmacology

Jaye Jacquelyn Stricker and
Charles E. Laurito

The word *narcotic* is derived from the Greek word *narko,* which means stupor or to be numb. It also refers to analgesics, such as morphine, that have the ability to produce dependency. The term *opioid* came into use with the development of synthetic agents with actions similar to that of morphine. Opium is a powder derived from the dried seed pods of the poppy *Papaver somniferum* and is actually a mixture of naturally occurring alkaloid compounds. The primary compound is morphine; however, there are more than twenty compounds in all. Morphine is the prototype of compounds in this category and the model to which all drugs discussed in this chapter are compared. The term *opioid* refers to numerous compounds, both synthetic and natural, that have some morphinelike actions and properties mediated by binding to opioid receptors. The ideal opioid is one that binds to its receptor in a highly specific way, produces only the desired analgesia, and causes no side effects.

The naturally occurring opium alkaloids are divided into two distinct classes. The phenanthrene group includes morphine, codeine, and thebaine, and the benzyloquinolone group includes papaverine. Papaverine has no opioid activity. These compounds have been used for centuries; however, morphine was first isolated in 1803, followed by codeine in 1832 and papaverine in 1848. Semisynthetic opioids (codeine and heroin) are synthesized by making relatively small modifications to the morphine molecule, while entirely synthetic opioids are produced by complex, multistep, rather than the simple, chemical modification of a preexisting compound.

Opioids are currently used by anesthesiologists as premedicants, sedatives, antitussives, pain relievers, adjuncts to anesthesia, and primary anesthetics. They all act at opioid receptors, which are located throughout the central nervous system.

☐ OPIOID RECEPTORS

The many agents in the opioid receptor group produce a variety of effects. A multiple receptor theory was originally postulated to explain these different responses, and it is now known that several different receptor populations exist in both the brain and the spinal cord. Receptors in the brain are concentrated in the periaqueductal gray matter, amygdala, corpus striatum, and hypothalamus. Spinal cord receptors are concentrated at the dorsal horn at the area termed the *substantia gelatinosa*. Each type of receptor shows specific effects when activated by an opioid agonist.

The μ-receptor is primarily located in the brain and is responsible for supraspinal analgesia. Two subpopulations of this receptor exist. The μ_1-receptors exclusively mediate supraspinal analgesia, while stimulating μ_2-receptors produces the undesired effects of hypoventilation, bradycardia, euphoria, and physical dependence. The endogenous ligand for these two receptors is β-endorphin. Other μ-receptor agonists include morphine, fentanyl, alfentanil, sufentanil, and codeine. Naloxone is a specific μ-receptor antagonist and reverses the effects of μ activation. The delta receptor modulates μ-receptor activity. Leuenkephalin is an endogenous agonist for this receptor. Naloxone also acts as its antagonist.

The κ-receptor mediates analgesia, but a greater number of these receptors are located in the spinal cord than in the brain. Sedation and miosis are also produced by κ-receptor activation with little or no effect on respiratory drive. Dynorphin is its endogenous agonist. Many of the agonist-antagonist opioid agents act specifically at the κ-receptor. Naloxone is a receptor antagonist here as well.

The σ-receptor causes unwanted excitatory effects: hallucinations, mydriasis, tachypnea, tachycardia, dysphoria, and hypertonia. No specific endogenous agonist is known.

☐ SYSTEMIC EFFECTS

Morphine is the prototype opioid agonist. Its systemic effects characterize those of all agents in this group. However, the specific character and magnitude of effects varies among agents.

CARDIOVASCULAR EFFECTS

In healthy, normovolemic patients, clinical doses of morphine produce little effect on the cardiovascular system. Direct myocardial depression is not significant, and decreases in blood pressure are unlikely in supine normovolemic patients. Orthostatic hypotension may occur with position changes, such as moving from supine to sitting, or standing. This is due to a blunting of two important compensatory responses. Morphine causes both bradycardia and peripheral vasodilation. Vasodilation results from diminished venous sympathetic tone and causes venous pooling and a decreased venous blood return to the heart. Bradycardia follows morphine's direct stimulation of the vagal nucleus in the medulla. This central effect can be abolished by prior atropine administration. The sinoatrial node is also directly depressed by morphine injection with an additional slowing of electrical conduction through the atrioventricular node.

An additional effect on blood pressure related to the administration of morphine is the release of histamine from the mast cells. The release of histamine is unrelated to specific receptor binding and is therefore not inhibited by naloxone administration. Histamine release is variable, but its effects are diminished by slowing the administration of the opioid, maintaining the patient in the supine position, and optimizing the patient's volume status. H_1 and H_2 receptor antagonist administration does not alter the release of histamine but does blunt the effects on blood pressure and vascular resistance.

Morphine administration does not sensitize the myocardium to the effects of catecholamines, and large doses of opioid agonists will blunt the degree of change in heart rate and blood pressure that follow surgical stimulation. Combinations of morphine with other agents or anesthetics can produce exaggerated cardiovascular responses that do not occur following use of individual agents.

RESPIRATORY EFFECTS

Morphine and other opioid agonists cause a dose-dependent depression of ventilation. This is the result of a direct effect on the ventilatory centers in the brainstem. These centers also become less responsive to $PaCO_2$ as an administered respiratory stimulant. Respiratory rate is slowed and tidal volume is increased. Periodic breathing and apnea can occur with high doses of morphine, and patients can become apneic while retaining consciousness and the ability to breathe on command. The elderly are more sensitive to the apneic effects of these agents. Depression of ventilation can occur rapidly and persists for several hours. Ciliary activity along the respiratory tree is also depressed in a dose-dependent fashion.

CENTRAL NERVOUS SYSTEM EFFECTS

Analgesia is the desired clinical effect of opiates. Small doses of μ-receptor agonists given incrementally to patients with pain provide reliable pain relief without the loss of consciousness. When morphine is given to patients without pain, it can cause dysphoria, which manifests as fear and anxiety. Opioid agonists activate the body's ability to modulate the pain system by binding to opioid receptors in the central nervous system. Morphine acts centrally to interfere with transmission, integration, and interpretation of arriving neural impulses. This action occurs in the spinal periaqueductal gray matter, as well as medullary and thalamic nuclei. Morphine also alters the patient's affective perception of pain. This follows action on the limbic system, which also contains a high concentration of opioid receptors.

Cerebral blood flow and intracranial pressure are decreased following narcotic use. Miosis occurs due to an excitatory effect on the Edinger-Westphal nucleus of the third cranial nerve; this effect is antagonized by use of atropine. Electroencephalographic changes resemble those of normal sleep: appearance of a slower delta wave pattern. The central nervous system is generally depressed, resulting in drowsiness and sedation, depression of the cough reflex, and respiratory depression.

Nausea and vomiting are common side effects of morphine and other opioid agonists. The agents directly stimulate the chemoreceptor trigger zone in the floor of the fourth ventricle. Morphine can also stimulate the vestibular nerve, which provides an additional trigger for nausea and vomiting.

GASTROINTESTINAL EFFECTS

Opioids cause spasm of the smooth muscle of the biliary tract and can increase intrabiliary pressure. This can exacerbate biliary colic and is easily confused with the pain of angina pectoris. This pain is relieved by naloxone, whereas the pain of angina pectoris is not. Both types of pain respond to nitroglycerine. Spasm of the sphincter of Oddi caused by the intraoperative administration of opioids may mimic common bile duct stones on intraoperative cholangiogram. Intravenous glucagon reverses this biliary smooth muscle spasm but, unlike naloxone, does not affect opioid analgesia.

Opioids have other effects on gastrointestinal motility. Peristalsis in the large and small bowel is decreased, although the overall tone is increased. The tone of the pyloric and anal sphincters, as well as the ileocecal valve, is increased. The increased transit time through the large bowel results in greater water absorption from the stool, causing constipation. In contrast, lower esophageal sphincter tone is decreased after narcotic use, leading to increased frequency of acid reflux.

GENITOURINARY EFFECTS

Morphine increases both the tone and frequency of peristalsis of the ureter. Detrusor muscle tone and the tone of the bladder sphincter are also increased. The overall result is urinary retention with the sensation of urgency.

CUTANEOUS EFFECTS

The cutaneous vasodilation that results from morphine administration is in part due to histamine release. Urticaria and erythema are commonly seen in the area around the skin injection site. This is not an allergic reaction.

ENDOCRINE EFFECTS

Opioids in high doses modify the endocrine response to surgical stress. This is particularly seen with fentanyl and its derivatives. Plasma concentrations of catecholamines, cortisol, antidiuretic hormone, growth hormone, and insulin are all decreased following fentanyl use.

REPRODUCTIVE EFFECTS

Opioid agonists are nonteratogenic. However, the placenta is not a barrier to these agents and they will cross to the fetus. The neonate of a mother using opioids in an addictive manner will become addicted.

TOLERANCE AND DEPENDENCE

Tolerance and dependence are major factors to consider when prescribing opioid agonists. These phenomena occur with the repeated use of all of the agents. Tolerance is the need to increase the dosage of opioid medication over time in order to produce a similar analgesic result. Tolerance takes several weeks to develop and is often seen during hospitalization. Although tolerance to the analgesic and respiratory depressant effects of these agents occurs, smaller doses of opioid will still cause miosis and constipation.

Physical dependence occurs, in contrast, when both a psychological and physical need for the drug develops. Once dependence is present, discontinuing the drug can cause withdrawal. The sympathetic nervous system is activated to cause symptoms of abdominal cramping, nausea and/or vomiting, diarrhea, insomnia, and restlessness.

The mechanisms responsible for the development of tolerance and dependence are not fully known. Postulated mechanisms include the development of an upregulated system of receptors in the brain and a basic cellular adaptation to the prolonged presence of the agent. There is no evidence that enzyme induction or increased opioid metabolism results in increased dose requirements.

OVERDOSE

Respiratory depression is the most serious side effect of systemic overdose. This manifests as hypoventilation or apnea. Pupils become miotic until hypoxia ensues, which eventually causes mydriasis. Skeletal muscles become flaccid and coma develops. The overall result is hypercarbia and acidosis leading to hypotension and seizures. Initial treatment of opioid overdose is support of ventilation and administration of an opioid antagonist (naloxone).

☐ SPECIFIC CHARACTERISTICS BY AGENT See Table 4–1.

MORPHINE

Morphine is difficult to synthesize and is still obtained directly from opium processing (Fig. 4–1). Its structure consists of the three rings of the phenanthrene nucleus with a fourth piperidine ring containing a tertiary amine. This structure makes morphine water-soluble. It is well-absorbed after intramuscular (IM) injection (90%) with an onset of action of 15 to 30 min and a duration of action of 3 to 4 h. Peak effects occur at 20 min after intravenous (IV) injection and at 45 min after IM injection. Absorption from the gastrointestinal tract is unreliable. Plasma concentrations do not correlate well with the pharmacologic actions observed.

Only small amounts of morphine enter the central nervous system due to the high degree of ionization at physiologic pH (>90%) and relatively poor lipid solubility. Morphine has a large volume of distribution (>3 L/kg) and rapidly accumulates in skeletal muscle, kidney, and liver.

Metabolism of morphine occurs in the liver, where it is conjugated with glucuronic acid. The predominant metabolite (80%) is morphine-3-glucuronide. Morphine-6-glucuronide is also formed in smaller amounts (8%). A secondary metabolic pathway involves demethylation to normorphine. Morphine metabolites are then excreted in the urine (90%), with the remainder undergoing biliary excretion. Morphine-6-glucuronide is pharmacologically active and has analgesic effects. Accumulation of the metabolites of morphine may occur in patients with impaired renal function, causing unexpected depressant effects after relatively small doses of the drug.

Table 4–1
PHARMACOKINETICS OF OPIOID AGENTS

Agent	pK	Protein Binding, %	Volume Distribution, L/kg	Elimination Half-Time, min
Morphine	7.9	30	3.2	115
Fentanyl	8.3	85	5.0	190
Sufentanil	8.0	93	2.7	150
Alfentanil	6.5	92	0.8	85
Meperidine	8.5	60	3	200
Naloxone			1.8	75

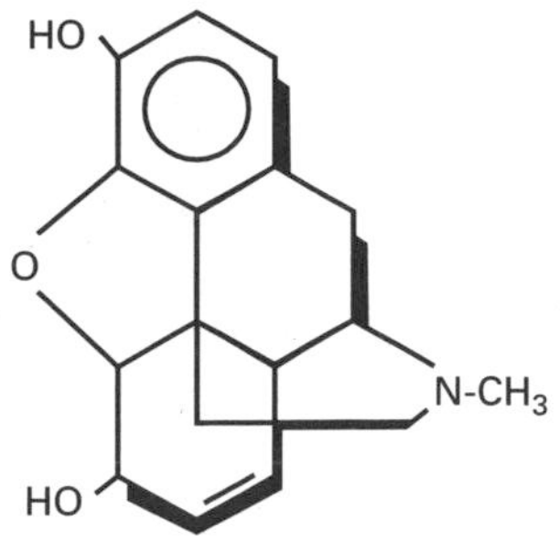

Figure 4–1 Morphine.

CODEINE

Codeine is another of the naturally occurring opium alkaloids. It has milder analgesic properties and has only one-tenth the potency of morphine. Most commonly it is administered orally, but is only two-thirds as effective when given orally, as compared to IV. Codeine will cause significant histamine release, which limits its IV usefulness.

MEPERIDINE

This is a synthetic phenylpiperidine derivative with a structure similar to atropine. It also has mild atropine-like effects. Meperidine has one-tenth the analgesic potency of morphine. It is well-absorbed from the gastrointestinal tract but is only half as effective by the oral route. Clinically important actions are similar to those of morphine, and both agents cause similar side effects at equianalgesic dosages. Orthostatic hypotension is more profound and frequent with meperidine than with morphine. Because of its atropinelike effects, tachycardia is seen, as opposed to the bradycardia caused by morphine. Meperidine is more highly bound to plasma proteins (60% versus 30%) than is morphine. The volume of distribution, however (3.0 L/kg), is similar to that of morphine. Duration of action is 3 to 4 h when given IM. Metabolism in the liver is to normeperidine by demethylation, which still provides 50% of the analgesic activity of the parent compound. Normeperidine has a prolonged elimination half-time of up to 40 h. It has stimulant effects on the central nervous system, which can lead to myoclonus and seizure. This is more likely following prolonged administration or administration to patients with impaired renal function who cannot readily eliminate the metabolite.

FENTANYL

Fentanyl is a synthetic phenylpiperidine derivative with a potency 100 times greater than that of morphine. When given intravenously, fentanyl has a more rapid onset (< 30 s) and a shorter duration of action than morphine. Its high lipid solubility explains its greater potency and rapidity of onset. Fentanyl redistributes to inactive sites such as skeletal muscle and fat. The lung also serves as a large storage site, with 75% of fentanyl undergoing first-pass uptake by the lung. The volume of distribution of fentanyl is greater than that of mor-

phine (up to 5.5 L/kg) and results in a longer elimination half-life. Fentanyl is more highly protein bound than morphine (85% versus 30%).

Metabolism of fentanyl in the liver occurs by several pathways to produce inactive metabolites that are excreted in the urine and bile. Fentanyl, unlike morphine, does not cause histamine release even in high doses. Bradycardia, however, is more profound. Chest wall rigidity can occur with high doses and make ventilation difficult. Equianalgesic doses of fentanyl and morphine cause a degree of respiratory depression similar to that found with meperidine. High-dose fentanyl decreases the stress response that occurs during cardiovascular surgery.

The clinical dosing range is wide for fentanyl, and higher doses seem to show fewer cardiovascular effects than other agents. Elderly patients may have reduced elimination. Cirrhosis does not affect the rate of fentanyl elimination.

SUFENTANIL

Sufentanil is a synthetic opioid agonist and an analog of fentanyl. It has a potency 1000 times greater than that of morphine and 10 times that of fentanyl. Its onset is quick (1 to 2 min). Sufentanil is highly lipophilic, and redistribution to inactive sites results in its brief duration of action. It is highly protein bound (93%), resulting in a smaller volume of distribution (2.7 L/kg) than that of morphine. Metabolism occurs rapidly in the liver to both inactive and weakly active metabolites. Sufentanil does not cause histamine release, and its preservation of cardiovascular stability is noteworthy. Chest wall rigidity can occur with rapid injections.

ALFENTANIL

Alfentanil is a synthetic opioid agonist and also a derivative of fentanyl. Its potency is 10 times greater than that of morphine. Onset is rapid (1 to 2 min), and effects are similar to those of morphine. Almost 90% of alfentanil is nonionized at physiologic pH due to a low pKa value of 6.5. Redistribution occurs to inactive sites, which results in a brief duration of action. The volume of distribution is quite small (< 1 L/kg), reflecting a lower lipid solubility. Hepatic metabolism to inactive metabolites is very efficient. Chest wall rigidity can occur. Cirrhosis prolongs the elimination half-life, but no change is seen with renal disease.

METHADONE

Methadone is a synthetic opioid agonist with a prolonged duration of action (24 h). It is highly effective and well-absorbed when given orally. It is frequently used for the control of withdrawal symptoms. Methadone is also often used to provide postoperative analgesia. Metabolism of the agent to inactive metabolites occurs in the liver. Side effects are similar to those produced by morphine, with significantly less euphoria and sedation.

☐ OTHER AGENTS

OPIOID RECEPTOR ANTAGONISTS

The opioid receptor antagonists have a high affinity for μ-receptors and are able to displace agonists from the receptors. They cause no opioid effects and are therefore classified as competitive antagonists. Naloxone is the prototype. Other agents include nalorphine, naltrexone, and levallorphan. Naloxone possesses no agonist activity and is more effective at the μ-receptor than at the κ- or σ-receptors. It is widely used in the operating room for reversal of the respiratory depression and sedation caused by opioid agonists. Naloxone exhibits no effects on its own in clinical doses. It is ineffective by the oral route. The duration of action is short (30 to 45 min), and repeated doses or an infusion is often necessary, since the agonist effects of morphine commonly outlast those of a single dose of naloxone. An unwanted side effect of naloxone use is reversal of the analgesic effects of the opioid. Nausea and vomiting are more likely following the rapid administration of IV naloxone. Also, an "overshoot" phenomenon may be observed with this agent, causing hypertension, tachycardia, ventricular dysrhythmia, and pulmonary edema. The cause of these reactions is unknown but may be due to a central release of catecholamines. A general rule for its use is slow titration. Use of antagonist agents can precipitate acute narcotic withdrawal in opioid-dependent patients.

Naltrexone is an antagonist agent that is highly effective by the oral route and longer-acting than IV naloxone. It is used more frequently in the treatment of narcotic addiction.

AGONIST-ANTAGONIST

There are many agents in the agonist-antagonist class. They bind to the μ-receptor and produce either antagonist or slight agonist effects. They also have actions at the other receptors (κ and σ) as agonists or antagonists. Agents included in this group are nalbuphine, pentazocine, butorphanol, and dezocine. The advantage of these agents is their ability to produce analgesia with less respiratory depression and less risk of dependence. They often exhibit a ceiling effect, however, meaning there is a dose above which further analgesia is not provided. The ceiling effect limits their usefulness in patients with severe pain.

Pentazocine is an analgesic agent similar in potency to morphine. It was the first agonist-antagonist agent used clinically. It is a weak antagonist at the μ-receptor and a strong agonist at the κ- and σ-receptors. Its antagonist activity is strong enough to precipitate withdrawal in opioid-dependent persons. Sedation is its most common side effect. No miosis, euphoria, or sense of well-being occur, as they do with the use of morphine. Hallucinations are a major side effect of pentazocine use and affect both visual and auditory systems. This complication is mediated via κ- and σ-receptor effects. Pentazocine also causes an increase in intracranial pressure, making its use dangerous in patients with altered intracranial dynamics.

Nalbuphine is also an agonist-antagonist. It is chemically related to naloxone and is equipotent to morphine. It is a partial agonist at the κ-receptor, with only weak agonist effects at the σ-receptor. It is a potent antagonist at the μ receptor. Onset of analgesia is similar to that provided by morphine in equipotent doses; however, a ceiling effect on the depression of respiration is seen because of antagonist effects of nalbuphine. Metabolism of the agent occurs in the liver.

☐ INTERACTIONS

The use of opioids with other respiratory depressants will cause an exaggerated effect. Another specific interaction involves the administration of meperidine and monoamine oxidase inhibitors. Patients receiving this combination may experience depression of their level of consciousness and severe hyperpyrexia. This reaction can be fatal. The mechanism for this complication following the concurrent use of these two drugs is unknown.

☐ CONCLUSIONS

Opioid agents have been used for millennia, and anesthesiologists currently use them in a variety of settings for many purposes. Morphine is the prototype opioid agonist to which all other agents are compared. Newer synthetic agents have broadened the armamentarium available. Familiarity with agonist, antagonist, and agonist-antagonist agents are imperative in clinical practice today.

BIBLIOGRAPHY

Ashburn MA et al: *Anesth Analg* 76:702–716, 1993.
Austin KL: *Anesthesiology* 53:460, 1980.
Bailey PL, Stanley TH: in Miller RD (ed): *Anesthesia,* 4th ed. New York, Churchill Livingstone, 1994.
Glass PSA et al: *Anesth Analg* 74:345–351, 1992.
Humphries HK: *Anesth Analg* 74:308, 1992.

McQauy HJ: *Pain* 36:111, 1989.
Pasternack GW: *JAMA* 259:1362, 1988.
Stoelting RK: *Pharmacology and Physiology in Anesthetic Practice,* 2d ed. Philadelphia, Lippincott, 1991.
Yaster M et al: *J Pediatr* 113:429, 1988.

Local Anesthetic Pharmacology

James R. Laidler, M.D.

☐ HISTORY

Use of the oldest anesthetic, cocaine, dates to pre-Colombian times, when the Incas ingested coca leaves. In 1855, the alkaloid mixture erythroxylin was extracted from the leaves, and 5 years later, in 1860, pure cocaine was extracted from this mixture by Albert Niemann. Niemann noted in passing that the bitter compound numbed his tongue when he tasted it. The utility of local anesthetic properties of cocaine remained unknown for an additional 24 years. Although cocaine rapidly gained popularity and was used in a variety of patent medicines and beverages (e.g., Coca-Cola), it was not until 1884 that Carl Koller rediscovered its local anesthetic properties. A year after Koller's discovery, William Halsted described the first nerve conduction anesthetic in humans, using cocaine and the newly invented hypodermic syringe. In 1889, August Bier used cocaine to perform the first subarachnoid anesthetic and incidentally discovered the spinal headache.

☐ SYNTHESIS OF ESTER LOCAL ANESTHETICS

Although cocaine had great utility as a local anesthetic, its toxicity and addictive properties were equally great. In the first 7 years after its introduction, 13 deaths were reported from medical use of cocaine. Following the elucidation of the structure of cocaine in 1895, the search for less toxic local anesthetics began. Many compounds with local anesthetic properties were synthesized, but few were of any clinical use. Most of the compounds were more toxic, more irritating, or less effective than cocaine. In 1904, procaine was synthe-

sized. Procaine is an effective, nonirritating local anesthetic with far less toxicity than cocaine. In addition, procaine has none of cocaine's addictive properties. All of the currently used ester local anesthetics (e.g., tetracaine) are derivatives of this parent compound.

☐ AMIDE LOCAL ANESTHETICS

In 1943, the first of the amide local anesthetics, lidocaine, was synthesized. Based on aniline, a precursor of petrochemical dyes, lidocaine shared the low toxicity of procaine and was more stable and far less likely to provoke allergic reactions. See Fig. 5–1.

☐ CHEMISTRY

ESTER AND AMIDE LINKAGES

Almost all local anesthetics in clinical use are composed of a hydrophilic group and lipophilic group joined by a carboxy linkage. The nature of the carboxy linkage, either ester or amide, gives a convenient means of separating the local anesthetics into two families. The carboxy linkage is planar (flat) and helps to keep the hydrophilic and lipophilic groups in the proper configuration for binding to the sodium channel, which is the site of action. In addition, the type of carboxy linkage influences the path of elimination. Ester-linked local anesthetics are readily hydrolyzed by plasma and tissue esterases, while amide linkages require more complex enzymatic modification before they can undergo hydrolysis.

Agent	Chemical Configuration			Physicochemical Properties			Pharmacologic Properties		
	Aromatic lipophilic	Intermediate chain	Amine hydrophilic	Molecular weight (base)	pK_a (36° C)	Octanol/buffer partition coefficient (25° C)	Onset	Relative Potency	Duration
Esters									
Procaine	H - N - ⬡ - COOCH$_2$CH$_2$ - N⟨C$_2$H$_5$ / C$_2$H$_5$ (H)			236	8.9	81	Slow	1	Short
Chloroprocaine	H - N - ⬡(Cl) - COOCH$_2$CH$_2$ - N⟨C$_2$H$_5$ / C$_2$H$_5$ (H)			271	9.1	720	Fast	1	Short
Tetracaine	H$_9$C$_4$N - ⬡ - COOCH$_2$CH$_2$ - N⟨CH$_3$ / CH$_3$ (H)			264	8.4	3615	Slow	8	Long
Amides									
Mepivacaine	⬡(CH$_3$/CH$_3$)-NHCO — N-piperidine(CH$_3$)			246	7.7	90	Fast	2	Moderate
Prilocaine	⬡(CH$_3$)-NHCOCH(CH$_3$) - N⟨C$_3$H$_7$ / H			220	7.8	129	Fast	2	Moderate
Lidocaine	⬡(CH$_3$/CH$_3$)-NHCOCH$_2$ - N⟨C$_2$H$_5$ / C$_2$H$_5$			234	7.8	30	Fast	2	Moderate
Ropivacaine	⬡(CH$_3$/CH$_3$)-NHCO — N-piperidine(H)(C$_3$H$_7$)			274	8.1	775	Moderate	8	Long
Bupivacaine	⬡(CH$_3$/CH$_3$)-NHCO — N-piperidine(C$_4$H$_9$)			288	8.1	2565	Moderate	8	Long
Etidocaine	⬡(CH$_3$/CH$_3$)-NHCOCH$_2$(C$_2$H$_5$) - N⟨C$_2$H$_5$ / C$_3$H$_7$			276	7.9	4900	Fast	6	Long

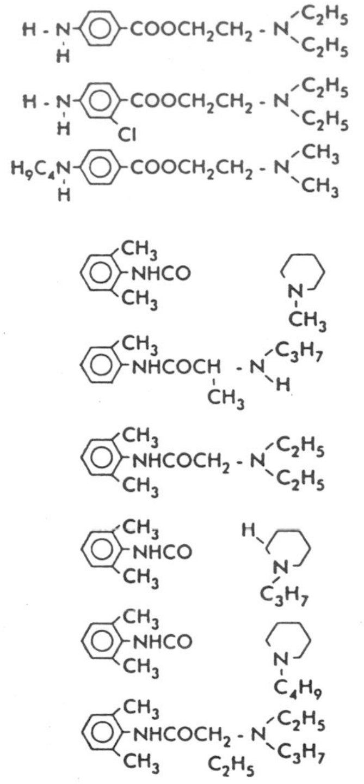

Figure 5-1 Characteristics of local anesthetics. (Reproduced with permission from Stricharz G, Sanchez V, Arthur G, Chafetz R, and Martin D. Fundamental properties of local anesthetics II. Measured octanol : buffer partition coefficients and pKa values of clinically used drugs. *Anesth Analg* 1990; 71:158–70.)

HYDROCARBON CHAIN LENGTH

The lipophilic component of the local anesthetic molecule is derived either from benzoic acid (ester local anesthetics) or aniline (amide local anesthetics). Both are bulky, planar aromatic ring structures. The hydrophilic component is much more variable but is usually a tertiary amine. Prilocaine and a few others have secondary amines as their hydrophilic component. The nitrogen atom in these tertiary and secondary amines readily accepts a proton (hydrogen ion), yielding a charged molecule that is much more water-soluble than the uncharged base. Benzocaine, a commonly used topical anesthetic, has an ester linkage with an ethyl group and therefore lacks an easily ionizable component. This accounts for its negligible solubility in water.

Since the discovery of the local anesthetic properties of cocaine, thousands of local anesthetics have been synthesized. Only a small number of these compounds have ever reached clinical use, and only a handful of these have remained in use. Those local anesthetics which have stood the test of time have certain structural features that help predict the characteristics of new compounds.

HYDROCARBON CHAIN LENGTH

Increasing the separation between the carboxy linkage and the amino nitrogen increases the lipid solubility of the local anesthetic. Lengthening and branching of the hydrocarbon chain also increase both the potency and the toxicity. The practical limits are the increasing toxicity and the decreasing water solubility. An optimum balance of potency, solubility, and toxicity can be found with hydrocarbon chains of one to three carbons. All local anesthetics currently in use have one or two carbons separating the carboxy and amino groups.

SUBSTITUTION ON LIPOPHILIC COMPONENT

Substitution of electron donor groups (e.g., $-NH_2$) at the para- position on the benzene ring tends to increase the potency of the local anesthetic while electron acceptors (e.g., $-NO_2$) reduce the potency. In para-amino substituted local anesthetics, lengthening the hydrocarbon chain of the para-amino group slows the hydrolysis. Procaine and tetracaine are both para-amino-substituted, with procaine having an unsubstituted amino group and tetracaine having a butyl-amino group.

Methyl substitution at the ortho- position on the benzene ring shields the carboxy linkage from hydrolysis, while substitution of chlorine in the same position accelerates hydrolysis. All of the amide local anesthetics have ortho-methyl substitution (all but prilocaine are 1,5 methyl-substituted, effectively a double ortho-substitution) and are very resistant to hydrolysis by tissue and plasma esterases. The ester local anesthetics are all hydrolyzed by these nonspecific esterases and chloroprocaine, which has an ortho-chlorine substitution, is hydrolyzed at an extremely rapid rate.

☐ NERVE CONDUCTION

INITIATION AND TERMINATION OF A NERVE IMPULSE

To understand how local anesthetics block nerve conduction, it is important to understand nerve conduction. A nerve impulse is carried along an individual neuron as a sequence of three events. First, the impulse is received by the neuron as a signal from outside the cell. In most cases, this signal is the arrival of a chemical neurotransmitter from a neighboring neuron across a synapse. However, sensory neurons can respond to other chemicals or to energy (e.g., light, heat, or pressure). Where the nerve enters the spinal cord, the impulse is converted to the release of a neurotransmitter. Between these two points, the impulse is carried as a unidirectional wave of depolarization along the cell membrane.

CELL MEMBRANE CHARACTERISTICS

The cell membrane consists of a double layer of long-chain fatty acids, arranged with the hydrophilic carboxylic acid group on the outside, facing the aqueous environment both inside and outside the cell. The center of the membrane consists of the long hydrocarbon "tails" of the fatty acids and is highly hydrophobic. This hydrophobic core of the membrane is essentially impermeable to charged molecules and acts as a good insulator. These properties allow the cell to develop an electrical potential across the membrane. This potential, known as the transmembrane potential, arises from the difference in intracellular and extracellular concentration of various ions and is essential to the function of all excitable membranes, such as those found in neural and cardiac tissue.

MEMBRANE POTENTIAL

Two facts are essential in understanding the transmembrane potential. The first is that the value of this potential depends on both the concentration of the individual ion and the permeability of the membrane to the ion. If the permeability of the membrane changes, the potential changes, even if there is no change in ion concentration. The second point is that the concentration differential at the membrane surface determines the transmembrane potential. Changing the concentration of the solution in contact with the membrane will change the transmembrane potential, even if the overall concentration of the solution changes only infinitesimally. These factors allow the transmembrane potential to change rapidly with only a small movement of ions.

INITIATION OF CELL MEMBRANE DEPOLARIZATION

Once the neuron receives the signal, either as a packet of neurotransmitter or energy, that signal causes a local reduction of the transmembrane potential from its normal resting value of -70 mV to a value more positive than -50 mV.

This causes the local sodium channels to dramatically increase their permeability by a factor of 500 to 5000. The local sodium concentration and the sodium permeability change. The transmembrane potential becomes less negative and briefly becomes positive as depolarization occurs.

PROPAGATION OF DEPOLARIZATION

The sodium channels are voltage-sensitive and open when the potential becomes more positive than 250 mV. This change in the potential occurs over a microscopic area, but it causes closed channels in the adjacent undepolarized areas to open and to spread the depolarization as a wave along the membrane. When the wave reaches the end of the cell, it triggers the release of neurotransmitter. As the wave of depolarization passes, the sodium channels again close, and the sodium-potassium ATPase pumps the additional sodium back out of the cell. Once the transmembrane potential is restored to its resting value, the neuron is ready to fire again. This scenario is slightly more complicated in myelinated neurons.

Myelinated neurons are wrapped in Schwann cells which are invested in a coating of myelin, a good insulator. This coating would completely stop impulse conduction if it were not for gaps in the insulation known as nodes of Ranvier. These gaps focus the electrical current of depolarization of the membrane and force the wave of depolarization to jump from node to subsequent node. The effect of this jumping speeds the conduction of nerve impulses. Rather than spreading slowly down the membrane, the impulse jumps from node to node, a process known as saltatory conduction.

The action potential and nerve conduction are both "all or none phenomena." If for any reason the degree of depolarization fails to raise the membrane potential to the point where the sodium channels open, the nerve impulse will stop. If enough sodium channels open to bring the transmembrane potential to the "threshold" value of approximately -50 mV, the impulse will be conducted. Anything that interferes with depolarization of the membrane can stop nerve conduction. At this point, a careful examination of the sodium channel is in order. See Fig. 5-2.

THE SODIUM CHANNEL

The primary known sites of action for local anesthetics are the membrane cation channels, primarily the calcium, potassium, and sodium channels. These channels are complex proteins spanning the cell membrane. Their purpose is to allow cations to cross the lipid bilayer of the cell membrane, which is otherwise impermeable to them. These ion channels are found in all cells, but the vast majority are in the membranes of excitable tissues, such as cardiac and neural cells, where rapid changes in transmembrane potential are needed for proper function.

Although local anesthetics have measurable effects on calcium and potassium channels, their greatest impact is on the functioning of sodium channels, and this is where the majority of research has focused. Much research on sodium chan-

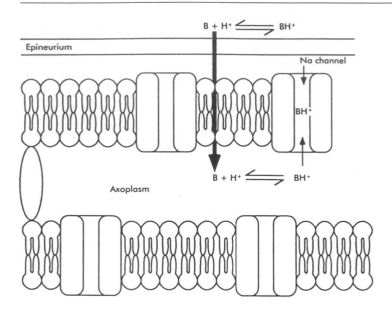

Figure 5–2 Interaction of sodium channel and local anesthetic. (Reproduced with permission from Rogers M, Tinker J, Covino B, and Longnecker D. *Principles and Practice of Anesthesiology.* Baltimore, Mosby-Year Book, 1993.)

nels has been done on the giant axons of squid. Fortunately, the sodium channel shows very little interspecies variation, so the results of experiments on invertebrate mollusks can be extrapolated to human nerve cells.

Sodium-Channel Specificity The sodium channel in neurons provides a voltage-gated pathway for ions to cross the cell membrane. The channel is remarkably specific for sodium. Its permeability to sodium (when the channel is open) is over a thousand times greater than that for other monovalent cations (Li^+, K^+, or Cs^+). Experimental data strongly suggest that the sodium channel exists in three different configurations: resting, open, and inactive. All configurations exist in equilibrium with each other; the predominant state is determined by local conditions.

"Gate" Model Despite many diagrams to the contrary, the sodium channel does not have a pair of "gates" or even one. It is a long glycoprotein that has extensive folding and hydrogen bonding that allow it to form a "pore" of variable size and geometry through the cell membrane. Changes in the transmembrane potential cause changes in the relationship of the various protein segments, thereby changing the configuration of the opening in the center of the channel. Although the idea of "gates" that open and close may help in imagining the action of the sodium channel, it is not an accurate representation.

Voltage-Dependent Configuration Changes At the resting transmembrane potential of -70 mV, almost all sodium channels are in the resting state and are essentially impermeable. If the transmembrane potential is made less negative, either artificially or through depolarization of the neuron, the equilibrium begins to change, slightly favoring the open configuration. When the potential reaches -50 mV,

there is a dramatic shift in the equilibrium favoring the open configuration, and most of the channels open. Sodium rushes into the cell through the open channels by moving passively down concentration and electrostatic gradients.

Since the transmembrane potential is determined in part by the sodium concentration differential across the membrane, the inrush of sodium causes the potential to drop even further, briefly becoming positive. At this point, the flow of sodium through the open sodium channels far exceeds the maximum capacity of the sodium-potassium ATPase pump. The process of depolarization that opens the sodium channel also initiates the process of inactivation. Within a few milliseconds, the open channel configuration "decays" into the inactivated state. This process is normally irreversible; that is, the inactive channels do not directly revert to the open configuration. In the inactive configuration, the sodium channels are impermeable, as they are in the resting state, but they cannot be opened. This provides the refractory period necessary for proper nerve and cardiac function. With the sodium channels impermeable, the sodium-potassium pump can begin to restore the normal sodium concentration differential and thereby return the transmembrane potential to its resting value. The inactive channels exist in equilibrium favoring the resting state as the potential returns to the resting value.

☐ LOCAL ANESTHETIC FUNCTION: MOLECULAR LEVEL

Local anesthetics block nerve impulse conduction by interfering with the normal function of the sodium channel. By binding to the sodium channel and preventing the passage of sodium ion, anesthetics stop the spread of cell membrane depolarization. The actual site and mechanism of the interaction between local anesthetics and the sodium channel is just now being elucidated.

SEARCHING FOR THE LOCAL ANESTHETIC SITE OF ACTION

When researchers first looked at the site of action for local anesthetics, they assumed that it was located on the extracellular opening of the sodium channel. This was consistent with the rapid onset of blockade when axons are bathed in a local anesthetic solution. Another clue was that previous studies showed conclusively that tetrodotoxin, an irreversible sodium channel blocker, binds to the exterior opening of the channel. Experiments using squid giant axons showed this not to be the site of action for local anesthetics used in clinical practice.

There are certain local anesthetics that, being quaternary amines, are almost completely ionized at physiologic conditions. Since ionized molecules cannot cross the intact cell membrane, these compounds cannot move from the bathing solution to the interior of the cell. When axons are bathed in these solutions, there is no change in the function of the sodium channel. However, when these solutions of local anesthetics are injected directly into the cytoplasm, the sodium channels are rapidly blocked. This suggests that the site of action is on the cytoplasmic side of the sodium channel.

An atypical local anesthetic, benzocaine lends further evidence for this site of action. Benzocaine has negligible solubility in water, so, although it readily crosses the cell membrane, it cannot enter the cytoplasm. Since benzocaine is an effective local anesthetic, it stands to reason that the site of action must be close enough to the cell membrane to allow the benzocaine molecule to reach it without having to enter the cytoplasm in any significant amount. This suggests that the binding site is in close proximity to the cytoplasm-membrane interface.

BINDING TO AN OPEN (OR CLOSED) CONFIGURATION

When the sodium channel changes configuration, a small transmembrane current is generated. Since this current occurs without any movement of ions, it can be separately measured independently of ion concentration. Using these small currents, researchers have found that the equilibrium of local anesthetic binding and dissociation favors binding the channel when it is in either the open or the inactive state. When the channel is in the resting state, the equilibrium favors dissociation.

PHASIC BLOCK

Phasic or "use-dependent" block is an interesting phenomenon. The speed of onset and degree of blockade has been observed to depend on the rate at which the axon is stimulated. The onset and degree of blockade are greater as the rate of stimulation is increased. This correlates with the clinical finding that local anesthesia has a faster onset when a patient is experiencing pain than when there is no pain. The faster firing rate of the sensory fibers in the patient in pain is thought to cause a more rapid onset of sodium-channel blockade.

Only ionizable local anesthetics exhibit phasic block and only to the degree that they exist in the ionized form in the cytoplasm. Unionizable local anesthetics, such as benzocaine, do not show phasic block. Phasic block implies that some aspect of the open sodium channel itself facilitates the binding of ionized local anesthetic. Perhaps it is the fact that the binding site is directly within the channel itself. Since benzocaine does not show phasic block, it apparently binds to a site that does not depend on the configuration of the channel for access. Perhaps uncharged molecules, such as benzocaine, have access to the binding site via an alternative route, possibly at the membrane-channel interface.

☐ LOCAL ANESTHETIC FUNCTION: NEURON LEVEL

MINIMUM INHIBITORY CONCENTRATION

An isolated neuron bathed in a nutrient solution is the standard model for studying local anesthetic action. As the concentration of local anesthetic in the solution increases, the number of functioning sodium channels decreases as they are progressively blocked. With fewer sodium channels able to respond to the action potential, less sodium moves into the cell and the amplitude of the action potential decreases. When a critical level of blockade is reached, the depolarization is inadequate to cause neighboring sodium channels to open. The concentration of local anesthetic at this point is called the minimum inhibitory concentration (MIC). Experiments using myelinated axons indicate that MIC is independent of axon thickness at the steady state. Although not as extensively studied, the evidence suggests that this holds for nonmyelinated neurons as well. Since steady-state conditions are rarely seen in clinical practice, thinner axons may be blocked before thicker axons, giving rise to the belief that thinner axons are blocked at lower anesthetic concentrations.

The MIC of local anesthetics is similar in many ways to the minimal alveolar concentration (MAC) of inhaled anesthetics; however the concept is not as useful clinically. Local anesthetics injected into the body are subject to absorption, dilution, and metabolism, and neurons are enveloped in tissue, muscle, and blood vessels. These factors limit our ability to estimate the concentration of local anesthetic at the axon. However, the MIC remains a useful standard for comparison of the potencies of local anesthetic agents.

CRITICAL LENGTH

If the neuron under study is placed in a bath that confines the local anesthetic exposure to a short length of the axon, an interesting phenomenon is noted. As the concentration of local anesthetic is increased, the action potential decreases in amplitude as it travels through the anesthetic bath. If the amplitude of the action potential drops below a critical point (approximately 3 to 5 mV), the impulse dies out. If, however, the action potential manages to traverse the anesthetic bath with enough amplitude, it is "revived" once it reaches the unblocked part of the axon.

If the local anesthetic exposure is limited to a portion of the axon, the concentration of local anesthetic needed to cause complete blockade of impulses is greater than when the entire axon is in contact. As the portion of the axon in contact with local anesthetic is decreased, higher concentrations of anesthetic are needed to cause blockade. When the length of axon in the bath decreases to a certain point, even extremely high concentrations of local anesthetic fail to halt impulse conduction. There is a critical length of axon that must be exposed to the local anesthetic in order to block conduction. Increasing the length of axon exposed to the bath decreases the anesthetic concentration needed, reaching a limit when approximately 25 to 30 mm of axon are exposed.

MYELINATED NEURONS AND CRITICAL LENGTH

Studies of myelinated axons show that thicker axons have a longer critical length than thinner axons. Since the distance between the nodes of Ranvier is greater in the thicker axon, there is a correlation. The critical length for myelinated neurons is two to three times the internodal distance. In the laboratory, impulses carried on myelinated axons have been shown to be able to "jump" over one or two nodes. To block conduction in myelinated neurons, at least two, and preferably, three nodes must be blocked with local anesthetic.

☐ LOCAL ANESTHETIC FUNCTION: NERVE LEVEL

Applying all of the experimental data to practical local or regional anesthesia is complicated by the realities of human anatomy. Unlike the situation in the laboratory, the neurons in the body are bundled into nerves, wrapped in fibrous tissue, surrounded by blood vessels, and buried in fat and muscle. All of these conditions and substances act to interfere with the efficacy of a local anesthetic.

DIFFUSION OF NERVE BUNDLES

Since most neurons are found in bundles, almost all local anesthetic blocks show a distinct progression in their onset and decay. The axons on the outside of the bundle are exposed to the local anesthetic earliest and in the highest concentrations. As the drug diffuses into the bundle, the concentration declines due to absorption by the axons and fibrous tissue. If sufficient local anesthetic is available, the central axons will be blocked after those on the outside are blocked. If the peak concentration of anesthetic attained at the center of the nerve bundle is insufficient for complete blockade, only a decrement in nerve conduction may occur. To achieve a state of dense anesthesia, the concentration throughout the bundle must be at or above

the MIC of the agent. In addition, the length of axon bathed by this concentration must be adequate to achieve blockade. This makes regional anesthesia somewhat unpredictable and helps explain partial sensory blockades.

In single-shot techniques, the local anesthetic begins to dissipate into the surrounding nonneural tissue as soon as it is injected. Uptake and redistribution by blood speeds the removal of drug from the site of action. As soon as the local anesthetic concentration in tissue surrounding the nerve falls below that measured at the outer axons, the drug begins to diffuse away from the nerve. At this point, the mechanics of diffusion are complex. Even as the drug begins to diffuse from the outer axons into the surrounding tissue, it may still be diffusing into the central axons. As the drug diffuses out of the core of the nerve, it moves into the outer layers, maintaining the local anesthetic concentration in those axons. Thus, nerve blocks normally decay in reverse order of their onset, such that the central axons recover first.

☐ EFFECTS OF CHEMICAL CHARACTERISTICS

DISSOCIATION CONSTANT (pK$_a$)

Local anesthetics are a group of compounds with subtle chemical differences that profoundly affect their specific biological actions. They are weak bases, meaning that they do not readily dissociate into charged ions when in aqueous solutions. Thus, a significant fraction of the molecules are in the uncharged or unionized state when in solution.

At equilibrium, the amount of the compound in the charged and uncharged states can be determined from the following equation:

$$K_a = \frac{[H^+]\,[base]}{[cation]} \qquad (1)$$

where the square brackets indicate concentration. K_a, the dissociation constant, is a characteristic of the individual compound. Since both $[H^+]$ and K_a are usually small numbers, they are more commonly expressed as the negative logarithms pH and pK$_a$. By taking the negative logarithm of both sides of this equation, the more common expressions appear:

$$pK_a = pH - \log\left[\frac{[base]}{[cation]}\right] \qquad (2)$$

Since pK$_a$ is a constant, the ratio of ionized to unionized local anesthetic is determined solely by the pH of the solution, and when the pH equals the pK$_a$, the concentration of base is equal to the concentration of cation. Table 5–1 lists dissociation constants for some local anesthetics.

pK$_a$ AND DIFFUSION ACROSS MEMBRANES

In the usual clinical uses of local anesthetics, the drug must first cross the cell membranes of the neuron and all interven-

Table 5–1
DISSOCIATION CONSTANTS FOR SELECTED LOCAL ANESTHETICS

Local Anesthetic	pK_a
Benzocaine	3.5
Mepivicaine	7.7
Lidocaine	7.8
Etidocaine	7.9
Bupivicaine	8.1
Ropivicaine	8.1
Tetracaine	8.4
Cocaine	8.6
Procaine	8.9
Chloroprocaine	9.1

ing layers of connective tissue, Schwann cell, and so on. Because of the lipid nature of these membranes, only the union-ized fraction of the drug will be able to diffuse in any appreciable amount. Although the ionized fraction has the measurable effect inside the cell, the penetration of the cell membranes by the anesthetic is the rate-limiting step.

Since the amount of drug in the unionized state has such a profound effect on the speed of onset of local anesthesia, it would follow that anesthetics that have a higher proportion of unionized drug would have a faster onset. This is exactly what is seen in clinical use. Local anesthetics with lower pK_a have a shorter onset time. Drugs such as lidocaine (pK_a 7.8) and mepivicaine (pK_a 7.7) have rapid onset, whereas drugs such as bupivacaine (pK_a 8.1) and procaine (pK_a 8.9) are much slower in onset. This phenomenon has practical limits, however. The unionized base of local anesthetics is usually very poorly soluble in water, which is why most are supplied as the salt (in solution of pH 4 to 5). If the pK_a is much lower than 6, the drug will not dissociate sufficiently to allow cation formation in the neuron. A classic example of this problem is benzocaine (pK_a 3.5), which, while it is an effective topical anesthetic, is worthless as an injectable drug.

LIPID SOLUBILITY

The lipid solubility of local anesthetics is given as a partition coefficient between water and a nonpolar solvent such as *n*-heptane, olive oil, octanol, or any of a variety of other liquids. Since neural tissue is rich in lipids and lipoprotein, the lipid solubility of a local anesthetic gives an indication of its affinity for the neurons. A local anesthetic that is highly lipid-soluble is readily absorbed by the lipids in nerve tissue (and other surrounding nonneural tissues) and is less able to diffuse away through the interstitial fluids. This absorbed local anesthetic also serves as a "depot" of drug, prolonging its action. The combination of decreased diffusion away from the site of injection and the "depot" effect leads to an increased potency for the more lipid-soluble local anesthetics. Bupivacaine (oil-water partition coefficient 130) and tetracaine (partition coefficient 80) are

more potent and have a longer duration of action than do lidocaine (partition coefficient 4) or mepivicaine (partition coefficient 12). Table 5–2 give oil-water partition coefficients for some local anesthetics.

PROTEIN BINDING

Like most drugs, local anesthetics bind to plasma and tissue proteins. Although local anesthetics bind to almost all proteins to some extent, most binding occurs to albumin and a1-acid glycoprotein (AAG). While the binding to albumin is not as strong as it is to AAG, the vast pool of albumin available for the agent to bind to is essentially impossible to saturate. Binding to AAG accounts for the greatest amount of plasma bound local anesthetic. It is responsible for the decrease in the plasma-bound fraction as the local anesthetic concentration is increased.

AAG is also an acute-phase reactant. Its concentration increases with trauma, infection, or surgery and decreases in pregnancy or cancer. Other drugs are also bound to AAG, as are the local anesthetics. Local anesthetics may displace them from these sites and raise the free fraction of these drugs in the blood.

Although there are marked differences between plasma proteins and the protein sodium channel, some have theorized that plasma protein binding is an indication of the strength of binding to the sodium channel. The basis of this theory is the observation that in most instances the duration of action of the local anesthetics is proportional to their degree of plasma protein binding.

ELIMINATION

Amide local anesthetics are metabolized in the liver; less than 5% of the drug is excreted unchanged by the kidneys. Even though urine testing for cocaine is one of the most common toxicologic tests done today, only 2 to 5% of the drug is excreted unchanged in the urine. Because of this dependence on hepatic alteration and clearance, elimination of local anesthetics is sensitive to cardiac output. As cardiac output drops, so does the clearance of amide local anesthetics. Hepatic dysfunction, as in alcoholic cirrhosis, will decrease clearance only in very advanced degrees of liver

Table 5–2
OIL-WATER PARTITION COEFFICIENTS FOR SELECTED LOCAL ANESTHETICS

Local Anesthetic	Partition Coefficient
Lidocaine	4
Mepivicaine	12
Etidocaine	191
Bupivicaine	130
Tetracaine	80

disease. The liver has sufficient functional reserve that only end-stage disease has any effect on elimination.

METABOLISM

Except for the very small amount that is excreted unchanged in the urine, amide local anesthetics are enzymatically altered in the liver prior to excretion in the urine and feces. As with other lipophilic drugs, the metabolites are generally more hydrophilic than the original compound. Although the toxicity of the metabolites is generally less than the parent compound, this is not always the case.

ESTER LOCAL ANESTHETICS

Ester-linked local anesthetics undergo hydrolysis of the linkage both in the plasma and in the liver. Local anesthetics based on para-aminobenzoic acid (PABA; e.g., procaine and tetracaine) are hydrolyzed more effectively by plasma esterases than by liver enzymes. Local anesthetics that are esters of other aromatic acids (e.g., piperocaine) are more effectively hydrolyzed by hepatic esterases. Cocaine, the only naturally occurring local anesthetic, is a double ester and requires both plasma and hepatic hydrolysis for metabolism.

AMIDE LOCAL ANESTHETICS

Amide local anesthetics are much more resistant to hydrolysis than are ester local anesthetics; they usually require enzymatic alteration before the amide bond can be hydrolyzed. The specific amide bond type determines how it is metabolized in the liver. The amide bond can be formed either by condensing an aromatic acid with an alkylamino alcohol or by condensing an aromatic amine with an alkylamino acid. The former results in an aminoalkyl amide bond, and the latter results in an aminoacyl amide bond. The two are decomposed in different ways. Aminoalkyl amide local anesthetics are not in common use at this time; the two drugs of this class in use today are procainamide and dibucaine. Of the two, procainamide has been more extensively studied. Both drugs are hydrolyzed so slowly that they are excreted largely unchanged in the urine. This makes the aminoalkyl amide local anesthetic an exception to the general rule of excretion for local anesthetics. The small amount of procainamide that is metabolized undergoes hydrolysis in the plasma. Dibucaine, despite its well-known affinity for plasma cholinesterase, is not hydrolyzed at all by this enzyme and undergoes little metabolism.

Aminoacyl amide local anesthetics include some of the most popular local anesthetics in use today. Lidocaine, bupivacaine, and ropivacaine are all aminoacyl amides. These drugs undergo extensive metabolism by hepatic mixed function oxidases and amideases in a multistep process. The oxidative pathways use the cytochrome P450 enzyme system.

☐ TOXICITY

CENTRAL NERVOUS SYSTEM TOXICITY

Local anesthetics are toxic to both the central nervous system (CNS) and cardiac tissue. CNS toxicity is generally seen at lower plasma concentrations. The early symptoms of CNS toxicity include sedation, disorientation, tinnitus, and perioral anesthesia. As higher blood levels of local anesthetic are reached, symptoms of excitation—restlessness, tremulousness, and anxiety—predominate, finally leading to seizures. As even higher blood levels are attained, excitation gives way to depression. Seizures stop, and respiratory depression and coma develop. Respiratory arrest ultimately occurs, often closely followed by cardiac arrest and circulatory collapse.

CARDIAC TOXICITY

The cardiac toxicity of local anesthetics has not been studied as much as the CNS toxicity because, until recently, investigators assumed that CNS toxicity would occur well before symptoms of cardiac toxicity. The plasma level at which CNS symptoms are seen are consistently lower than the point at which cardiac toxicity begins. A series of deaths among pregnant women receiving 0.75% bupivacaine epidurally brought the problem of cardiac toxicity to light.

TOXICITY OF 0.75% BUPIVACAINE

It was determined from the clinical history that all or much of the drug dose the women received was inadvertently injected intravascularly. The patients experienced sudden cardiovascular collapse and died despite aggressive efforts at resuscitation. The physicians involved noted no evidence of CNS toxicity preceding the cardiovascular collapse. The problem with using 0.75% bupivacaine in obstetric patients had little to do with the drug concentration and much to do with the nature of the drug itself.

Although the absolute plasma level needed for cardiac toxicity is higher than for CNS toxicity, the two levels are dangerously close with bupivacaine. The lidocaine dose needed to cause complete cardiac collapse (in dogs) is 7 times that needed to cause seizures. By contrast, the cardiac toxic dose of bupivacaine is only 4 times the dose needed for seizures. Bupivacaine in high serum concentrations will also produce severe cardiac dysrhythmia and profoundly depress myocardial contractility. This differs from lidocaine. The bupivacaine molecule is slower to enter and inhibit sodium channel activity in cardiac membranes, and it is also slower to exit. Bupivacaine depresses the rapid phase of depolarization both in the ventricular muscle cells and in the cells of the conduction system. The rate of recovery from the bupivacaine block is slower than that from lidocaine. The slower recovery causes an incomplete restoration of the depolarized state between successive action potentials. This effect is particularly noteworthy with rapid heart rates. The different recoveries from the two anesthetics explain the antidysrhythmic properties of lidocaine versus the propensity toward dysrhythmia with high doses of bupivacaine. In addition, pregnancy decreases the dose of local anesthetic needed to cause toxicity, in part because of altered protein binding. This would make a highly protein bound drug such as bupivacaine even more toxic.

MYOCARDIAL TOXICITY

In addition to their profound effect on the conduction system of the heart, local anesthetics cause direct myocardial depression. Although the mechanism is not yet clear, studies have shown that the agents inhibit the release of calcium from the sarcoplasmic reticulum, although increasing the extracellular calcium concentration does not reverse the effect. The negative inotropic effect of local anesthetics is dose-dependent. The more potent agents (e.g., tetracaine and bupivacaine) cause a greater decrease in contractility than do the less potent agents (e.g., lidocaine and procaine).

Although ventricular arrhythmias are not commonly seen with lidocaine, tetracaine, or mepivicaine, they are a feature of the cardiotoxicity of bupivacaine and, to a lesser extent, etidocaine. Premature ventricular contractions, ventricular tachycardia (similar to torsades de pointes), and ventricular fibrillation have all been seen in experimental animals and human patients. The mechanism of these dysrhythmias is not well-defined. Blockade of the fast sodium channels may be involved. It is notable that the injection of bupivacaine into the cerebral circulation and certain parts of the brain also causes similar dysrhythmia without toxic concentration of local anesthetic in the systemic circulation.

MISCELLANEOUS TOXICITIES

Allergy   True allergy to ester local anesthetics is a fairly common condition. Esters are all metabolized to para-amino benzoic acid (PABA), an allergen and sensitizing agent. Most patients who report an allergy to local anesthetics have a positive reaction (wheal and flare) to intradermal procaine, chloroprocaine, or tetracaine. However, PABA is found in a variety of household pharmaceuticals, and up to one-third of the American population have a positive reaction to intradermal ester local anesthetics. Most people who react to intradermal ester local anesthetics do not go on to develop systemic anaphylaxis if these agents are used for local or regional anesthesia.

Documented allergy to an amide local anesthetics is extremely rare. Intradermal testing with a variety of amide local anesthetics has shown infrequent reaction and none of the test subjects experienced anaphylaxis. Most adverse reactions to local anesthetics are either CNS toxicity or reaction to adrenergic stimulation from intravascular injection of epinephrine-containing solutions. Amide local anesthetic solutions may also contain the preservative methylparaben, which may cause allergic reactions due to its similarity to PABA.

BIBLIOGRAPHY

Bokesch PM, Raymond SA, Strichartz GR: Dependence of lidocaine potency on pH and PCO_2. *Anesth Analg* 66:9-17, 1987.

Butterworth JF, Strichartz GR: Molecular mechanisms of local anesthesia: a review. *Anesthesiology* 72:711-734, 1990.

Courtney KR, Strichartz GR: Structural elements which determine local anesthetic activity, in Strichartz GR et al (ed): *Handbook of Experimental Pharmacology:* 81:53–94, 1987.

Cousins MJ, Bridenbaugh PO (eds): *Neural Blockade in Clinical Anesthesia and Management of Pain,* 2d ed. Philadelphia, Lippincott, 1988.

Covino BG, Vassalo HG: *Local Anesthetics: Mechanisms of Action and Clinical Use.* New York, Grune & Stratton, 1976.

Lee AG: Model for action of local anesthetics, *Nature* 262: 545–548, 1976.

Raymond SA, Steffensen SC, Gugino LD, Strichartz GR: The role of length of nerve exposed to local anesthetics in impulse blocking action. *Anesth Analg* 68:563-70, 1988.

6

Muscle Relaxant Pharmacology

Maria DeCastro

A thorough understanding of the pharmacology of muscle relaxants is essential to safe anesthetic practice. Neuromuscular blocking agents are frequently used to facilitate laryngoscopy and to provide muscle relaxation necessary for optimal surgical conditions. Thus, muscle relaxants are among the most common drugs used in providing anesthetic care.

☐ ANATOMY OF THE NEUROMUSCULAR JUNCTION

The neuromuscular junction is the major site of action of the commonly used muscle relaxants (Fig. 6–1). It consists of an unmyelinated nerve ending that lies in a synaptic trough. Within the nerve terminal are a large number of acetylcholine-containing vesicles that line up in active zones where transmitter release occurs. Each vesicle contains roughly 10,000 molecules of acetylcholine. The enzyme choline-O-acetyltransferase, which is responsible for the synthesis of acetylcholine from choline and acetylcoenzyme A, is also present in the nerve terminal. Directly opposite the active zones of the nerve terminal are specialized folds of the postjunctional membrane of skeletal muscle that form the motor endplate. Nicotinic cholinergic receptors occupy these endplates in very high concentrations, typically more than twenty million receptors in a single motor endplate. The nerve terminal and endplate are separated by the synaptic cleft, a 50 to 70 nm wide gap which contains basement membrane material. Acetylcholinesterase is present in the folds of the synaptic cleft.

The postjunctional nicotinic cholinergic receptor is a pentameric, ligand-gated ion channel with a total molecular weight of 250,000 daltons. The postjunctional receptor in adult skeletal muscle is composed of two alpha, and one each, beta, delta, and epsilon subunits. These traverse the postjunctional membrane with one-half of the composite molecule extending from the extracellular surface (Fig. 6–2). The subunits are arranged to form a central pore, which comprises the ion channel (right panel, Fig. 6–2). The natural ligand of this receptor is acetylcholine and the open conformation is triggered when acetylcholine molecules bind to both of the alpha subunits. This increases cationic conductance, allowing sodium entry which causes depolarization of the endplate.

The resting nerve randomly releases small packets of acetylcholine, called quanta, each containing about 1,000 molecules of acetylcholine. Quantal release causes the mini-endplate potential which is insufficient to depolarize the adjacent muscle membrane. However, a propagated action potential results in the release of approximately 50 acetylcholine vesicles from the nerve terminal. The resulting endplate potential then depolarizes the adjacent muscle membrane and triggers excitation-contraction coupling (see Chap. 8). Both random, quantal release of acetylcholine and that initiated by the action potential are calcium dependent. Note that the amount of acetylcholine released from the nerve terminal following an action potential is more than ten times the number of molecules necessary to generate an endplate potential. This excess quantity of acetylcholine is responsible for the "margin of safety" in neuromuscular transmission and accounts for the fact that competitive inhibitors of acetylcholine binding, like the nondepolarizing muscle relaxants, must bind more than 80 percent of available receptors before twitch tension is reduced.

Nondepolarizing muscle relaxants compete with acetylcholine by binding to either or both α subunits, which prevents the open channel conformation. Succinylcholine binds to both α subunits, leading to sustained depolarization of the muscle membrane. As cations, neuromuscular blockers can

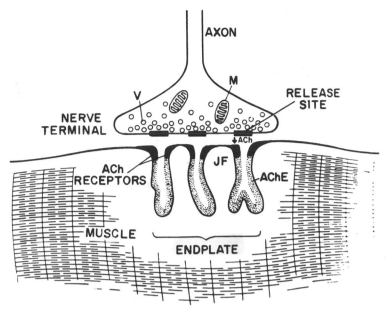

Figure 6-1   The neuromuscular junction. V, vesicle; M, mitochondria; ACh, acetylcholine; JF, junctional fold; AChE, acetylcholinesterase. Reproduced with permission of Massachusetts Medical Society from Drachman DA. Myasthenia gravis. *N Engl J Med* 1978; 298:136-142.

also enter the channel of the open cholinergic receptor, preventing normal ion influx. This phenomenon can be seen clinically with larger doses of nondepolarizing muscle relaxants and may result in a block that is more difficult to antagonize with acetylcholinesterase inhibitors.

Prejunctional cholinergic receptors are present in the nerve terminal and influence the mobilization of acetylcholine. Prejunctional receptors differ from postjunctional receptors in their binding characteristics. Blockade of prejunctional receptors appears to occur preferentially during high-frequency stimulation. Extrajunctional nicotinic cholinergic receptors are normally scattered throughout adult muscle membrane in very small numbers. These are identical to receptors in fetal skeletal muscle and differ from those in the adult endplate only by substitution of the epsilon subunit with a gamma subunit. Extrajunctional receptors proliferate in denervated or atrophied muscle and mediate the abnormal response to depolarizing muscle relaxants in these situations.

The number of individual muscle fibers supplied by a given neuromuscular junction is variable. Muscles involved in fine motor movements have fewer muscle fibers innervated by a given neuromuscular junction. The extraocular muscles characteristically have multiple innervation, in which each muscle fiber is supplied by several neuromuscular junctions. Muscles with multiple innervation exhibit a contracture response to depolarizing neuromuscular blockade. This phenomenon may explain the rise in intraocular pressure that occurs with the administration of succinylcholine.

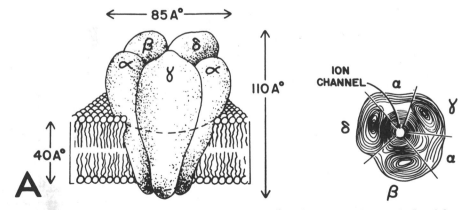

Figure 6-2   The fetal, or extrajunctional, nicotinic cholinergic receptor (see text). In adult muscle, the normal endplate receptor is identical except that the gamma subunit is replaced with an epsilon subunit, which is coded by a different gene. Reproduced with permission from Taylor P. *Anesthesiology* 1985; 63:1-3.

☐ STRUCTURE-ACTIVITY RELATIONS

Acetylcholine (Fig. 6–3) is a positively charged quaternary ammonium compound that attaches to the negatively charged nicotinic cholinergic receptor. Acetylcholine also binds to other types of cholinergic receptors (cardiac muscarinic and nicotinic receptors at the autonomic ganglia). The pharmacologic properties of the various neuromuscular blockers depend on their relative affinities for the various cholinergic receptors. These properties can be explained by certain chemical features.

All neuromuscular blockers share some structural similarity to acetylcholine. Succinylcholine resembles two molecules of acetylcholine linked together. The nondepolarizers are bulkier molecules but also contain an acetylcholine-like moiety. The nondepolarizers have one to three quaternary ammonium groups. Specificity for the nicotinic cholinergic receptor at the neuromuscular junction has been attributed to an optimum distance (1.2 to 1.4 nm) between nitrogen molecules of the bisquaternary compounds. However, the varying distances between nitrogen molecules in various clinically effective neuromuscular blockers and the recognition of the monoquaternary structures of D-tubocurarine and vecuronium have challenged this tenet.

A shorter distance between the two nitrogen molecules of bisquaternary compounds promotes affinity for nicotinic receptors at the autonomic ganglion. Hexamethonium and fazadinium (a nondepolarizing muscle relaxant that is not available in the United States) have shorter distances between ammonium atoms than do the steroidal muscle relaxants (pancuronium, pipecuronium, and vecuronium).

Muscarinic blockade is a feature of the trisquaternary compound gallamine. Muscarinic blockade has also been an important side effect of the steroidal muscle relaxant pancuronium. Removal of the methyl group on the A ring of pancuronium forms vecuronium. This minor chemical adjustment reduces its ability to produce muscarinic blockade.

Benzoisoquinolone compounds (D-tubocurarine, metocurine, atracurium, and mivacurium) tend to cause histamine release. The methylated compounds metocurine and atracurium exhibit less histamine release than does D-tubocurarine.

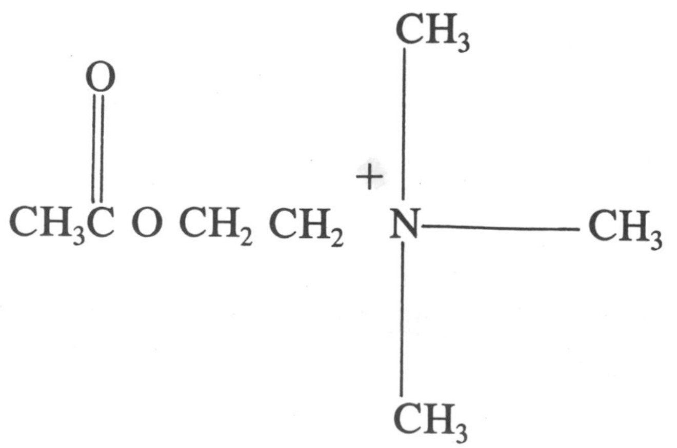

Figure 6–3   Acetylcholine.

☐ MONITORING THE NEUROMUSCULAR JUNCTION

The response to neuromuscular blocking agents is variable and is altered by various factors, including coexisting disease states and administration of other medications. Most commonly, the neuromuscular junction is monitored at the ulnar nerve in the forearm. A motor response at the adductor pollicis brevis muscle in the hand can be assessed by tactile or visual evaluation. Evoked tension or electromyographic measurements are much more sensitive monitors of neuromuscular function and are useful research tools. Other sites that can be monitored include the median, posterior tibial, peroneal, and facial nerves.

Various muscles recover from neuromuscular blockade at various rates. Muscles of the jaw, orbicularis oculi, larynx, and diaphragm appear to recover from neuromuscular blockade faster than does the adductor pollicis brevis. This relationship indicates that adequate conditions for laryngoscopy may be achieved before abolition of a twitch response at the thumb. Monitoring of neuromuscular function at the relatively resistant orbicularis oculi muscle may lead to overdosage of nondepolarizing neuromuscular blockers, while monitoring at the adductor pollicis should provide a margin of safety (as the diaphragm and the muscles of airway protection should recover more quickly from neuromuscular blockade).

Patterns of stimulation that are used in monitoring the neuromuscular junction include single-twitch, train-of-four, tetanic, posttetanic, and double-burst stimulation. Depolarizing and nondepolarizing muscle relaxants exhibit various responses to stimulation.

Depolarizing blockade (phase I type) is characterized by a decreased amplitude of response to single-twitch stimulus. The response to repeated single-twitch stimulus and tetanic stimulus is sustained. Train-of-four stimulation does not fade (T1:T4 ratio >0.7), and there is no posttetanic potentiation during depolarizing blockade. Depolarizing blockade is antagonized by nondepolarizing drugs, and it is potentiated by administration of anticholinesterase agents. Muscle fasciculations at the onset also characterize depolarizing block.

Nondepolarizing blockade is characterized by train-of-four fade (T1:T4 ratio <0.7). Tetanic fade and posttetanic potentiation characterize nondepolarizing blockade. Double-burst stimulation may be a more sensitive indicator of recovery during nondepolarizing neuromuscular blockade than train-of-four ratio. Nondepolarizing block is antagonized by depolarizing drugs. Synergism may occur with concomitant administration of various nondepolarizers. Antagonism by anticholinesterase agents is characteristic. Muscle fasciculations do not occur at the onset of nondepolarizing blockade.

Phase II type depolarizing block occurs with higher doses of depolarizing muscle relaxants. It resembles nondepolarizing neuromuscular blockade. Fade and decreased train-of-four ratio are characteristic, and it is reversible with anticholinesterase agents. This feature distinguishes it from phase I block, which is potentiated by anticholinesterase agents.

☐ DEPOLARIZING MUSCLE RELAXANTS

Depolarizing muscle relaxants include succinylcholine and decamethonium. Decamethonium is used infrequently. Despite a multitude of current controversies, succinylcholine is still frequently used to provide rapid, intense, short-lasting neuromuscular blockade. Much of the research in nondepolarizing neuromuscular blocking pharmacology has been directed toward finding a substitute for succinylcholine. To date, none exists.

The ED_{90} for succinylcholine in adults during nitrous oxide anesthesia is 0.27 mg/kg intravenously. An intubating dose of succinylcholine of 0.5 to 1 mg/kg has an onset of action of 30 to 60 s and a duration of action of 3 to 5 min. Diffusion away from the neuromuscular junction into extracellular fluid leads to the termination of succinylcholine's effect.

Succinylcholine is very rapidly metabolized by plasma cholinesterase (also termed pseudocholinesterase) to succinylmonocholine, and this compound is then metabolized by the same enzyme to succinic acid and choline. Plasma cholinesterase is present in the liver and in plasma but is not present at the neuromuscular junction. Atypical plasma cholinesterase enzymes and deficiencies of normal plasma cholinesterase may prolong succinylcholine neuroblockade by allowing more succinylcholine to reach the neuromuscular junction. Many coexisting conditions, including liver disease, pregnancy, and cancer, have been found to reduce levels of plasma cholinesterase. In addition, many medications, including acetylcholinesterase inhibitors, metoclopramide, and others, may decrease plasma pseudocholinesterase. However, clinically significant prolongation of succinylcholine blockade is not seen in patients with even very low levels (20% of normal values) of the qualitatively normal plasma cholinesterase enzyme.

The atypical plasma cholinesterase variants can lead to marked prolongation in succinylcholine blockade. These genetic variants are of several types, including the dibucaine-related and the flouride-sensitive genes. The dibucaine-related variants are the most important (Table 6–1). The dibucaine test is a qualitative test of the plasma cholinesterase enzyme. The local anesthetic dibucaine inhibits the activity of normal plasma cholinesterase by 80%, while the homozygous atypical cholinesterase is inhibited by only 20%. In cases of prolonged blockade from succinylcholine, reversal with acetylcholinesterase inhibitors is unreliable. Administration of fresh-frozen plasma, which contains plasma cholinesterase, is effective in reversing the prolonged block. Supportive care with mechanical ventilation is the recommended therapy, since the risks of blood-product administration are not justified. Purified human plasma cholinesterase, which is a heat-treated derivative of normal plasma, has been utilized in reversing prolonged succinylcholine neuromuscular blockade due to the atypical cholinesterase enzyme. The risks of transmission of blood-borne pathogens are minimal in comparison with those associated with fresh frozen plasma and are comparable to the risks associated with administration of albumin.

Table 6–1
CORRELATION OF PSEUDOCHOLINESTERASE GENOTYPE, SUCCINYLCHOLINE SENSITIVITY AND DIBUCAINE NUMBER (DN)*

Genotype	DN	Duration of Paralysis
Homozygous normal	80	Normal
Heterozygous	50	Slightly prolonged
Homozygous atypical	20	Very prolonged

* Adapted with permission from Miller, RD and Savarese, J. Pharmacology of Muscle Relaxants and their Antagonists, in Miller RD (ed): *Anaesthesia* 3d ed., New York: Churchill-Livingstone, 1990.

Initial depolarization of the neuromuscular junction reflects the agonist activity of succinylcholine at the nicotinic receptor on skeletal muscle. This property is noted clinically by the presence of muscular fasciculations and leads to several important complications of succinylcholine use. Muscular fasciculations may lead to myalgias, myoglobinuria, and variable increases in intragastric pressure. Prior administration of a nondepolarizing muscle relaxant may attenuate myalgias and the elevation in intragastric pressure. A tonic contracture response may follow the administration of succinylcholine in some muscles. In the extraocular muscles of the eye, this may result in increases in intraocular pressure. Masseter spasm may result from tonic contracture of the muscles of the jaw. The increases in intracranial pressure seen with succinylcholine are also presumed to be a reflection of agonist activity, although the mechanism is not clearly understood.

The most serious complication of agonist activity at the nicotinic receptor is the potential for an exaggerated hyperkalemic response to succinylcholine with resultant cardiac arrest. Patients susceptible to this phenomenon include those with burn injuries, severe infections, skeletal muscle trauma or atrophy, upper motor neuron lesions or neuromuscular disease, including children with undiagnosed myopathies. The tendency to develop a hyperkalemic response has been noted as early as 4 days after a denervation injury and continues indefinitely. There is no evidence that cerebral palsy predisposes patients to a hyperkalemic response to succinylcholine. The increased number of extrajunctional receptors in denervated muscle provides more sites for succinylcholine binding and subsequently more sites for potassium leakage. The hyperkalemic response cannot be blocked by prior administration of a nondepolarizer.

Cardiovascular effects of succinylcholine include a variety of bradydysrhythmias, which reflect agonist activity at the cardiac muscarinic receptors. They are more common with repeated doses of succinylcholine and may reflect activity of succinylmonocholine. Succinylcholine also exhibits agonist activity at nicotinic receptors at the autonomic ganglia, which results in tachycardia and hypertension.

Rare complications of succinylcholine use include anaphylaxis and triggering of malignant hyperthermia. The nondepolarizing muscle relaxants are not triggers for malignant hyperthermia.

NONDEPOLARIZING MUSCLE RELAXANTS

Nondepolarizing muscle relaxants are all highly ionized. Their volumes of distribution are therefore limited to the extracellular fluid. Since they are water-soluble compounds, they do not cross the blood-brain barrier or the placenta. The nondepolarizing muscle relaxants can be divided by their durations of action into short-, intermediate-, and long-acting agents. Nondepolarizers differ in their potency, onset, mechanism of elimination, and duration. The various classes of nondepolarizers also vary in their cardiovascular effects, which include antimuscarinic and histamine-releasing properties.

SHORT-ACTING NONDEPOLARIZERS

Mivacurium Mivacurium is the only short-acting nondepolarizing muscle relaxant. It is a benzylisoquinoline compound. The ED_{95} of mivacurium is 0.08 mg/kg. An intubating dose of 0.2 mg/kg has an onset of approximately 2 min. Its clinical duration of action is 15 to 20 min. Like other nondepolarizers, its duration of action is prolonged at higher doses. Mivacurium is metabolized by plasma cholinesterase very quickly. Other minor secondary pathways for its elimination through the kidney and liver do exist. Duration of action is prolonged in patients with liver and kidney failure. In patients who are homozygous for the atypical plasma cholinesterase gene, this drug behaves as a long-acting agent, since it then depends entirely on the secondary elimination pathways for the termination of its effect. Administration of anticholinesterase agents to reverse a mivacurium block is controversial, since spontaneous recovery is so rapid. Anticholinesterase can potentially inhibit the plasma cholinesterase enzyme, but both neostigmine and edrophonium are better inhibitors of acetylcholinesterase than of plasma cholinesterase. It does appear that anticholinesterase agents accelerate recovery from mivacurium neuroblockade and that reversal of deep mivacurium block occurs more quickly than reversal of other nondepolarizers. Mivacurium can cause histamine release, since it is a benzoisoquinolone. This effect is more significant at larger doses and when the drug is administered rapidly.

INTERMEDIATE-ACTING NONDEPOLARIZERS

Atracurium Atracurium is an intermediate-acting nondepolarizing muscle relaxant. It is a benzylisoquinoline compound. Its ED_{95} is 0.15 to 0.3 mg/kg. An intubating dose of 0.4 to 0.5 mg/kg has an onset time of 3 to 5 min. After administration of ED_{95}, the time to 25% recovery of twitch height is 25 to 35 min. Spontaneous recovery to 95% twitch height occurs after 44 min.

Atracurium undergoes spontaneous degradation at normal body temperature and pH (Hofmann elimination) to laudonosine and acrylate. This spontaneous degradation also occurs at room temperature, but much more slowly. For this reason atracurium is stored refrigerated. This reaction is nonenzymatic and is not dependent on renal or hepatic function. It is slowed by hypothermia and acidosis. The byproduct laudanosine is a tertiary amine that crosses the blood-brain barrier. Laudanosine acts as a stimulant in the central nervous system and as a vasodilator. These effects are dependent on blood concentrations. It is unlikely that the levels of laudanosine achieved during routine intraoperative dosing have significant clinical effects. During prolonged continuous infusion in the intensive care unit or in the presence of liver dysfunction, accumulation of laudanosine may be of some theoretic concern. Atracurium is also eliminated by ester hydrolysis. The nonspecific esterases that catalyze these reactions are distinct from plasma cholinesterase.

Atracurium can cause histamine release, since it is a benzylisoquinoline. This response becomes clinically significant at higher dosage ranges (3 times the ED_{95}). It can be attenuated by slow administration.

Vecuronium Vecuronium is a steroidal muscle relaxant of intermediate duration. It is much more lipid-soluble than its analog pancuronium and is unstable in solution. Its ED_{95} is 0.04 to 0.07 mg/kg. An intubating dose of 0.07 to 0.1 mg/kg has an onset time of 3 to 5 min. Like atracurium, time to 25% recovery of twitch height after administration of ED_{95} is 25 to 35 min. The onset time can be shortened by administration of larger doses (0.2 mg/kg or greater), but this leads to longer recovery times (> 120 min). Onset time can also be shortened by administration of 10% of the intubating dose of vecuronium 3 to 6 min prior to the remainder of the dose. This technique is termed priming and may be associated with some risk of loss of airway protective reflexes.

Lipid solubility facilitates vecuronium's rapid metabolism in the liver and allows it to be excreted in the bile. Vecuronium is deacetylated in the liver, and some of its metabolites (especially 3-hydroxyvecuronium) have weak neuromuscular blocking properties. With larger doses of vecuronium (> 0.2 mg/kg), elimination may be prolonged in patients with liver disease. Vecuronium also undergoes some renal elimination (10 to 20%). Modest prolongation of duration of action is seen in patients with renal failure and is more pronounced with larger doses. Prolonged neuromuscular blockade following infusion of vecuronium in the intensive care unit has been reported. Accumulation of active metabolites of vecuronium is the presumed mechanism.

The steroidal muscle relaxants have antimuscarinic properties. This property has been eliminated in the synthesis of vecuronium by demethylating the A ring of the steroidal nucleus of pancuronium. The result is that vecuronium is devoid of cardiovascular effects. In combination with drugs that increase vagal tone (such as opiates), vecuronium has been reported to cause severe bradydysrhythmias.

Rocuronium   Rocuronium is the newest of the intermediate-acting nondepolarizers. It is a steroidal muscle relaxant. Rocuronium is less potent and has a shorter onset time than vecuronium. Its ED_{95} is 0.4 mg/kg. With a dose of 1.5 to 3 times the ED_{95} (0.6 to 1.2 mg/kg), onset time can be reduced to 60 to 90 s. It is important to reiterate that neuromuscular blockade of the laryngeal muscles appears to occur earlier than blockade of the adductor pollicis; therefore, adequate intubating conditions may be achieved before adductor pollicis twitch abolition. Recovery indices are similar to vecuronium when equipotent doses are administered.

Rocuronium depends on the kidney and liver for elimination but is not metabolized to a significant degree. Duration of action is prolonged in the presence of hepatic dysfunction.

As a steroidal muscle relaxant, rocuronium does have mild antimuscarinic properties. This tachycardia is less than that seen with pancuronium. It is dose-dependent, and it is more likely to occur with administration of the larger doses (0.6 to 0.9 mg/kg) recommended for rapid intubation.

LONG-ACTING NONDEPOLARIZERS

D-Tubocurarine   D-Tubocurarine is a long-acting benzylisoquinoline compound with an ED_{95} of 0.5 to 0.6 mg/kg. Its onset time is 3 to 5 min, and its duration is 60 to 90 min. It does not undergo significant metabolism. It is partially dependent on renal elimination. Forty to sixty percent of the drug is excreted in the urine. Its elimination half-life is prolonged in elderly patients due to the progressive decline in creatinine clearance and in patients with renal failure. D-Tubocurarine does undergo hepatic metabolism but can be excreted unchanged in the bile.

D-Tubocurarine has important cardiovascular side effects. Rapid administration can lead to histamine release. Significant hypotension (greater than 20% decline in mean arterial pressure) can occur with its administration. This decrease in blood pressure is not associated with a decrease in cardiac output but instead reflects only a decrease in systemic vascular resistance. In addition, at higher doses, D-tubocurarine can act as ganglionic blocker, contributing to its hypotensive effect.

Metocurine   Metocurine is a long-acting benzylisoquinoline similar to D-tubocurarine. Its ED_{95} is 0.28 mg/kg. Its onset time of 3 to 5 min and its duration of 60 to 90 min are the same as those of D-tubocurarine. Metocurine depends primarily on renal elimination; 80 to 100% of metocurine is excreted in the urine. It is not metabolized in the liver and is not excreted in the bile. Although metocurine can cause histamine release and act as a weak ganglionic blocker, these

effects are much attenuated when compared to D-tubocurarine.

Pancuronium   Pancuronium is a steroidal muscle relaxant with a long duration of action. Its ED_{95} is 0.07 mg/kg. Its onset time and duration are similar to those of D-tubocurarine and metocurine, with an onset of 3 to 5 min and a duration of 60 to 90 min. It is highly dependent on renal excretion. Sixty to eighty percent of this drug is eliminated by the kidneys. Its duration of effect is significantly prolonged in renal failure. Pancuronium does undergo some hepatic metabolism, although less than vecuronium. The half-life of pancuronium is increased in patients with hepatic failure, although a larger initial dose may be required in these patients due to a larger volume of distribution. Pathways for deacetylation are the same for pancuronium as for vecuronium, and the 3-hydroxypancuronium metabolite does exhibit neuromuscular-blocking properties.

Administration of pancuronium is associated with a modest rise in heart rate (10 to 15% increase), due mostly to its selective blockade of cardiac muscarinic receptors. There is also evidence that pancuronium may block other types of muscarinic receptors that act as inhibitors of sympathetic outflow. This feature may explain pancuronium's proarrhythmic effect, especially when administered in conjunction with halothane and tricyclic antidepressants. This tachycardia is associated with a mild increase in blood pressure and cardiac output, although there is no evidence that pancuronium is a positive inotrope. Pancuronium is not a ganglionic blocker and does not cause histamine release.

Gallamine   Gallamine is a methonium compound (related to decamethonium) with an ED_{95} of 1 mg/kg. Its onset and duration are similar to those of the previously discussed long-acting nondepolarizers. It is eliminated exclusively by the kidney. Gallamine is associated with a more pronounced blockade of cardiac muscarinic receptors than pancuronium. Blockade of inhibitory sympathetic influences may contribute to the tachycardia. Gallamine is not a ganglionic blocker. It does not release histamine.

Doxacurium   Doxacurium is a very potent, long-acting benzylisoquinoline with an ED_{95} of 0.025 mg/kg. Onset time for a dose of 0.04 mg/kg is 4 min since potency is inversely related to onset time. An intubating dose of two times the ED_{95} lasts 90 to 100 min. The elimination of doxacurium is primarily through the kidney. It does not undergo metabolism in the liver and is recovered in the bile only to a small degree. It does not release histamine and has no cardiovascular side effects.

Pipecuronium   Pipecuronium is a long-acting steroidal muscle relaxant with an ED_{95} of 0.04 mg/kg. Onset time of an intubating dose of 0.08 mg/kg is 4 to 6 min, and duration is similar to that of doxacurium. It is excreted primarily by the kidney (60 to 90%) and to a much smaller extent by the

Table 6-2
RECOMMENDED REVERSAL DOSES ACCORDING TO TRAIN-OF-FOUR RESPONSE (TOF)*

TOF Visible Twitches	Fade	Reversal Agent	Dose, mg/kg
None[a]			
≤2	++++	Neostigmine	0.07
3-4	+++	Neostigmine	0.04
4	++	Edrophonium	0.5
4	±	Edrophonium	0.25

[a] Postpone reversal until some evoked response is detected.
* Reproduced with permission from Beran, DR, Donati, F and Kopman, A. *Anesthesiology* 77:785-805, 1992.

liver. It does not undergo significant metabolism. Like doxacurium, it is free of significant cardiovascular effects.

ANTAGONISM OF NONDEPOLARIZING NEUROMUSCULAR BLOCKADE

Antagonism by acetylcholinesterase inhibitors is one of the characteristic features of nondepolarizing neuromuscular blockade. Edrophonium is a competitive inhibitor of the acetylcholinesterase enzyme. Neostigmine and pyridostigmine carbamylate the acetylcholinesterase enzyme, which inhibits its ability to hydrolyze acetylcholine. Edrophonium has a more rapid onset of action than neostigmine, which has a more rapid onset of action than pyridostigmine. The clinical duration of these drugs is 1 to 2 h. Their elimination is prolonged in renal failure. Although neostigmine has been reported to cause neuromuscular blockade, this effect occurs at much larger doses than those used clinically. One type of dosing strategy, using ulnar-adductor pollicis monitoring, is shown in Table 6-2.

The intensity of block and the drug used to achieve block (short-, intermediate-, or long-acting agents) have significant impact on the reversibility of the block. Neostigmine appears to be more capable of reversing very deep blocks (single twitch height <10% or one twitch visible on train of four) than either edrophonium or pyridostigmine. The time to adequate reversal can be shortened by administering a larger dose of anticholinesterase agent. Antagonism of intermediate-acting drugs is faster than that of the long-acting agents because the intermediate-acting drugs are metabolized, which increases their spontaneous recovery rates. As would be predicted in situations in which there is impairment of metabolism and excretion of these drugs, reversal may be slower. Their reversibility profile becomes more like that of the long-acting nondepolarizing agents.

Reversal of mivacurium neuromuscular blockade, which has been discussed, is controversial, since spontaneous re-

covery is so rapid. In patients who are homozygotes for the atypical plasma cholinesterase enzyme, mivacurium neuroblockade resembles blockade with a long-acting nondepolarizer. Recently, mivacurium blockade in patients who are homozygotes for the atypical plasma cholinesterase enzyme has been reversed with purified human plasma cholinesterase enzyme and neostigmine. The duration of action of this drug is prolonged from 10 to 20 min in patients who are homozygous for the normal enzyme to over 3 h in patients who are homozygous for the atypical enzyme. In patients who are heterozygous, block is prolonged to 20 to 30 min. Once spontaneous recovery of prolonged block is documented, antagonist can be administered to accelerate recovery. This recommendation is different than in prolonged neuromuscular blockade from succinylcholine, in which supportive care is recommended.

INTERACTION WITH OTHER DRUGS AND CONDITIONS

Many drugs interact with nondepolarizing muscle relaxants. Among the most important of these interactions is prolongation of neuromuscular blockade by several types of antibiotics. The aminoglycosides, tetracyclines, and clindamycin have all been reported to prolong neuromuscular blockade. The penicillins and cephalosporins are notable because they do not appear to prolong neuromuscular blockade.

The local anesthetics and type I cardiac antidysrhythmic agents can depress conduction at the neuromuscular junction. Potential mechanisms include block of release of acetylcholine at the prejunctional membrane and stabilization of the postjunctional membrane.

Magnesium has significant depressant effects at the neuromuscular junction. Prolongation of succinylcholine and nondepolarizing block are associated with its use. Lithium carbonate, which acts as a sodium analog, may interfere with neuromuscular transmission and has been associated with prolonged depolarizing and nondepolarizing blocks. The volatile anesthetics enhance nondepolarizing neuromuscular blockade. This effect is greater with enflurane and isoflurane than with halothane. Hypothermia, respiratory acidosis, and hypokalemia may also prolong nondepolarizing neuromuscular blockade.

The diuretic furosemide at low dosages (10 μg/kg) appears to inhibit the prejunctional release of acetylcholine and may enhance nondepolarizing neuromuscular blockade when administered in low doses. In higher doses (1 to 4 mg/kg), it antagonizes neuromuscular blockade.

Patients receiving phenytoin exhibit resistance to nondepolarizing neuromuscular blockade. The immunosuppressant azathioprine may also antagonize nondepolarizing block.

In summary, many drugs affect synaptic transmission at the neuromuscular junction or alter the actions of muscle relaxants at the neuromuscular junction. Monitoring of neuromuscular function is essential to allow safe dosing of relaxants in these situations.

BIBLIOGRAPHY

Bevan DR: Clinical pearls: muscle relaxants. 1995 IARS Review Course Lectures. *Anesth Analg* Suppl:89–92, 1995.

Bevan DR, Donati F, Kopman AF: Reversal of neuromuscular blockade. *Anesthesiology* 77:785–805, 1992.

Drachman DA: Myasthenia gravis. *N Engl J Med* 298:136–142, 1978.

Katz RL (ed): *Muscle Relaxants: Basic and Clinical Aspects.* Orlando, FL, Grune & Stratton, 1985.

Lien CA: Rational use of muscle relaxants. 1994 IARS Review Course Lectures. *Anesth Analg* Suppl:66–72, 1994.

Miller RD: Use of muscle relaxants in non-operating room locations. 1993 IARS Review Course Lectures. *Anesth Analg* Suppl:6–9, 1993.

Miller RD, Saverese JJ: Pharmacology of muscle relaxants and their antagonists, in Miller RD (ed): *Anesthesia.* New York, Churchill Livingstone, 1990.

Milligan KR, Beers HT: Vecuronium-associated cardiac arrest. *Anesthesia* 40:385, 1985.

Ostergaard D, Jensen FS, Viby-Mogensen J: Reversal of intense mivacurium block with human plasma cholinesterase in patients with atypical plasma cholinesterase. *Anesthesiology* 82:1295–1298, 1995.

Savarese JJ: New, newer, newest and imaginary muscle relaxants. 1992 IARS Review Course Lectures. *Anesth Analg* Suppl:62–67, 1992.

Savarese JJ: Reversal and monitoring of neuromuscular blockade: changing attitudes. 1994 IARS Review Course Lectures. *Anesth Analg* Suppl:100–106, 1994.

Stoelting RK: Neuromuscular Blocking Drugs, in Stoelting RK: *Pharmacology and Physiology in Anesthetic Practice,* 2d ed. Philadelphia, J. B. Lippincott, 1991.

Taylor P: Are neuromuscular blocking agents more effective in pairs? *Anesthesiology* 63:1–3, 1985.

Viby-Mogensen J: Succinylcholine neuromuscular blockade in subjects homozygous for atypical plasma cholinesterase. *Anesthesiology* 55:429–434, 1981.

Anatomy, Physiology, and Pharmacology of the Autonomic Nervous System

Bruce James and
Timothy VadeBoncouer

☐ ANATOMY OF THE AUTONOMIC NERVOUS SYSTEM

The autonomic nervous system regulates vital body systems that are not under voluntary control, including circulation, respiration, temperature regulation, metabolism, and hormone secretion. There are two subdivisions of the autonomic nervous system: the sympathetic and the parasympathetic nervous systems.

The sympathetic nerve fibers arise from the thoracic and first and second lumbar segments of the spinal cord. The sympathetic preganglionic neurons, which have their cell bodies in the spinal cord, leave the cord with the ventral nerve roots and proceed to 1 of the 22 pairs of ganglia of the paravertebral sympathetic chain. The cervical, lower lumbar, and sacral sympathetic ganglia receive preganglionic fibers that have not synapsed in ganglia adjacent to the spinal segments from which they emerged. The preganglionic fibers synapse with postganglionic fibers, and the postganglionic fibers emerge from the paravertebral ganglia to the various effector organs. The preganglionic fibers are mainly myelinated, while the postganglionic fibers are usually unmyelinated. The distribution of the sympathetic fibers differs from that of the spinal nerves. This distribution is related to the embryologic origin of the various organs and fibers:

Fiber Origination	Innervation
T1	Head
T2	Neck
T3–6	Upper extremities and thorax
T7–11	Abdomen
T12–L2	Lower extremities

The parasympathetic nervous system is cranial and sacral in origin. The preganglionic cells arise from the brainstem and the second through fourth sacral segments of the spinal cord (occasionally with contribution from the first sacral segment). In contrast to the sympathetic nervous system, the parasympathetic nervous system is confined to the viscera. The preganglionic fibers run from their origin to synapse with their postganglionic fibers in or near the viscera they supply.

The cranial segment of the parasympathetic nervous system arises from cranial nerves III, VII, IX, and X. Cranial nerve III (oculomotor) supplies the ciliary and sphincter muscles of the lens and iris in the eye (causing pupillary constriction). Cranial nerve VII (facial) supplies and stimulates the secretion of the nasal, lacrimal, submaxillary, submandibular, and sublingual glands. Cranial nerve IX (glossopharyngeal) supplies the parotid gland and also stimulates its secretion. Cranial nerve X (vagus), which accounts for approximately 75% of all parasympathetic outflow, supplies the thorax and abdomen. This includes supplying the pulmonary, cardiac, and esophageal plexuses in the thorax and the stomach, small intestine, liver, and pancreas in the abdomen. The primary pulmonary effect is bronchoconstriction and the main cardiac effect is bradycardia. The effect on the gastrointestinal system is to stimulate secretion and motility.

The sacral portion of the parasympathetic nervous system supplies the descending colon, rectum, bladder, distal ureters, and genitals. These nerves promote gastrointestinal motility and secretion as well as urination and erection.

☐ PHYSIOLOGY OF THE AUTONOMIC NERVOUS SYSTEM

The effects of the autonomic nervous system are caused by the release of neurotransmitters at the pre- and postganglionic nerve terminals. In the sympathetic and parasympathetic nervous systems, all preganglionic fibers release acetylcholine and are therefore cholinergic fibers. The postganglionic fibers of the sympathetic nervous system secrete norepinephrine as their neurotransmitter, while the postganglionic fibers of the parasympathetic nervous system release acetylcholine. There are some exceptions to this rule. Though part of the sympathetic system, at sweat glands and some blood vessels, the postganglionic transmitter is acetylcholine.

The fibers that utilize norepinephrine as their neurotransmitter are usually referred to as adrenergic. The synthesis of norepinephrine occurs with a number of enzyme-controlled steps in the nerve endings. The norepinephrine is stored in synaptic vesicles and is released in response to action potentials. Adrenergic nerve fibers can sustain the output of norepinephrine during prolonged periods of stimulation. Norepinephrine also inhibits its own release by virtue of its stimulation of α_2 presynaptic receptors. The termination of action of norepinephrine is by two mechanisms: diffusion from receptor sites and reuptake into the nerve terminal. The latter is the more predominant, accounting for about 80% of termination of effect. The transport system for norepinephrine reuptake can be blocked by many drugs, including cocaine and tricyclic antidepressants. There is also metabolism of norepinephrine by monoamine oxidase (MAO) and catechol-O-methyltransferase (COMT). MAO is responsible for metabolism during uptake. COMT in the liver and kidneys will metabolize norepinephrine that diffuses away from the nerve terminal. The combination of these mechanisms accounts for the short duration of action of norepinephrine.

The fibers that utilize acetylcholine as their neurotransmitter are usually referred to as cholinergic. Choline and acetyl coenzyme A combine with the enzyme choline acetyltransferase to form acetylcholine in the cytoplasm of preganglionic fibers and in the postganglionic parasympathetic fibers. The acetylcholine is stored in vesicles until it is released in response to an action potential. Calcium is needed for acetylcholine release. The calcium influx occurs with the initial depolarization prior to the action potential, and calcium binds to the vesicle membranes, resulting in the release of the acetylcholine. The short effect that acetylcholine has on receptors is secondary to its rapid hydrolysis by acetylcholinesterase (true cholinesterase) to choline and acetate.

THE ADRENAL MEDULLA

Considered part of the sympathetic nervous system, the adrenal medulla is directly innervated by preganglionic sympathetic fibers. The adrenal medulla is derived embryologically from neural tissue and therefore acts as a sympathetic ganglion. Approximately 80% of the catecholamine released by the adrenal medulla is epinephrine.

In the adrenal medulla, norepinephrine is converted to epinephrine by the enzyme phenylethanolamine N-methyltransferase. Since phenylethanolamine N-methyltransferase

activity is increased by cortisol, any stress that releases glucocorticoids results in the increased synthesis and release of epinephrine. Glucocorticoids also increase the activity of the enzyme tyrosine hydroxylase, which is the rate-limiting step in the formation of norepinephrine (and thus epinephrine).

The release of acetylcholine from the preganglionic nerve fibers causes an influx of calcium, which in turn induces the release of adrenal medullary vesicles containing epinephrine and norepinephrine into the bloodstream. This release produces a response similar to but of a longer duration than that of direct sympathetic nervous system stimulation. The longer duration reflects the time needed for COMT metabolism of epinephrine and norepinephrine ($\sim$10 to 30 s).

MOLECULAR STRUCTURE AND FUNCTION OF THE ADRENERGIC RECEPTORS

The adrenergic receptors are specific proteins on the cell membrane. The receptors interact with a catecholamine or other adrenergic receptor agonist. This interaction causes stimulation of a number of regulatory proteins that bind guanine nucleoside triphosphate (GTP). These are referred to as G proteins, since they regulate the interaction between the receptor and adenyl cyclase or phospholipase C. The β receptors all stimulate adenyl cyclase by way of the G protein called Gs (stimulatory G protein). The α_2 receptor inhibits adenyl cyclase through the G protein called Gi (inhibitory G protein). The α_1 receptor stimulates phospholipase C by way of another less well-known G protein: Gp (another stimulatory G protein). Adenyl cyclase is a catalyst for conversion of adenosine triphosphate (ATP) to cyclic adenosine monophosphate (cAMP). The increase in cAMP stimulates protein kinase A. Phospholipase C catalyzes the hydrolysis of phosphatidylinositol 4,5-diphosphate to form diacylglycerol (DAG) and inositol triphosphate (IP3). DAG and IP3 both may cause release of intracellular calcium. The calcium activates calmodulin and protein kinase C. DAG may also directly activate protein kinase C. The activation of protein kinase A and/or protein kinase C sets off a chain of phosphorylation that produces the characteristic cellular response seen with the stimulation of that receptor (see Figure 7–1).

THE ADRENERGIC RECEPTORS

The major adrenergic receptor types are α, β, and dopaminergic.

There are two types of α receptors: α_1 and α_2. The α_1 receptors are postsynaptic. This α_1 stimulation results in vasoconstriction, mydriasis, relaxation of gastrointestinal tract smooth muscle, salivation, sweating, and contraction of gastrointestinal and bladder sphincters. The α_2 receptors are pre- and postsynaptic, with the presynaptic α_2 receptors causing an inhibition of norepinephrine release. The postsynaptic α_2 receptors mediate platelet aggregation, inhibit insulin and renin release, and cause a hyperpolarization of the central nervous system, resulting in a decreased anesthetic requirement and sedation.

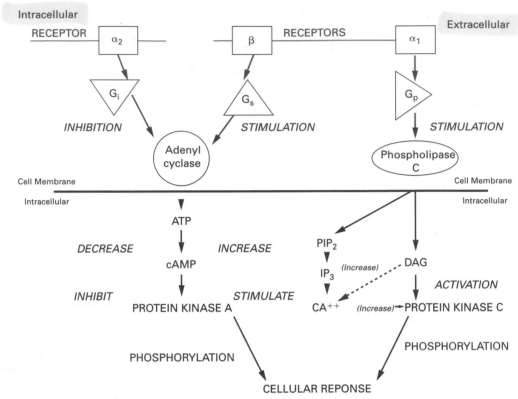

Figure 7–1 The structure and function of adrenergic receptors

There are also two β receptor types: β_1 and β_2. The β_1 receptors are postsynaptic. Their stimulation causes an increase in myocardial contractility, automaticity, heart rate, and conduction velocity. The β_2 receptors are postsynaptic and generally noncardiac. Activation of β_2 receptors stimulates lipolysis and glycogenolysis, and produces smooth muscle relaxation (vasodilation, bronchodilation, and gastrointestinal, bladder, and uterine relaxation).

Dopamine is a neurotransmitter found in the central and peripheral nervous systems. There are two types of dopamin-

ergic receptors: DA_1 and DA_2. The DA_1 receptors are postsynaptic and are found in the smooth muscle of the renal, mesenteric, cerebral, and coronary blood vessels. Their activation results in vasodilation of the renal and mesenteric vasculature. The DA_2 receptors are primarily presynaptic and inhibit release of norepinephrine. Stimulation of DA_2 receptors also results in vasodilation.

The overall effect of each sympathetic agonist is equal to the sum of its α, β, and dopaminergic receptor stimulation (see Table 7–1).

Table 7–1
RECEPTOR INTERACTIONS, DOSES, AND CLINICAL EFFECTS OF SEVERAL ADRENERGIC AGONISTS

| Drugs | RECEPTORS | | | | | | CARDIOVASCULAR EFFECTS | | | Mechanism of Action | IV Bolus Dose | Continuous Infusion Dose |
	α_1	α_2	β_1	β_2	DA_1	DA_2	CO	HR	SVR			
Epinephrine	+	++	+++	++	0	0	+++	++	+/−	Direct	2–8 μg	1–20 μg/min
Norepinephrine	+++	+++	++	+	0	0	−	−	+++	Direct	Not used	2–16 μg/min
Dopamine	++	0	++	++	+++	?	++	+	+	Direct	Not used	0.5–20 μg/kg/min
Isoproterenol	0	0	+++	+++	0	0	+++	+++	−−	Direct	1–4 μg	1–5 μg/min
Dobutamine	0	0	++	++	0	0	++	+	−	Direct	Not used	2–10 μg/kg/min
Ephedrine	+	0	+	+	0	0	+	+	+	Indirect (some direct)	5–15 mg	Not used
Phenylephrine	++	0	0	0	0	0	−	−	++	Direct	20–200 μg	0.15–0.7 μg/kg/min
Methoxamine	+++	0	0	0	0	0	−	−	+++	Direct	1–5 mg	Not used

THE CHOLINERGIC RECEPTORS

There are two types of cholinergic receptors. The first type is the nicotinic receptor, with its subtypes: N_1 and N_2. These receptors are found on the plasma membranes of parasympathetic and sympathetic postganglionic cells in autonomic ganglia as well as on the plasma membranes of the muscles innervated by somatic motor fibers. Stimulation of N_1 receptors initiates depolarization and firing of postganglionic cells and in the adrenal medulla leads to catecholamine release. Stimulation of the N_2 receptor results in skeletal muscle contraction.

Muscarinic receptors (M_1, M_2, and M_3) are the second type of cholinergic receptor. The M_1 receptors are located in the autonomic ganglia, the central nervous system and secretory glands. The M_2 receptors are found primarily in the heart. The M_3 receptors are found in exocrine glands and smooth muscle. The M_1 receptors create a slow excitatory response, the M_2 have an inhibitory effect on the heart, and the M_3 stimulate secretion from exocrine glands and contraction of smooth muscles.

☐ PHARMACOLOGY OF THE SYMPATHETIC AGONISTS

EPINEPHRINE

Epinephrine is an endogenous catecholamine released from the adrenal medulla. The effects seen from epinephrine come from its direct stimulation of α and β receptors. The effects include an increase in myocardial contractility, heart rate, vascular and smooth muscle tone, glandular secretions, glycogenolysis, and lipolysis. At the α receptor, epinephrine is 2 to 10 times more potent than norepinephrine, and it has 100 times greater effect at the β_1 and β_2 receptors than does isoproterenol.

The cardiovascular effects of epinephrine are, as mentioned, α and β effects. At intravenous doses of 1 to 2 μg/min, β_2 effects predominate; at 4 μg/min β_1 effects predominate; and in doses of 10 to 20 μg/min, both α and β stimulation occurs, with α effects predominating over the peripheral β effects, especially in the skin and renal vasculature. A bolus dose of 2 to 8 μg produces cardiac stimulation for 1 to 5 min. The β_1 effects cause an increase in systolic blood pressure, heart rate, and cardiac output (CO). The β_2 stimulation causes a decrease in diastolic blood pressure secondary to dilation of vascular smooth muscle. The increase in heart rate is from the accelerated rate of spontaneous phase IV depolarization, which also increases the likelihood of dysrhythmias. Systole is shortened and strengthened by epinephrine, with the systole being shortened more than diastole, increasing the time of diastolic perfusion and coronary blood flow. The α_1 effects cause intense vasoconstriction of the skin, mucosa, and hepatorenal vasculature. When β_2 and α_1 effects occur simultaneously, the net effect is a decrease in systemic vascular resistance (SVR), with redistribution of blood flow to the skeletal muscles. The α effect causes a decrease in renal blood flow. There is no significant effect of epinephrine on the cerebral arterioles. The β_2 stimulation caused by epinephrine produces bronchiolar smooth muscle relaxation from an increase in intracellular cAMP.

The metabolic effects of epinephrine include inhibition of insulin release (α_1 effect), stimulation of liver glycogenolysis and adipose tissue lipolysis (β_1 effect), and resulting hyperglycemia. From β_2 stimulation, there is a pseudohypokalemia from skeletal muscle Na^+/K^+ pump activation and shifting of potassium from the extracellular to the intracellular space.

Epinephrine is added to local anesthetics to prolong their duration and the intensity of their effect. This prolongation is presumably caused by local perineural vasoconstriction and a reduced rate of systemic absorption.

NOREPINEPHRINE

Norepinephrine is the neurotransmitter released from postganglionic sympathetic nerves. It is structurally similar to epinephrine, differing only by the absence of the methyl substitution on the amino group. The primary effect of norepinephrine is as a potent α_1 stimulant, which causes intense arterial and venous vasoconstriction. Renal, hepatic, cerebral, and muscle blood flows are all decreased. With the increase in systemic vascular resistance, there is an increase in systolic, diastolic, and mean arterial pressures, as well as a baroreceptor-mediated decrease in heart rate. Norepinephrine may reduce tissue blood flow to a point where a metabolic acidosis is produced. At the β receptor, norepinephrine has little β_2 effect and has a β_1 effect approximately equivalent to that of epinephrine (weak β_1 activity).

Norepinephrine is used for treatment of refractory hypotension. It is infused through a central venous access (range 2 to 16 μg/min) to avoid possible extravasation and resultant local vasoconstriction and tissue necrosis.

DOPAMINE

Dopamine, a natural catecholamine, is a metabolic precursor of norepinephrine and epinephrine. It acts as a neurotransmitter in the central and peripheral nervous systems. The DA_1 receptors are located postsynaptically in the renal, cerebral, mesenteric, and coronary arterial beds. The DA_1 effects are first seen at infusion rates of 0.5 to 1.0 μg/kg/min and are maximal at 2 to 3 μg/kg/min. The DA_2 receptors are presynaptic and inhibit release of norepinephrine. At doses in the 2 to 6 μg/kg/min range, cardiac β stimulation is seen with an increase in CO. These β effects are observed up to approximately 10 μg/kg/min. In doses as low as 5 μg/kg/min and more frequently at doses greater than 10 μg/kg/min, one sees primarily α_1 stimulation. This α_1 stimulation overrides the DA_2 effects of dopamine.

The DA_1 receptor stimulation produces an increase in renal blood flow (RBF) by renal vasodilation. The β_1 effect of increased CO also produces an increase in RBF. These dopaminergic effects are important in low CO states and maximize CO, RBF, glomerular filtration rate (GFR), and urine output.

Accompanying the increase in CO are an elevated heart rate, SVR, and arterial blood pressure. Part of the inotropy achieved with dopamine is secondary to the release of norepinephrine. With the α_1 stimulation and lack of β_2 activity, there may be no change or an increase in ventricular filling pressures.

ISOPROTERENOL

Isoproterenol is a synthetic catecholamine that has primarily β_1 and β_2 agonist properties. At usual clinical doses, isoproterenol has no significant α effect. At the β receptor, isoproterenol increases heart rate, contractility, and automaticity. Its β_2 effects cause a decrease in SVR in all vascular beds. There may be an increase in systolic blood pressure due to the increase in CO, but mean and diastolic blood pressures will decrease from the fall in SVR. Isoproterenol may cause tachyarhythmias from its direct effects on the sinoatrial and atrioventricular nodes, or from a baroreceptor-mediated reflex response to peripheral vasodilation. The dysrhythmias and increase in heart rate may cause a decrease in CO secondary to impaired filling. Isoproterenol is generally avoided in patients with coronary artery disease because it increases myocardial oxygen consumption and decreases coronary blood flow. It is most frequently used in the treatment of bradyarrhythmias and atrioventricular heart block because it stimulates myocardial pacemaker cells. Isoproterenol acts as a pulmonary vasodilator and is therefore useful in the treatment of right heart failure and pulmonary hypertension. It also is the inotrope of choice to increase conduction and contractility in the post-cardiac-transplant patient. The usual dose for isoproterenol intravenously is 1 to 5 μg/min.

Isoproterenol also produces significant bronchodilation from stimulation of β_2 receptors. It may be used intravenously or in aerosolized form to treat bronchoconstriction, but the undesirable tachycardia from β_1 stimulation has limited its use.

DOBUTAMINE

Dobutamine is a synthetic isoproterenol derivative. Its primary mode of action is to increase contractility, stroke volume, and CO via stimulation of β_1 receptors. The inotropic effect is more evident than the chronotropy (compared to isoproterenol) because of the prominent β_1 activity and lesser β_2 and α_1 stimulation. There is a small increase in heart rate compared to isoproterenol, and a slight decrease in SVR. Dobutamine causes an increase in conduction velocity through the atrioventricular node, which predisposes patients in atrial fibrillation to a more marked increase in heart rate. Dobutamine is very useful for low-output cardiac failure, especially if the heart rate and SVR are already increased. Renal blood flow is also increased as a result of the increase in cardiac output.

The usual dobutamine dosage range is 2 to 10 μg/kg/min via continuous intravenous infusion. At doses >10 μg/kg/min, there is a predisposition to tachycardia and dysrhythmias.

EPHEDRINE

Ephedrine is a noncatecholamine synthetic sympathomimetic amine. It stimulates both α and β receptors and exerts its activity both directly and indirectly. Its indirect action is mediated through the release of norepinephrine from nerve terminals. It also stimulates adrenergic receptors directly. Since it is a noncatecholamine it has a longer effect because it is not metabolized by COMT.

Its effects are similar to epinephrine: there is an increase in CO, heart rate, systolic and diastolic blood pressure, and pulse pressure. Uterine blood flow effects are minimal, making it a good choice for restoring maternal blood pressure to normal in an obstetric patient who has received an epidural or spinal anesthetic. Renal and splanchnic blood flow are decreased, but cerebral, coronary, and muscular blood flow are increased. There is a mild β_2 effect, causing some bronchodilation. Because of its indirect action, tachyphylaxis may occur with repeat doses. Ephedrine can be given orally (15 to 50 mg), intramuscularly (10 to 50 mg), or intravenously (5 to 15 mg).

PHENYLEPHRINE

Phenylephrine, a strong α_1 agonist with minimal β-agonist activity, is a direct-acting synthetic noncatecholamine. It is structurally similar to ephedrine. Phenylephrine causes an increase in both systolic and diastolic blood pressure, producing a reflex slowing of the heart rate (secondary to baroreceptor stimulation). The increase in blood pressure is the result of α-receptor-mediated peripheral arterial vasoconstriction, which in turn decreases the CO. Renal, splanchnic, and cutaneous blood flows are all reduced, but coronary and pulmonary blood flows are increased.

Phenylephrine can be given intramuscularly or intravenously. Intravenous doses of 20 to 200 μg or intramuscular doses of 5 to 10 mg may be used to treat vasodilation (e.g., during spinal or epidural anesthesia). It may also be given by continuous infusion, usually in the range of 0.15 to 0.7 μg/kg/min, but the infusion is generally titrated to the blood pressure response.

METHOXAMINE

Methoxamine is a synthetic noncatecholamine that acts directly on α receptors. It is not metabolized by COMT or MAO. Methoxamine is more α-selective than phenylephrine and, in contrast to phenylephrine, has no β activity, even at high doses. It causes an increase in both systolic and diastolic blood pressure as well as a baroreceptor-mediated reflex bradycardia. There may be a decrease in CO secondary to the resulting bradycardia and increased SVR. Renal blood flow is decreased more with methoxamine than with similar doses of norepinephrine. Coronary blood flow may increase from the combination of bradycardia and increases in coronary perfusion pressure. Methoxamine is used in the treatment of hypotension and has been used to treat paroxysmal atrial tachycardia.

Methoxamine can be given intravenously (1 to 5 mg) or intramuscularly (10 to 20 mg). When given intravenously, the duration of action is longer than that of phenylephrine and may be a disadvantage, since it cannot be titrated as easily as phenylephrine. The intramuscular dose lasts approximately 1 to 1.5 h.

CLONIDINE

Clonidine is a selective α_2 agonist with a 200:1 preference for α_2 receptors over α_1. Clonidine acts both centrally and peripherally. Its central action, seen because it is lipid-soluble and able to cross the blood-brain barrier, is to decrease sympathetic outflow from the medulla. This accounts for its use as an antihypertensive. Other central effects include sedation, anxiolysis, and analgesia. Clonidine also acts peripherally by decreasing the release of norepinephrine.

Clonidine decreases anesthetic and opioid requirement, blunts the hemodynamic response to laryngoscopy, decreases extremes in blood pressure during anesthesia, decreases intraocular pressure, decreases perioperative catecholamine levels, and decreases postoperative analgesic requirements. Clonidine has also been used to treat withdrawal symptoms of alcohol, benzodiazepines, and opioids. When given intrathecally, clonidine is an analgesic, presumably through activation of noradrenergic descending inhibitory systems.

Clonidine has an elimination half-life of between 6 and 12 h. It is approximately 50% metabolized in the liver. The remaining 50% is excreted unchanged in the urine.

The side effects of clonidine administration include dry mouth, hypotension, bradycardia, and sedation. Since clonidine withdrawal (with chronic use) may precipitate a hypertensive crisis, it should be continued through the perioperative period.

DEXMEDETOMIDINE

Dexmedetomidine is an α_2 agonist. It is a second-generation α_2 agonist in that it is more α_2-selective than is clonidine (1600:1). Dexmedetomidine stimulates presynaptic and postsynaptic α_2-adrenergic receptors both centrally and peripherally. Like clonidine, dexmedetomidine decreases anesthetic requirements, decreases catecholamine levels, blunts the hemodynamic response to laryngoscopy, and reduces postoperative narcotic requirements. Because of its increased selectivity, side effects such as bradycardia and hypotension are decreased.

Table 7-2
DIFFERENTIAL EFFECTS OF THREE ANTICHOLINERGIC DRUGS

Drugs	EFFECTS			
	Antisialagogue	Sedation	Heart rate	Mydriasis
Atropine	+	+	+++	+
Scopolamine	++	+++	+	++
Glycopyrrolate	+++	0	+	0

☐ THE ANTICHOLINERGIC DRUGS

The anticholinergic drugs competitively inhibit acetylcholine at the cholinergic postganglionic receptors and thus block the muscarinic effects of acetylcholine. The anticholinergics have little or no effect at the nicotinic receptors.

Of the classic anticholinergics, two are naturally occurring and one is synthetic. Scopolamine and atropine are natural alkaloids of the belladonna plant, and glycopyrrolate is a synthetic derivative.

The anticholinergics are nonspecific in their antagonism of all muscarinic receptors. Their effects on the muscarinic receptors include increased heart rate, decreased salivation, decreased gastric acid production, mydriasis and cycloplegia, decreased lower esophageal sphincter tone, bronchodilation, and biliary and ureteral smooth muscle relaxation. Scopolamine, and to a much lesser extent atropine, have a sedating effect because, as tertiary amines, they may cross the blood-brain barrier. This tertiary amine structure also accounts for their ability to cross the placental barrier. Glycopyrrolate is a quaternary ammonium and is unable to cross either the placental or blood-brain barrier, and has no sedative effect.

The anticholinergics have a wide variety of clinical uses. Their lack of selectivity means that side effects usually accompany the desired effect (see Table 7-2). Clinical uses include use as an antisialogogue, prevention or treatment of bradycardia, as prophylaxis against motion sickness, as a sedative/amnestic, as a mydriatic, and for preventing the muscarinic effects produced by anticholinesterase drugs during antagonism of nondepolarizing neuromuscular blockade.

Pharmacogenetic Disease

Jeffrey E. Fletcher,
Timothy VadeBoncouer,
and Guy Weinberg

☐ MALIGNANT HYPERTHERMIA

Malignant hyperthermia (MH) is an inherited disorder of skeletal muscle triggered most frequently by the halogenated volatile anesthetics and succinylcholine. The mode of transmission is autosomal dominant with variable penetrance. The disease appears to be heterogeneous and any one of at least three proteins could be causative. A major locus for MH susceptibility (MHS-1) has been localized to chromosome 19q13.1, close to or on the gene encoding the skeletal muscle ryanodine receptor, or sarcoplasmic reticulum calcium release channel. This locus has been found to be tightly linked to MH in about 30 to 50% of the susceptible families, with the actual percentage depending on the geographic location of the patient population examined. Evidence exists for other potential loci on chromosome 17q (MHS-2, gene candidate α subunit of sodium channel) and 7 q (MHS-3, gene candidate $\alpha_2\delta$ subunits of dihydropyridine receptor). It is clear that one or more modulators are essential for expression of the syndrome. The incidence of MH is estimated at 1 in 12,000 pediatric anesthetics to 1 in 40,000 adult anesthetics. There is a higher incidence when the volatile anesthetics and succinylcholine are used in combination. While the age range for MH cases is 2 months to 70 years, there is a high male-to-female predominance (3:1) and a far greater incidence of MH cases reported in subjects under the age of 15. MH is most often associated with otolaryngologic surgeries, followed by orthopedic surgeries. About two-thirds of patients with a genetic predisposition to MH manifest signs during their first anesthetic exposure, whereas about one-third have up to three uneventful episodes before signs of MH are noted. With a greater awareness of the syndrome, better monitoring, and the use of dantrolene, the overall mortality

from MH has decreased from between 70 to 80% to as low as 5 to 20%.

PATHOPHYSIOLOGY

Background The term MH will be reserved for the inherited anesthesia-induced hypermetabolic syndrome in humans. The syndrome most likely can be a common final pathway for any one of several different defects. The analogous syndrome in pigs will be specifically referred to as the porcine stress syndrome (PSS). We will not address the MH-like syndrome reported in horses and dogs. The reasons for differentiating between MH and PSS syndromes include the following: (1) one mutation in the ryanodine receptor gene, is possibly associated with all PSS (thymine for cytosine substitution at nucleotide 1843 results in a cysteine[615] for arginine[615]), but the analogous mutation in humans has not convincingly been demonstrated to cause the human MH syndrome, even in the very few MH families in which it is present; (2) stress, which readily elicits PSS, is not generally thought of as a triggering stimulus for human MH; (3) Ca^{2+} regulation in human MH muscle is not affected in the same way by the primary defect as in PSS muscle; and (4) unlike PSS, a defect in any one of several different proteins can cause the human MH syndrome.

The pathophysiology of human MH has been difficult to elucidate for several reasons. In most cases, humans who are MH-susceptible appear perfectly normal in the absence of anesthetics and have no histologic evidence of a muscle disorder. It is difficult to phenotype those individuals based on only mild signs suggestive of MH during anesthesia, since these signs could result from a number of perioperative complications unrelated to MH. The only convincing case is a full-blown life-threatening episode of MH, and such cases are rare due to the discontinuation of triggering anesthesia upon early signs of MH. A second complicating factor is an age dependence of MH and PSS and other variability in presentation that is probably due to up- and downregulation of one or more modulating processes, resulting in what is termed variable penetrance. Third, the functions of several proteins are altered indirectly in MH, and their state of altered function probably varies with the state of the modulating processes.

The main triggering agents are the halogenated volatile anesthetics (halothane, enflurane, isoflurane, methoxyflurane, and desflurane) and depolarizing neuromuscular-blocking agents (primarily succinylcholine). Cyclopropane and ether are also regarded as triggering agents. Halothane and succinylcholine act synergistically in vivo to increase serum creatine kinase values and in vitro to induce contractures in skeletal muscle. Caffeine is used for diagnostic testing. While halothane and caffeine both cause release of Ca^{2+} from the sarcoplasmic reticulum, they do not act by identical mechanisms. Ryanodine has also been reported to be more effective in inducing contractures in MH than in normal muscle, although these studies are in the early stages. Dantrolene is the most effective antagonist of the MH syndrome. In isolated muscle preparations, dantrolene antagonizes halothane- and caffeine-induced contractures. Although dantrolene blocks Ca^{2+} release from the sarcoplasmic reticulum, its mechanism has not been exactly identified. Dantrolene does not affect membrane potentials but does reduce excitability of the muscle to some extent at clinically effective concentrations.

Association of MH with Muscle Disorders   A number of muscle disorders have been associated with MH. Two appear highly related: central core disease and King-Denborough syndrome. Recently, data have suggested that central core disease and MH are allelic in some families and that both disorders are caused by the same defect in the ryanodine receptor. All patients with central core disease in an MH-susceptible family have been believed to be susceptible to MH; however, this association has become less clear. Some families with central core disease do not have any members testing positive for MH susceptibility, and, even within families in which the two disorders appear to be coinherited, cosegregation of MH and central core disease is not absolute. Duchenne type and Becker's muscular dystrophy seem to present a unique response to anesthetics that is now being considered a clearly distinct variant form of MH characterized by hyperkalemia and cardiac arrest. While often a response to triggering anesthesia, myotonia is only rarely associated with more convincing hypermetabolic signs of MH. There is growing evidence of an association between exertional heat stroke and MH. The association between neuroleptic malignant syndrome and MH has been difficult to clarify. In general, neuroleptic malignant syndrome appears to be centrally mediated, but some subjects have abnormal diagnostic contracture test results for MH.

Information Derived from the Contracture Test for Diagnosis of Human MH   Considerable variability between fiber bundles from the same biopsy specimen suggests that the MH mutation is not homogeneously spread throughout the skeletal muscle mass. The contracture response to halothane exhibits a curious temperature dependence that is difficult to explain. That is, the contractures to halothane observed in MH muscle at 37°C are greatly attenuated or abolished at 25°C. There appears to be no association between the magnitude of the contracture response in the diagnostic test and the severity of an MH episode, since a positive contracture test result can be obtained at a time when PSS-susceptible swine will not exhibit a response to triggering anesthetics. Halothane-induced contractures are dependent on extracellular Ca^{2+}.

Tissues Expressing the MH Defect   The MH and PSS defects are expressed in skeletal muscle, as evidenced by the in vitro contracture test for MH susceptibility. There seems to be a difference between swine and humans in the extent to which the MS or PSS defect is expressed outside skeletal muscle. This is not completely surprising, since the primary defects and the patterns of inheritance are not identical. In the pig, the defect is manifest in red and white blood cells. Evidence exists for primary expression of the defect in cardiac muscle in PSS-susceptible individuals, but this has been controversial. Hepatic cells are also affected in PSS-susceptible subjects. In humans, the expression of the defect appears to be restricted to skeletal muscle in most cases. Therefore, we will focus on mechanisms in that tissue.

Organelles in Skeletal Muscle Expressing the MH Defect

Sarcoplasmic Reticulum
Elevated myoplasmic Ca^{2+} levels appear to play a crucial role in MH. The mechanisms for controlling Ca^{2+} levels reside primarily in the sarcoplasmic reticulum (Fig. 8–1). Several investigators have identified altered function of the sarcoplasmic reticulum in PSS. This alteration is manifested as a low threshold of Ca^{2+}-induced Ca^{2+} release (less added Ca^{2+} is required to open the Ca^{2+}-regulated Ca^{2+} release channel) and an enhanced rate (not amount) of Ca^{2+} release. The rate or amount of Ca^{2+} uptake is not believed to be significantly affected in MH or PSS muscle. In human MH muscle, the Ca^{2+} release process appears to be normal in the absence of anesthetics. Regarding the effects of anesthetics on Ca^{2+} release, the rate of halothane-induced Ca^{2+} release is abnormally high in PSS-susceptible subjects. It is believed that the differences observed in halothane-induced Ca^{2+} release are actually due to an acceleration in Ca^{2+}-induced Ca^{2+} release by halothane. There is no effect of temperature on the rate of halothane-induced Ca^{2+} release, as is observed with halothane-induced contractures of MH muscle and fatty acid-enhanced halothane-induced Ca^{2+} release (see next page).

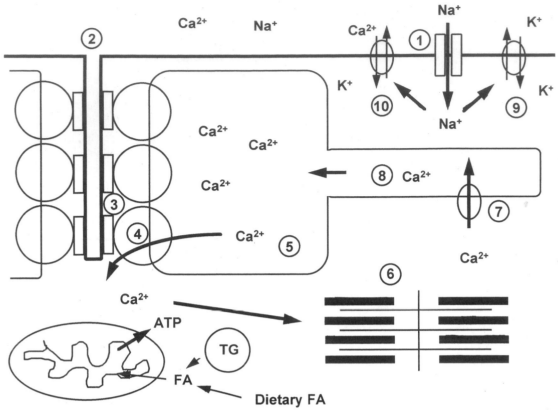

Figure 8–1 Excitation-contraction coupling and MH. The action potential generated at the endplate region of the neuromuscular junction is propagated down the sarcolemma (muscle plasma membrane) by the opening of voltage-dependent Na^+ channels (1). The action potential continues down into the t tubules (2) to the dihydropyridine receptors (3). The dihydropyridine receptors in skeletal muscle function as voltage sensors and are coupled to the Ca^{2+}-release channels (4). Through this coupled signaling process, the Ca^{2+}-release channels are opened, a portion of the available terminal cisternae Ca^{2+} stores (5) are released, and the levels of myoplasmic Ca^{2+} are elevated. The Ca^{2+} then diffuses to the myofibrils (6) and interacts with the troponin-tropomyosin complex associated with actin (thin lines) and allows interaction of actin with myosin (thick lines) for mechanical movement. The Ca^{2+} diffuses away from the myofibrils, and this Ca^{2+} signal is terminated by an ATP-driven Ca^{2+} pump (7), which pumps Ca^{2+} into the longitudinal sarcoplasmic reticulum (8). The Ca^{2+} diffuses from the longitudinal sarcoplasmic reticulum to the terminal cisternae, where it is concentrated for release by Ca^{2+}-binding proteins. Na^+ entering during the action potential is subsequently extruded from the cell by the Na,K-ATPase (9) and possibly through Na^+-Ca^{2+} exchange (10). The latter process would elevate intracellular Ca^{2+} and could result from delayed inactivation of Na^+ currents. A major form of energy for supplying cellular ATP for the ion pumps and numerous other energy-consuming processes is fatty acid (FA) derived from the serum (dietary FA) or from intramuscular triglyceride (TG) stores. Therefore, a defect in the intracellular Ca^{2+}-regulating processes (increased Ca^{2+} release or decreased Ca^{2+} uptake) or a defect in the sarcolemma could account for an increase in myoplasmic Ca^{2+}.

Mitochondria

Mitochondria oxidize a variety of substrates to generate the form of energy (ATP) most useful for driving cellular reactions. Defects in mitochondrial function do not appear to initiate the MH syndrome but have provided an interesting model in which to examine some biochemical consequences of the MH defect, and they may participate as the syndrome progresses. A low threshold for uncoupling Ca^{2+}-stimulated succinate oxidation in the absence of ADP is observed in PSS and human MH muscle at 40°C and is not observed at 25°C. Therefore, the mitochondria may become uncoupled as the syndrome progresses and then would not generate enough ATP to sustain the ATP-driven Ca^{2+} pump. Fatty acids have been suggested to be involved in Ca^{2+}-stimulated uncoupling of mitochondria. Accelerated skeletal muscle triglyceride-associated metabolism appears to be the source of free fatty acids in MH and PSS. Under nonanesthetic con-

ditions, this greater fatty acid flux may be required as fuel to keep ATP levels from being lowered by the ATPase-driven Ca^{2+} and Na^+-K^+ pumps removing calcium and sodium from the myoplasm.

Sarcolemma

The sarcolemma maintains the membrane potential of the muscle cell and acts as a permeability barrier to Na^+, K^+, Cl^-, and Ca^{2+}. Although skeletal muscle does not require extracellular Ca^{2+} for contractility, halothane-induced contractures for in vitro diagnosis do require extracellular Ca^{2+}. A breakdown in the sarcolemma could result in a large influx of Ca^{2+} from the extracellular medium. Also, opening specific Ca^{2+} channels (e.g., dihydropyridine receptors) in the sarcolemma would allow the entry of extracellular Ca^{2+}. There are reports of altered dihydropyridine receptor binding, altered Na^+ channel function, and diminished maximum sarcolemmal Ca^{2+} accumulation and ATP-stimulated Ca^{2+} uptake in PSS.

General Membrane Defect

The MH and PSS defects are manifest in several membranes in many ways. Various probes used to detect membrane fluidity or microviscosity have detected differences between PSS and control skeletal muscle. Since the functions of a large number of proteins are altered, perhaps due secondarily to altered physical characteristics of the membrane, the nondescript term *general membrane defect* has been used to characterize this pervasive influence of the MH defect. It is important to consider that at least some of the changes in function may occur only on physical or chemical perturbation of the tissue.

Specific Proteins with Altered Function in MH
The Calcium-Release Channel

The Ca^{2+}-release channel is an extremely large homotetramer in which the subunits have a molecular weight of about 560,000 each. The Ca^{2+}-release channel has a binding site for the contracture-inducing plant alkaloid ryanodine and is therefore also referred to as the ryanodine receptor. The function of the Ca^{2+}-release channel is definitely altered in PSS muscle, most likely due to the genetic mutation, and this may account directly for the altered Ca^{2+} release in PSS muscle described under "Sarcoplasmic Reticulum." Binding studies have revealed that, although the number of binding sites is unaltered in PSS, the K_d (a measure related to binding affinity) of ryanodine binding to the Ca^{2+}-release channel is reduced in PSS muscle, and this value appears to be an average of ryanodine binding to two or more interconvertible states (differing in affinity) of the channel. Subtle functional changes have been observed in the Ca^{2+}-release channel from PSS and MH muscle using planer bilayer approaches. These differences relate primarily to an increased probability of the Ca^{2+}-release channel being in an open state in MH muscle. As with the sarcoplasmic reticulum studies, differences between normal and PSS-susceptible subjects have been reported in the absence of halothane or caffeine. Also in agreement with the sarcoplasmic reticulum studies, human MH muscle requires the presence of caffeine or halothane to detect abnormalities. In human MH muscle, there appear to be two populations of ion channels: halothane-insensitive and halothane-sensitive. The halothane-sensitive channels have an increased probability of opening in the presence of clinically relevant concentrations of halothane. They do not occur in all MH muscle, and both types (or states) of channels can coexist in the same muscle biopsy sample.

The Sodium Channel

Skeletal muscle sodium channels have two subunits: α, with a molecular weight of 220,000, and β, with a molecular weight of 40,000. The α subunit contains the ion channel. The "adult" sodium-channel α subunit in skeletal muscle is encoded on chromosome 17, and the β subunit is encoded on chromosome 19. Sodium channels in skeletal muscle are of two types, and they can be differentiated by their sensitivity to tetrodotoxin (TTX), which blocks the channel pore. The first is an "embryonic," or TTX-insensitive, type, which is identical to the cardiac sodium channel, and the second is the adult, or TTX-sensitive, type. Defects in the sodium channel have been implicated as the cause of other disorders of skeletal muscle, including hyperkalemic periodic paralysis and paramyotonia congenita. The function of the sodium channel is abnormal in primary cultures of human MH skeletal muscle. Intracellular injection of fatty acids into primary cell cultures of normal human skeletal muscle having primarily embryonic Na^+ currents introduces additional adult Na^+ currents. In contrast, the Na^+ channels in primary cultures of skeletal muscle from MH-susceptible humans are primarily in the adult state even without injected fatty acid, and the intracellular injection of fatty acids has no further effect. This phenomenon may be related to the elevated fatty acid flux in MH muscle (see below).

Dihydropyridine Receptor

The involvement of the dihydropyridine receptor (DHPR calcium channel) in excitation-contraction coupling has made it an actively investigated protein in MH. The DHPR is comprised of five subunits: α_1, α_2, β_1, γ, and δ. The α_1 subunit is the ion pore structure. The α_1 and δ subunits are encoded by a single gene. In PSS muscle, there are reports of altered DHPR receptor binding.

Lipids: Potential Modulators of the Syndrome There is a difference between carrying the MH mutation and having the full potential for expressing an MH episode. An MH episode is not observed on every challenge even within the same humans with MH and even in PSS-susceptible swine who are homozygous for the [615]Arg to [615]Cys ryanodine receptor mutation. Therefore, the primary MH defect may be essential, but it is not sufficient, for the MH syndrome. Lipids have been proposed as involved in modulating the syndrome.

Fatty acid production is elevated in mitochondrial fractions and whole muscle homogenates from PSS- and MH-susceptible individuals. There is an age-related increase in fatty acid production in skeletal muscle that parallels an age-related increase in susceptibility of the PSS-susceptible pigs. When only free fatty acids are examined, they are found to be at normal levels in human MH and PSS muscle. Perhaps the enhanced utilization of fatty acids is a compensatory response to replace ATP utilized to drive the Ca^{2+}-ATPase-associated Ca^{2+} pump in an effort to remove chronically elevated levels of Ca^{2+}. The addition of fatty acids to sarcoplasmic reticulum preparations markedly (~20- to 30-fold) decreases the concentration of halothane required for the sustained opening of the Ca^{2+}-release channel. This suggests that a defect in the excitation coupling process per se is not a requirement for the MH syndrome. Unlike all the previous studies of Ca^{2+} release, there is an absolute temperature-dependence (which occurs at 37°C, not at 25°C) of the fatty acid enhancement of halothane-induced Ca^{2+} release, which is consistent with the temperature-dependence of halothane-induced contractures of MH muscle.

Phosphatidylinositol phospholipids have become of interest since one specific metabolite of phospholipase C action, IP_3 (inositol 1,4,5-trisphosphate) has been demonstrated to be elevated in human MH and PSS muscle. The elevation of all products of phosphatidylinositol hydrolysis suggests that phospholipase C activity may be elevated in MH.

The antioxidant defense abnormality in PSS is especially interesting, since it could be either the cause or the effect of accelerated fatty acid production. In either case, it provides a novel target site for prophylactic and therapeutic intervention. Despite an antioxidant defense abnormality, the levels of skeletal muscle antioxidants and antioxidant enzymes are normal. Excessive peroxidation could contribute to the loss of Ca^{2+} regulation in MH muscle.

Conclusions While some of the pieces of the puzzle regarding PSS are falling into place, we have much to learn about human MH. The Ca^{2+}-release channel mutation resulting in a conversion of ^{615}Arg to ^{615}Cys appears to account for susceptibility to most or all of the PSS. While some human MH families may also have a defect in the Ca^{2+}-release channel, there is convincing evidence that a defect in any one of several proteins (including the Na^+ channel and DHPR) may account for the syndrome. Fatty acids and/or phospholipase C, or an antioxidant abnormality, have been suggested to modulate the expression of the syndrome. The functions of many proteins are altered indirectly in MH and PSS, and sorting out cause-effect relationships is difficult, especially with an overriding modulator and activation of second messenger systems, which further confuse the puzzle.

SIGNS AND SYMPTOMS

The clinical features of MH are variable. Tachycardia and metabolic and respiratory acidosis are often seen. Extreme hypercarbia is usually seen. Central venous oxygen desaturation may also occur. Since the central venous oxygen and carbon dioxide (CO_2) levels change more markedly than do those in arterial blood, expired CO_2 or central venous CO_2 levels are a more accurate reflection of whole-body CO_2 stores. Skin signs vary from flushing to blanching and skin mottling. An increase in body temperature may occur at rates of 0.5 to 1°C every 15 min and, in rare uncontrolled cases, may reach levels of 45°C. Heat is liberated during the continued synthesis and utilization of ATP and appears to originate in the liver and skeletal muscle. Skeletal muscle rigidity, the most frequent sign of MH, may involve the entire body and/or be manifested only as masseter muscle spasm. Approximately 50% of patients who demonstrate only masseter muscle spasm have positive muscle biopsy results for susceptibility to MH. In addition, masseter muscle spasm occurs in approximately 1 in 100 children who do not have MH who are anesthetized with halothane followed by succinylcholine.

Numerous laboratory findings may aid in the diagnosis of MH, but none is considered to be pathognomonic. MH is associated with increased transaminase levels after the onset of an attack. There is an increase in creatine kinase levels, which peaks at 12 to 24 h after onset of a MH attack. A postoperative creatine kinase level >20,000 international units after succinylcholine-induced masseter rigidity is often indicative of either MH susceptibility or an underlying myopathy. Plasma and urine myoglobin levels increase secondary to massive rhabomyolysis. Hyperkalemia as well as hypercalcemia, may also be seen.

Late complications include disseminated intravascular coagulation, which may be due to hemolysis, or increased release of tissue thromboplastins, secondary to an increased permeability in tissues or overt tissue damage. Disseminated intravascular coagulation also may be secondary to shock due to inadequate capillary perfusion. Other late complications include pulmonary edema and acute renal failure. Central nervous system damage may include blindness, seizures, coma, and paralysis.

During convalescence after an episode of MH, the patient may complain of muscle weakness, tenderness, and/or swelling.

DIFFERENTIAL DIAGNOSIS

The differential diagnosis of MH includes light anesthesia, thyroid storm, sepsis, pheochromocytoma, drug and pyrogen reactions, temporomandibular joint dysfunction, muscle diseases (e.g., myotonic muscular dystrophy and disuse myopathy), and neuroleptic malignant syndrome.

TREATMENT WITH DANTROLENE

Dantrolene, a hydantoin derivative, is the only drug reliably effective for treatment of MH. Use of this drug has decreased mortality from roughly 80% to as low as 5%. Dantrolene is used orally in the treatment of chronic skeletal muscle spasticity associated with upper motor neuron diseases, such as stroke, cerebral palsy, and spinal cord injury.

The half-life of dantrolene is approximately 12 h when given intravenously. Its effect begins in 2 to 3 min and reaches a peak in 5 to 10 min. Dantrolene is metabolized in the liver by oxidative and reductive pathways. Its metabolites are excreted in the urine. Side effects include sedation, skeletal muscle weakness, nausea, transient dizziness, local thrombophlebitis, diplopia, dysarthria, swelling of the tongue, and, rarely, hepatic dysfunction.

The dose of dantrolene is 1 to 2 mg/kg intravenously (mixed with sterile water), which is repeated every 5 to 10 min to a maximum dose of 10 mg/kg, depending on the patient's clinical response. Dantrolene should be continued in the postoperative period to prevent possible recrudescences. In the postoperative period, dantrolene should be given intravenously 1 to 2 mg/kg every 4 to 6 h up to 24 h or by mouth 4 mg/kg every day for 2 to 4 days.

Dantrolene may be given preoperatively 2 to 3 mg/kg intravenously 10 to 30 min prior to the onset of anesthesia. Dantrolene may also be given preoperatively by mouth at a dose of 4 mg/kg to 2 to 4 h prior to induction of anesthesia, but preanesthetic use of dantrolene is not a universally accepted practice.

Dantrolene is not antagonized by calcium at clinical doses. Dantrolene has no effective antidote but can be antagonized transiently by germine monoacetate, anticholinesterase agents, and 4-aminopyridine. Germine monoacetate reversal follows no direct pharmacologic antagonism. It is the result of the fact that germine monoacetate causes repetitive firing of muscle in response to single stimulation such that repetitive myoplasmic-free calcium release occurs.

SYMPTOMATIC TREATMENT

When the diagnosis of MH is known, prudent practice is the avoidance of triggering agents.

With the onset of signs and symptoms of MH, the first measure is to discontinue all triggering agents and hyperventilate with 100% oxygen to normocarbia. If time and the availability of personnel permit, flush the anesthesia circuit and change the breathing circuit and CO_2 absorber or the entire anesthesia machine. The surgeon should be immediately advised of the problem. Sodium bicarbonate should be administered to correct any acidosis. Dantrolene should be administered. Calcium antagonists are not effective for treatment of MH and should be avoided, since they can cause hyperkalemia in the presence of dantrolene. The patient should be hydrated with cooled intravenous fluids. Surface cooling should take place. Gastric, peritoneal, or bladder lavage with cold fluids should take place if possible. Pump bypass with a heat exchanger can also be used to cool the patient. Cooling should be discontinued when the temperature is approximately 38°C to avoid hypothermia. During the steps described above, additional vascular access should be secured with intravenous and arterial catheters. A urinary catheter and nasogastric tube should also be inserted. Blood samples should be sent for analysis. This analysis should include assessments of arterial blood gas, glucose, serum osmolarity, blood urea nitrogen, creatinine, creatine kinase, LDH, liver function, serum myoglobin, lactate levels, and mixed venous CO_2 as well as a complete blood count. Blood samples should also be sent for clotting studies, including measurements of prothrombin time, partial prothrombin time, and fibrinogen and fibrin degradation products. Urinalysis should also be performed, and hemoglobin as well as myoglobin should be checked for (however, elevations in these substances usually occur approximately 4 to 8 h after the onset of a MH episode). Urine output should be monitored and maintained with adequate intravenous fluids, which may be supplemented with mannitol and/or furosemide. Urine output should be maintained in an effort to avoid acute renal failure secondary to deposition of myoglobin in the renal tubules. Glucose and insulin may be needed to correct hyperkalemia. The patient should be monitored closely for any dysrhythmias, and procainamide should be given as needed. Lidocaine is not as effective as procainamide.

Postoperatively, the patient should remain in the intensive care unit. Follow-up should concentrate on any residual muscle damage as well as any acid-base and/or electrolyte abnormalities. Dantrolene therapy should also be continued for a minimum of 1 to 2 days.

Follow-up counseling should occur with the patient and family. A muscle biopsy may be warranted in patients in whom a confirmation of the diagnosis is desired. A bracelet indicating MH susceptibility should be worn by the patient.

IDENTIFICATION OF MH-SUSCEPTIBLE PATIENTS

In identifying and assessing the MH-susceptible patient, a thorough patient and family history should be obtained. Previous anesthetic experiences should be questioned with regard to fever, rigidity, cardiac dysrhythmias, prolonged awakening, muscle pain, dark urine after anesthesia, and muscle swelling and/or weakness after anesthesia.

The patient's or family's response to physical exertion should also be elucidated, because environmental stress may, in rare cases, be an associated trigger of MH. Patients and families should be questioned with regard to excessively high temperature with infections and/or a history of heat intolerance.

MH is associated with various musculoskeletal disorders, such as Duchenne's muscular dystrophy, osteogenesis imperfecta, paramyotonia congenita, myelomeningocele, central core disease, periodic paralysis, mitochondrial myopathy, myoadenalate deaminase deficiency, and King Denborough syndrome. Patients with ptosis, strabismus, weakness, increased muscle bulk, muscle cramping, recurrent dislocations, hernia or back trouble, kyphoscoliosis, or hyperextensible joints may have an increased susceptibility to MH. Other conditions associated with MH susceptibility include Burkitt's lymphoma and neuroleptic malignant syndrome.

Many laboratory studies have attempted to assist in the diagnosis of MH. Most have not been found to be reliable enough for routine use. Skeletal muscle biopsy is the only accepted test for diagnosing MH susceptibility. This test is an in vitro isometric contracture test of muscle often taken from the vastus lateralis muscle. The muscle is subjected to isometric contracture testing under the influence of caffeine or halothane. Caffeine causes contracture of skeletal muscles by stimulating the release of calcium by the sarcoplasmic reticulum. MH-susceptible individuals show exaggerated contractures of skeletal muscle under the influence of caffeine or halothane. Results of skeletal muscle biopsy in vitro isometric contracture testing may indicate three possible results: (1) MH-susceptible (MHS), which indicates a clearly abnormal response either to halothane or caffeine; (2) MH-nonsusceptible (MHN), which indicates normal results of both tests; and (3) MH-equivocal (MHE), which indicates borderline results. The MHE outcome is treated clinically as MHS.

MANAGEMENT OF THE ANESTHETIC

Some authors suggest that, prior to induction of anesthesia in a MH-susceptible patient, the patient should be given dantrolene, as noted previously. Adequate sedation should be given in an effort to avoid stress. Phenothiazines should be avoided, since they have the potential to cause the related neuroleptic malignant syndrome. Other preoperative medications should not include anticholinergics, since they may interfere with normal body heat loss and also may increase heart rate.

No studies confirm that MH can be triggered by residual concentrations of volatile anesthetics, especially halothane, delivered from previously used anesthesia machines. The dose of halothane necessary to trigger a reaction in a patient susceptible to MH is unknown. The lowest concentration of any potent inhaled anesthetic that can trigger a MH crisis is also unknown.

Precautionary measures should include use of a disposable anesthesia breathing circuit, use of new CO_2 absorbent, removal of volatile agent vaporizers, replacement of the fresh gas flow outlet hose, and continuous flow of oxygen at 10 L/min for 5 min preceding machine use.

Regional anesthesia can be employed successfully using ester and amide local anesthetics. However, regional anesthesia may not protect the susceptible patient from stress.

DRUGS THAT MAY TRIGGER MH

The inhalation agents halothane, enflurane, isoflurane, sevoflurane, desflurane, methoxyflurane, cyclopropane, and ether should not be used. Succinylcholine and decamethonium (depolarizing agents) should also not be used.

DRUGS CONSIDERED SAFE FOR MH-SUSCEPTIBLE PATIENTS

Nitrous oxide may be used safely. However, it may stimulate the sympathetic nervous system, which may confuse the diagnosis of MH. Barbiturates, propofol, opioids, benzodiazapines, etomidate, and droperidol can be used safely. Ketamine can be used, although it may cause an increase in blood pressure as well as heart rate and temperature, which, again, may be confused with signs of MH. The nondepolarizer neuromuscular blocking agents pancuronium, atracurium, and vecuronium may be used safely. Anticholinesterase and anticholinergics may also be used. Anticholinergics, however, may cause increases in heart rate as well as temperature. Local anesthetics, as noted previously, can be used, although regional anesthesia may not eliminate stress that may trigger MH.

☐ PLASMA CHOLINESTERASE VARIANTS

The enzyme plasma cholinesterase, also referred to as pseudocholinesterase or butyrylcholinesterase, is a homotetramer of molecular weight 324,000. It is synthesized in the liver and found in many tissues, but in particularly high concentration in the plasma. Plasma cholinesterase has no known natural substrate or function, since patients without detectable enzyme activity are virtually symptom free, until they receive a dose of succinylcholine, or mivacurium.

SUCCINYLCHOLINE AND PLASMA CHOLINESTERASE

The brief duration of succinylcholine's action results from its extensive and very rapid hydrolysis by plasma cholinesterase. This occurs in two steps: succinylcholine is first hydrolyzed to succinylmonocholine and choline and then to succinic acid and choline. Only a small fraction of any intravenous dose normally reaches the neuromuscular junction. Neuromuscular block is then terminated by diffusion of succinylcholine away from the endplate. Thus, plasma cholinesterase activity is the primary determinant of duration of succinylcholine paralysis. Deficient plasma cholinesterase activity results in a much higher percent of a given dose of succinylcholine reaching the endplate and therefore an abnormally prolonged paralysis.

VARIATIONS IN PLASMA CHOLINESTERASE ACTIVITY

Plasma cholinesterase activity can differ between patients, and vary over time in a given patient. The activity of plasma cholinesterase is, for instance, age dependent. It gradually increases from birth, when the activity is approximately 50% that of normal adults, to puberty, when adult levels are achieved. Pregnancy is associated with a 25 to 30% reduction in activity, which begins at week 10 and lasts through post partum week 6. In addition to pregnancy, various pathologic states, such as liver disease, and certain drugs, such as echothiophate, can reduce plasma cholinesterase activity. Despite theoretical concerns that such patients will demonstrate prolonged paralysis after succinylcholine administration, these conditions almost never result in clinically significant sensitivity to succinylcholine, since even 20% of normal enzyme activity leads to only minimal prolongation of succinylcholine paralysis. Certain genetic variants, however, can demonstrate substantially prolonged weakness after a single dose of succinylcholine or mivacurium.

GENETICS OF PLASMA CHOLINESTERASE ACTIVITY

Deficiency in plasma cholinesterase activity can result from mutations that affect either quality or quantity of the enzyme, or both. The specific mutations are well worked out for at least nine different clinically relevant plasma cholinesterase mutations, however, all except the classical atypical allele first described by Kalow in 1957, are extremely rare. The three best known mutant alleles are 1) atypical, which produces an enzyme resistant to dibucaine inhibition (see below); 2) fluoride-resistant, this gene product is resistant to fluoride inhibition; 3) silent, which is the null allele, meaning the gene produces no enzyme. Clinically significant plasma

Table 8–1
DISTRIBUTION, SUCCINYLCHOLINE SENSITIVITY, AND THE BIOCHEMICAL CHARACTERISTICS OF PSEUDOCHOLINESTERASE VARIANTS IN A BRITISH POPULATION*

Genotype	Relative Mean Enzymatic Activity	DN		FN		Frequency	Succinylcholine Prolongation
		Mean	Range	Mean	Range		
$E_1^u E_1^u$	100	80	77–83	61	56–66	96%	?1/2500 moderately sensitive
$E_1^a E_1^a$	43	21	8–28	19	10–28	1/2000	All very sensitive
$E_1^f E_1^f$	74	67	64–69	36	34–43	1/154,000	All moderately sensitive
$E_1^s E_1^s$	Enzymatic activity nil or too low to measure					1/100,000	All very sensitive
$E_1^u E_1^a$	77	62	48–69	50	44–54	1/25	?1/500 moderately sensitive
$E_1^u E_1^f$	86	74	70–83	52	46–54	1/200	?1/100 moderately sensitive
$E_1^u E_1^s$	50	80	77–83	61	56–68	1/190	?1/1000 moderately sensitive
$E_1^a E_1^f$	59	53	45–59	33	28–39	1/20,000	All moderately sensitive
$E_1^a E_1^s$	22	21	8–28	19	10–28	1/29,000	All very sensitive
$E_1^f E_1^s$	37	67	64–69	36	34–43	1/150,000	All moderately sensitive

* Reproduced with permission from Whittaker M. Plasma cholinesterase variants and the anesthetist. *Anaesthesia* 35:174, 1980.

cholinesterase deficiency is autosomal recessive for all these mutations, since heterozygotes with a normal allele will generate enough plasma cholinesterase to metabolize standard succinylcholine doses. However, a wide variety of allele combinations are possible, as shown in Table 8–1. Homozygous atypical plasma cholinesterase is by far the most common form of clinically significant cholinesterase deficiency, occurring at a frequency of roughly 1 in 2500. Though homozygotes produce normal quantities of this enzyme, it has virtually no capacity for hydrolyzing succinylcholine.

DIBUCAINE NUMBER

The standard assay of plasma cholinesterase measures hydrolysis of a benzylcholine substrate. This reaction is normally inhibited by the local anesthetic, dibucaine, and Kalow first demonstrated that the atypical plasma cholinesterase enzyme is resistant to this effect. The dibucaine number (DN) is given by the percent inhibition by dibucaine of benzylcholine hydrolysis; DN is about 80 in normal homozygotes, while atypical homozygotes have a DN of 20, and heterozygotes have intermediate values. The DN is a very good screening test for diagnosing carriers or homozygotes for the atypical cholinesterase (Table 8–1). A different variant allele produces an enzyme resistant to another inhibitor of the assay, fluoride ion. Measuring this effect yields the fluoride number (FN, see Table 8–1). Total cholinesterase quantity is unaffected in homozygotes for the normal, atypical and fluoride variants. However, the enzyme is very low to undetectable in homozygotes for the silent allele. Unlike the other variants, this is a quantitative, not a qualitative abnormality. For the vast majority of plasma cholinesterase deficient patients, genotype can be determined by combining quantification of total enzyme, and determination of DN and FN.

MANAGEMENT OF PATIENTS WITH PLASMA CHOLINESTERASE DEFICIENCY

The primary consideration in patients homozygous for a clinically relevant mutation in the plasma cholinesterase gene is sensitivity to the muscle relaxants normally metabolized by this enzyme, succinylcholine and mivacurium. This sensitivity manifests itself in the case of both relaxants, as significant prolongation of paralysis. Intubating doses of these drugs in patients homozygous for the common, atypical variant, results in roughly 3 to 4 h of paralysis in the case of mivicurium, and 6 to 12 h for succinylcholine. Assuming the diagnosis is not known beforehand, this becomes a diagnosis of exclusion, pending a DN determination, in patients with reversal resistant neuromuscular blockade. The best treatment in the case of succinylcholine paralysis is conservative management with mechanical ventilation until the patient's strength returns. Fresh frozen plasma, whole blood, or purified enzyme can theoretically reverse the enzyme deficiency and the paralysis, but this approach is not generally warranted by risk-benefit analysis. In the case of mivicurium, paralysis can be safely reversed with the standard neostigmine and antimuscarinic combination provided a twitch monitor demonstrates return of some function at the neuromuscular junction. Notably, there is some concern that these patients are at increased risk for toxicity or abnormal prolongation of nerve block when using local anesthetics with an ester linkage. The risk is probably more theoretical than clinically relevant, but it is certainly worth considering an alternative local anesthetic in patients known to be homozygous for a cholinesterase variant.

☐ THE PORPHYRIAS

The porphyrias are a heterogeneous group of disorders caused by disruption of the heme synthetic pathway. The

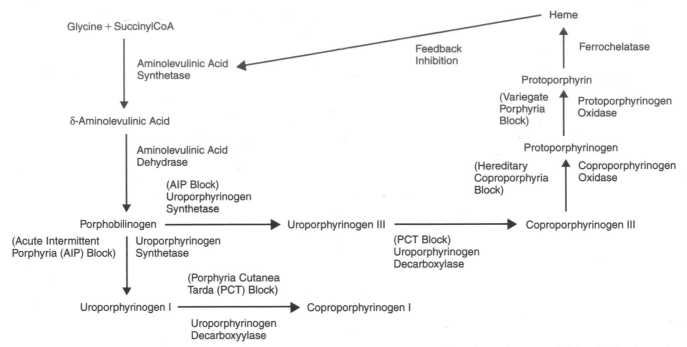

Figure 8-2 The biochemical pathways involved in heme synthesis. Enzymatic steps and locations of enzyme deficiencies for the various porphyrias are depicted. Courtesy of Richard Berlin, MD.

first, and rate-limiting, step in heme synthesis (Fig. 8–2) is the reaction of succinylCoA with glycine to form delta-aminolevulinic acid (ALA). This reaction is catalyzed by ALA synthetase which is feedback inhibited by heme, the product of the final reaction in this scheme. Obviously, a total deficiency in heme synthesis is not compatible with life and most of the porphyrias result from genetic mutation in a synthetic enzyme that causes only a partial disruption of this pathway. This leads to failure of feedback inhibition and accumulation of the heme synthetic intermediates which are considered responsible for the clinical picture of porphyria. The pathway can be disrupted at any of several points, and the resulting patterns of metabolite accumulation allow one to predict the corresponding clinical manifestations for a specific porphyria.

The porphyrias can be classified by several means: the organ system location of the primary metabolic defect; the organ system most affected by the disease; whether the symptoms are inducible; and whether the disease course is typically acute or chronic. The classic distinction is between those porphyrias where the affected enzyme is primarily in the liver or hematopoietic system: the hepatic versus the erythropoietic porphyrias. As a whole, the porphyrias generally affect either the nervous system or skin, or both and it is useful to know the particular pattern of a given disease for a patient one is treating. By far the most important distinction among the porphyrias for the anesthesiologist is whether the clinical state is inducible, meaning that specific drugs or conditions can precipitate an attack of porphyria.

The erythropoietic porphyrias, uroporphyria and protoporphyria, cause skin friability and photosensitivity but no neurologic symptoms. They are not inducible. The nonacute he-

patic porphyria, porphyria cutanea tarda, is also a "skin only" porphyria and is not inducible. For all these, the anesthesiologist must be aware of any history of cutaneous fragility in preparing a plan for patient positioning and other aspects of perioperative management.

The remaining hepatic porphyrias are all inducible and "acute": acute intermittent porphyria (AIP), hereditary coproporphyria, variegate porphyria and the recently described plumboporphyria. Neurologic symptoms are common to all these and hereditary coproporphyria and variegate porphyria share cutaneous manifestations as well. Other than an isolated population in South Africa where variegate porphyria is common, AIP is easily the most common porphyria and its clinical picture provides the canon for diagnosis and treatment of an acute, inducible porphyric crisis.

ACUTE INTERMITTENT PORPHYRIA

Acute intermittent porphyria affects the central nervous system as well as the peripheral nervous system. One of the primary mechanisms for the observed signs and symptoms may be deprivation of the porphyrins that play a role in either the impulse conduction mechanism or in the maintenance of myelin. Demyelination is seen histologically.

Acute intermittent porphyria is inherited as an autosomal dominant trait with an onset usually after 15 years of age. The worldwide incidence is approximately 1 in 80,000 individuals. The defect is due to a deficiency in uroporphyrinogen synthetase activity. This leads to an increase in activity of ALA synthetase and a resultant accumulation of porphobilinogen.

Diagnosis is made in the presence of increased urinary excretion of ALA and porphobilinogen. Decreased levels of uroporphyrinogen synthetase in red blood cells are also noted. In acute intermittent porphyria, the urine will turn black on standing from an increased urinary excretion of porphobilinogen. A DNA analysis technique that examines markers on the porphobilinogen deaminase gene has been described, permitting early detection of porphyria carriers.

CLINICAL MANIFESTATIONS

Signs and symptoms in acute intermittent porphyria are numerous. Acute episodes may last days to weeks, and periods of "remission" (low-grade disease activity) may separate them. A patient with acute intermittent porphyria will have variable neurological problems. The principal neurologic lesion is demyelinization, leading to motor weakness, decreased peripheral reflex responses, and dysfunction of the autonomic nervous system, central, peripheral and including the cranial nerves. Cranial nerve involvement may result in aphonia, respiratory paralysis, and/or dysphagia. Bulbar paralysis as well as cerebellar dysfunction may also be seen. Central nervous system involvement may also manifest as psychiatric disturbances, alterations of consciousness, stupor, confusion, seizures, or psychoses, which may persist between attacks. Central hypothalamic disturbance may be manifested as a decrease in serum sodium secondary to inappropriate ADH secretion. Hypokalemia and hypomagnesemia may also be observed. Quadriplegia or hemiplegia secondary to this demyelinating injury can occur. Peripheral neuropathies may involve sensory and/or motor components. The patients may also complain of pain in the limbs. Dysfunction of the autonomic nervous system may appear as labile hypertension, orthostatic hypotension, diaphoresis, hyperpyrexia, and/or tachycardia. The patient may also complain of abdominal pain, which may be secondary to an autonomic neuropathy, resulting in areas of spasm and dilatation in the intestines. This severe abdominal pain may simulate appendicitis, intestinal obstruction, and renal or biliary colic. Nausea and vomiting may also be observed.

Prevention of the signs and symptoms of acute intermittent porphyria may be accomplished by avoiding triggering agents. Triggering agents, most frequently barbiturates, increase the activity of ALA synthetase and can therefore increase porphyrin synthesis sufficiently to precipitate an acute attack in susceptible individuals. Typically, the triggering agents are lipid-soluble drugs that can induce synthesis of the cytochrome P-450 enzyme system. It is believed that this may stoke the heme synthetic pathway by consuming heme in the accelerated cytochrome synthesis, resulting in loss of feedback inhibition of ALA activity. Endogenous triggering factors include fasting, dehydration, infection, estrogens, emotional stress, acute alcohol abuse, and acute sunburn. It should be noted that there is an increased incidence in young to middle-aged females, which suggests a role of female hormones in the exacerbation of acute intermittent porphyria. This role of hormones is also suggested by the total absence

of acute intermittent porphyria before puberty and an exacerbation during pregnancy.

The treatment of acute attacks of porphyria includes withdrawal of triggering agents, symptomatic therapy, and methods aimed at reversing the disease process. Administration of β blockers, hydration, glucose, and exogenous heme are treatment mainstays. Propranolol controls tachycardia and may actually decrease enzyme activity. Hydration with a glucose-containing solution is necessary up until the time of and during the surgical procedure. The infusion of a glucose solution aids in suppressing the activity of enzymes involved in the production of ALA and porphobilinogen. In addition, an infusion of hematin (3 to 4 mg/kg/day) may also be used. The hematin provides a substrate for cytochrome production and suppresses activity of ALA synthetase. Problems associated with hematin use include renal failure, coagulopathy, and thrombophlebitis. A newer heme preparation, heme arginate, is more stable in solution, has a longer shelf life, and is not associated with the morbid side effects of hematin. Heme arginate currently is not approved for use in the United States, pending clinical trials.

Management involves avoidance of agents capable of provoking an attack. Drugs that induce cytochrome enzyme production can trigger symptoms. Most notable of these are barbiturates, all of which are contraindicated in patients with porphyria. Other drugs can be classified as either probably safe, or unsafe, for use in patients with an acute inducible porphyria. However, the porphyrias are rare enough, and perioperative experience with these patients so infrequent, that such classification of most drugs is still somewhat conditional. Agents commonly used by anesthesiologists that are generally considered safe in patients with inducible porphyria include: morphine, fentanyl and its derivatives, beta blockers, atropine, neostigmine, succinylcholine and nitrous oxide. In addition to the barbiturates, which are strictly contraindicated, anesthetic agents that may be dangerous for such patients include: benzodiazepines, enflurane, halothane, calcium channel blockers, animophylline, meperidine, lidocaine, cimetidine, dilantin, clonidine, hydralazine, ketamine, and etomidate. Certain synthetic anticholinesterase drugs that are used as insecticides can produce demyelinization themselves. Therefore, related drugs, such as neostigmine, should be avoided. There is a relative contraindication against the use of regional anesthesia, since the neurologic deficits produced by porphyria might be incorrectly attributed to the anesthetic technique. Intraoperatively, it is necessary to pad all skin contact points due to the friable nature of the porphyric patient's skin.

Diagnosis preoperatively should involve an extensive family as well as personal history. A history of past episodes of acute abdominal pain and/or paralysis and whether these were known to be drug-precipitated are important to elicit. The presence of skin involvement should be noted. The patients often have an increased susceptibility to minor trauma, which results in development of blisters or erosions. Luxuriant eyebrows associated with temporal hirsutism, which may also involve the face, can be seen. Finally, acute attacks and/or cutaneous involvement, which may occur in a patient's immediate relatives, should be investigated.

VARIEGATE PORPHYRIA

In variegate porphyria, both sexes are affected, with an onset after 10 years of age. Inheritance is autosomal dominant. The defect involves a decrease in the enzyme activity of protoporphyrinogen oxidase. There is an increase in urinary ALA as well as porphobilinogen levels.

Signs and symptoms include photosensitivity as well as fragile skin with numerous bullae. Neurologic sequelae, as seen in acute intermittent porphyria, can occur. Prophylaxis, treatment, and management are analogous to those for the patient with acute intermittent porphyria.

HEREDITARY COPROPORPHYRIA

Hereditary coproporphyria is an autosomal dominant disease. Onset can occur at any age. The defect involves a decrease in the enzyme activity of coproporphyrinogen oxidase. There is an increased fecal excretion of coproporphyrinogen III as well as an increase in urinary ALA and porphobilinogen levels.

Signs and symptoms, as well as prophylaxis, treatment, and management, are similar to those for acute intermittent porphyria. Hereditary coproporphyria tends to have a less severe course in terms of motor neuron injury.

ALA DEHYDRATASE DEFICIENCY PORPHYRIA

ALA dehydrastase deficiency porphyria, also known as plumboporphyria (PLP), is autosomal dominant. The defect,

as the name implies, occurs in the enzyme responsible for converting ALA to porphobilinogen.

Signs and symptoms and prophylaxis and treatment are similar to those for acute intermittent porphyria.

PORPHYRIA CUTANEA TARDA

Porphyria cutanea tarda is not associated with neurologic involvement. It is inherited as an autosomal dominant trait. There is decreased activity of uroporphyrinogen decarboxylase with an increase in urinary excretion of uroporphyrin.

Signs and symptoms are often noted in males after 35 years of age. Alcohol abuse is frequently present. Photosensitivity and friable skin are commonly seen. Hepatocellular necrosis secondary to porphyrin accumulation in the liver can occur.

Drugs used in the management of anesthesia do not present a hazard to the patient with porphyria cutanea tarda. It is important to avoid ultraviolet light as well as excessive pressure on the skin. Consideration should be given to coexisting liver disease.

ERYTHROPIETIC UROPORPHYRIA

Signs and symptoms often involve photosensitivity, vesicular eruptions, urticaria, and edema. Cholelithiasis due to increased protoporphyrin excretion may occur. Survival to adulthood is likely. Again, the anesthetic agents that are a hazard to those patients with the inducible porphyrias do not pose a problem to patients with erythropoietic protoporphyria.

BIBLIOGRAPHY

Malignant Hyperthermia

Beebe JJ, Sessler DI: Preparation of anesthesia machines for patients susceptible to malignant hyperthermia. *Anesthesiology* 69:395–400, 1988.

Britt BA: Dantrolene. *Can Anaesth Soc J* 31:61–75, 1984.

Brownell AKW: Malignant hyperthermia: relationship to other diseases. *Br J Anaesth* 60:303–308, 1988.

Gronert GA, Schulman SR, Mott J: Malignant hyperthermia, in Miller RD (ed): *Anesthesia*, 3d ed. New York, Churchill Livingstone, pp 935–956, 1990.

Miller JD, Lee C: Muscle diseases, in Katz J, Benumof JL, Kadis LB (eds): *Anesthesia and Uncommon Diseases,* 3d ed. Philadelphia, Saunders, pp 626–636, 1990.

Rosenberg H: Clinical presentation of malignant hyperthermia. *Br J Anaesth* 60:268–273, 1988.

Rosenberg H, Fletcher JE, Seitman D: Pharmacogenetics, in Barash PG, Cullen BF, Stoelting RK (eds): *Clinical Anesthesia*. 3rd Edition Philadelphia, Lippincott, in press 1996.

Smith RJ: Preoperative assessment of risk factors. *Br J Anaesth* 60:317–319, 1988.

Plasma Cholinesterase Variants

Kalow W, Genest K: A method for the detection of atypical forms of human serum cholinesterase: determination of dibucaine numbers. *Can J Biochem Physiol* 35:339–346, 1957.

Rosenberg H, Fletcher JE, Seitman D: Pharmacogenetics, in Barash PG, Cullen BF, Stoelting RK (eds): *Clinical Anesthesia*. 3rd Edition Philadelphia, Lippincott, in press 1996.

VanBeck JO: Pseudocholinesterase pharmacology, in Faust RJ (ed): *Anesthesiology Review*. New York, Churchill Livingstone, pp 112–113, 1991.

Viby-Mogensen J: Succinylcholine neuromuscular blockade in subjects heterozygous for abnormal plasma cholinesterase. *Anesthesiology* 55:231–235, 1981.

Viby-Mogensen J: Correlation of succinylcholine duration of action with plasma cholinesterase activity in subjects with the genotypically normal enzyme. *Anesthesiology* 53:517–520, 1980.

Viby-Mogensen J: Succinylcholine neuromuscular blockade in subjects homozygous for atypical plasma cholinesterase. *Anesthesiology* 55:429–434, 1981.

Whitaker M: Plasma cholinesterase variants and the anaesthetist. *Anesthesiology* 35:174–197, 1980.

Porphyrias

Eales L: Porphyria and the dangerous life-threatening drugs. *S Afr Med J* 56:914–917, 1979.

Elder GH, Gray CH, Nicholson DC: The porphyrias: a review. *J Clin Pathol* 25:1013–1033, 1972.

Harrison GG, Meissner PN, Hift RJ: Anaesthesia for the porphyric patient. *Anesthesiology* 48:417–421, 1993.

Jackson SH, Millar WM: Genetic and metabolic diseases, in Katz J, Benumof JL, Kadis LB (eds): *Anesthesia and Uncommon Diseases,* 3d ed. Philadelphia, Saunders, pp 84–99, 1990.

Jensen NF, Fiddler DS, Striepe V: Anesthetic considerations in porphyrias. *Anesth Analg* 80:591–599, 1995.

Roizen MF: Anesthetic implications of concurrent diseases, in Miller RD (ed): *Anesthesia,* 3d ed. New York, Churchill Livingstone, pp 847–849, 1990.

Rosenberg H, Fletcher JE, Seitman D: Pharmacogenetics, in Barash PG, Cullen BF, Stoelting RK (eds): *Clinical Anesthesia.* 3rd Edition Philadelphia, Lippincott, in press 1996.

Respiratory Physiology and Pathophysiology

James Christon and Phillip Factor

This chapter presents the core elements of respiratory physiology and pathophysiology. Understanding these principles is important for prevention and treatment of perioperative pulmonary complications.

☐ STRUCTURE AND FUNCTION OF THE RESPIRATORY SYSTEM

The primary function of the lung is gas exchange between venous blood and inspired air. The anatomy and structure of the lung are ideally suited for this task.

AIRWAYS: THE TRACHEOBRONCHIAL TREE

The tracheobronchial tree begins with the trachea and divides into an estimated 23 generations of increasingly smaller airways (Fig. 9–1). The trachea divides into the right and left mainstem bronchi, which subsequently divide into lobar, segmental, and subsegmental bronchi. From subsegmental bronchi, the airways further divide into bronchioles and eventually into terminal bronchioles, which are the smallest airways without alveoli. Airways without alveoli constitute the conducting zone; this region is also referred to as anatomic dead space, since it does not take part in gas exchange. It has a volume of about 150 mL in a normal adult.

The terminal bronchioles divide into respiratory bronchioles (generations 17 through 19), which are the first airways that contain alveoli. The respiratory bronchioles give rise to alveolar ducts and finally alveolar sacs, which contain an average of 17 alveoli, each about 0.3 mm in diameter. There are approximately 150 million alveoli in each average adult lung. The area of the lung that contains alveoli, where gas exchange occurs, is referred to as the respiratory zone. The re-

spiratory zone accounts for the largest portion of total lung volume, approximately 3000 mL.

With each successive division down the tracheobronchial tree, the mucosa changes from ciliated columnar to cuboidal and finally to flat alveolar epithelial cells in the alveoli, where gas exchange occurs. The walls of the upper airway gradually lose their cartilaginous support and then their smooth muscle. Without cartilaginous or muscular support, the smaller airways are dependent on airway pressure to maintain patency.

ALVEOLI

The alveoli are the gas exchange units of the lung. Each alveolus is in close contact with a network of pulmonary capillaries. Oxygen and carbon dioxide move between air and blood by simple diffusion driven by partial-pressure gradients. According to Fick's law of diffusion, the amount of gas that moves across a sheet of tissue is proportional to the area of the sheet and inversely proportional to its thickness. The alveolar-capillary membrane is exceedingly thin, less than 0.4 mm, and extremely large, between 50 and 100 m². Because of the small size of the alveoli, alveolar surface tension is high, which promotes alveolar collapse. This problem is overcome by the production of lipoprotein complexes (surfactant) by type II pneumocytes, which lower the surface tension of the alveoli and counter their tendency to collapse.

THE CHEST AND MUSCLES OF RESPIRATION

Inspiration is initiated by the dome-shaped diaphragm, which is innervated by the phrenic nerve from cervical segments 3 through 5. Contraction of the diaphragm forces the abdominal contents downward and forward while the ribs are lifted

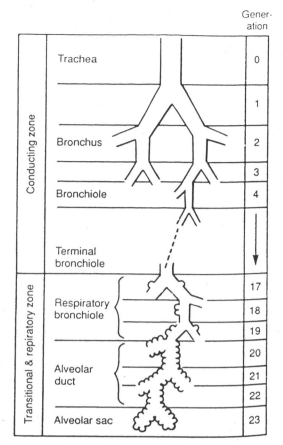

Generation

Figure 9–1   Diagrammatic representation of the human airways. Generations 1 through 16 comprise the conducting zone. Generations 17 through 23 constitute the respiratory zone. (With permission from Weibel ER: *Morphometry of the Human Lung.* Berlin, Springer-Verlag, 1963.)

up and out, increasing the volume of the chest (Fig. 9–2). The expansion of the thorax lowers intrapleural and intraalveolar pressure, generating a pressure gradient that favors movement of air into the lungs. During a normal breath, the diaphragm may descend about 1 cm, while with forced inspiration, diaphragmatic excursion can be 10 cm. The external intercostals also aid in inspiration by pulling the ribs up and out. With increasing respiratory effort, the other accessory muscles of inspiration are recruited. These muscles include the scalene muscle, which elevates the first two ribs and the sternocleidomastoid, platysma, and pectoralis muscles, which raises the sternum. The alae nasi, which flare the nostrils, also augment inspiration by maintaining upper airway patency.

When the diaphragm is paralyzed or fatigued (after prolonged tachypnea or synchronized intermittent mechanical ventilation), it may not function properly. In these settings, the diaphragm cannot mechanically fix the thorax, since the generation of negative intrathoracic pressure may cause cephalad movement of the diaphragm and inward movement of the abdomen with inspiration. This is known as paradoxical breathing, and upper thoracic and neck accessory muscles are then required to expand the chest. In contrast, patients

with hyperinflated lungs (e.g., asthma and chronic obstructive pulmonary disease) may have flat diaphragms that pull the chest inward rather than outward with inspiration (Hoover's sign).

Expiration in the absence of airway obstruction is a passive process. The lung and chest wall are elastic and return to their baseline positions to maintain pressure equilibrium. During exercise, voluntary hyperventilation, and certain disease states, expiration becomes an active process. The most important muscles for active expiration are the rectus abdominis, transverse abdominis, and internal and external oblique muscles. Contraction of these muscles pulls the sternum down and increases intraabdominal pressure, forcing the diaphragm upward. The internal intercostal muscles also may help in active expiration by pulling the ribs down and out.

PULMONARY CIRCULATION

The lungs are supplied by two arterial circulations, the pulmonary and bronchial. The pulmonary circulation receives the entire output of mixed venous blood from the right heart via the main pulmonary artery. The blood travels through the alveolar capillary bed to the pulmonary veins, which drain into the left atrium. The large cross-sectional area of the pulmonary arterial circulation results in low arterial pressures compared to the mean systemic arterial pressure (15 mmHg versus 90 mmHg). The diameter of a capillary segment is about 10 μm, which is just large enough for a red blood cell. Blood in the capillaries usually passes through two to three alveoli, which takes about three-quarters of a second, before it reaches the pulmonary venous circulation.

The bronchial circulation is systemic in nature and arises from the left heart. It supplies the metabolic needs of the tracheobronchial tree to the level of terminal and respiratory bronchioles. This blood returns to the left heart via the pulmonary venous system. The amount of blood in the bronchial circulation is small compared to that in the pulmonary circulation. Most cases of massive hemoptysis are secondary to erosion into high-pressure bronchial arteries, not pulmonary arteries. The lung can function normally without the bronchial circulation, as it does after lung transplan-

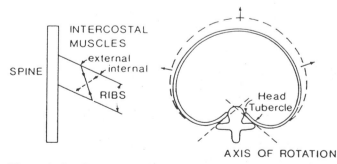

Figure 9–2   Contraction of the external intercostals pulls the ribs upward and outward, increasing intrathoracic volume. The internal intercostals pull the ribs downward and inward and facilitate forced expiration. (With permission from West JB: *Respiratory Physiology: The essentials,* 4th ed. Baltimore, Williams & Wilkins, 1990.)

tation or after therapeutic arterial embolization for massive hemoptysis.

PULMONARY LYMPHATIC SYSTEM

When fluid leaves the capillary network due to hydrostatic and oncotic pressures, it passes into the interstitium of the alveolar wall and into the perivascular and peribronchial spaces within the lung. Within these spaces the pulmonary lymphatic vessels run alongside the airways and eventually lead into the hilar lymph nodes. Lymphatic drainage channels from both lungs communicate along the trachea in the mediastinal lymph nodes. Pulmonary lymph flow is normally only a few milliliters per hour but can increase dramatically in the presence of pulmonary edema when there is engorgement of the perivascular and peribronchial interstitial spaces.

☐ VENTILATION, MECHANICS OF BREATHING, AND CONTROL OF BREATHING

VENTILATION

Tidal volume is the amount of gas exhaled during a normal breath. Tidal volume multiplied by the respiratory rate is total ventilation (or minute volume). In an average adult, tidal volume is typically 500 mL (5 to 8 mL/kg), and respiratory rate is normally 12 breaths per minute, yielding a total ventilation of 6.0 L/min. Not all of this gas participates in gas exchange; some remains in the conducting zone of the lung. This volume is referred to as the anatomic dead space; this volume multiplied by the respiratory rate gives dead space ventilation. The volume of gas that actually reaches the alveoli (respiratory zone) and is involved in gas exchange is known as alveolar gas. Alveolar gas volume multiplied by respiratory rate yields alveolar ventilation. In an average adult with a tidal volume (V_T) of 500 mL, 150 mL is dead space (V_D), giving 350 mL of alveolar gas (V_A).

Total ventilation can be measured by collecting expired gas in a bag. Alveolar ventilation is more difficult to determine unless the dead space fraction is known (see below) and can be subtracted from total ventilation. Another way to measure alveolar ventilation is to measure the carbon dioxide concentration in expired gas. Since all expired CO_2 comes from alveolar gas (and not dead space), we assume

$$V_{CO_2} = V_A \times \%CO_2/100 \tag{1}$$

$$V_A = (V_{CO_2} \times 100)/\%CO_2 \tag{2}$$

The $\%CO_2/100$ is the fractional concentration of CO_2 and is proportional to the partial pressure of CO_2. Thus,

$$V_A = (V_{CO_2}/P_{CO_2}) \times K \tag{3}$$

This equation shows that alveolar ventilation and the partial pressure of carbon dioxide are inversely related. For the P_{CO_2} to double, alveolar ventilation must be cut in half.

Anatomic Dead Space   Dead space can be measured using Fowler's single-breath nitrogen method. Following a single inspiration of 100% O_2, N_2 concentration measured during exhalation rises as the dead space gas (which should be 100% O_2) is washed out by alveolar gas, which contains N_2 from previous inhalation of air. The N_2 concentration will plateau when alveolar gas is exhaled (alveolar plateau). The dead space is found by plotting N_2 concentration against expired volume and drawing a vertical line such that areas A and B are equal. The dead space or anatomic dead space is the volume of gas expired up to the vertical line, which is the midpoint of the transition from dead space to alveolar gas.

Physiologic Dead Space   Physiologic dead space consists of both anatomic dead space and alveolar dead space (the volume of gas that does not eliminate CO_2 and is not part of the conducting airways). The Bohr method assumes that all expired CO_2 comes from alveolar gas and none from dead space. Assuming that no CO_2 is lost, the amount of CO_2 present before expiration (concentration $\times$ volume) $C_1V_A + C_2V_D$ is equal to the amount of CO_2 after expiration C_3V_T. Since the partial pressure of a gas is proportional to its concentration, we can replace C with P_{CO_2}:

$$P_{A_{CO_2}} \times V_A = P_{E_{CO_2}} \times V_T \tag{4}$$

However,

$$V_T = V_A + V_D \text{ and } V_A = V_T - V_D \tag{5}$$

Therefore,

$$P_{A_{CO_2}}(V_T - V_D) = P_{E_{CO_2}} \times V_T \tag{6}$$

$$P_{A_{CO_2}}V_T - P_{A_{CO_2}}V_D = P_{E_{CO_2}} \times V_T \tag{7}$$

$$P_{A_{CO_2}} - P_{A_{CO_2}}V_D/V_T = P_{E_{CO_2}} \tag{8}$$

$$P_{A_{CO_2}}V_D/V_T = P_{A_{CO_2}} - P_{E_{CO_2}} \tag{9}$$

$$V_D/V_T = (P_{A_{CO_2}} - P_{E_{CO_2}})/P_{A_{CO_2}} \text{ (the Bohr equation)} \tag{10}$$

In spontaneously breathing patients, normal V_D/V_T is approximately 0.33 (0.2 to 0.4). Because the Bohr equation measures the volume of the lung that does not eliminate CO_2, this volume is referred to as physiologic dead space. In disease states, anatomic dead space changes little, and thus most effects are due to increases in alveolar dead space.

MECHANICS OF BREATHING

In order for active inspiration to occur, the respiratory muscles contract to expand the lung and generate negative intraalveolar pressure. The work these muscles must perform is a reflection of the forces they must overcome to expand the lung and chest wall. These mechanical forces fall into two categories: the elastic properties of the lung and chest wall, and airway resistance.

Elastic Properties of the Chest Wall   The lung is an elastic organ that recoils inward, or collapses, when not supported. The chest wall is also an elastic structure; however, when unrestrained, it recoils outward. At the end of a passive exhalation, lung volume is determined by the balance between the tendency of the lungs to collapse and the chest wall to expand. Thus, if air enters the intrapleural space (pneumothorax) and the intrapleural pressure becomes zero, the lung collapses inward and the chest wall springs out. After a full inspiration, the inward force of the respiratory system (lung + chest wall) exceeds the outward force of the lungs, and passive expiration results.

Elastic Properties of the Lung
The Pressure-Volume Curve
If the lungs are slowly inflated and deflated, the pressure-volume curve during inflation differs from that obtained during deflation. This behavior is known as hysteresis (Fig. 9–3). The lung volume at any given pressure is larger during deflation than during inflation.

Compliance
Lung compliance ($\Delta V/\Delta P$) can be determined from the slope of a pressure-volume (PV) curve. Normal breathing occurs on the steepest portion of this curve, where compliance is the greatest (e.g., small changes in pressure produce large changes in lung volume). At higher expanding pressures, the pressure-volume curve is flattened as the elastic fibers of the lung are stretched, causing the lung to stiffen and compliance to fall. Normal compliance is about 200 mL/cm water. In restrictive disease (Fig. 9–4), the pressure-volume curve shifts to the right and the slope becomes depressed, reducing lung compliance and functional residual capacity (FRC). Because of the lower compliance, it takes a much larger change in pressure to change lung volume. In patients with restrictive diseases, such as pulmonary edema or atelectasis, continuous

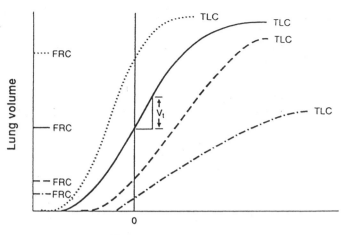

Transpulmonary pressure

Figure 9–4 The solid line is a normal pulmonary pressure-volume curve, ignoring hysteresis. Humans normally breathe on the linear, steep portion of this curve (region of greatest compliance). The vertical line at 0 transpulmonary pressure is FRC. Mild restrictive disease (dashed line) shifts the curve right with little change in slope. With restrictive disease, patients breathe at a lower FRC, at a point where the slope of the curve (i.e., compliance) is less. Severe restrictive disease significantly depresses FRC and reduces the slope of the entire curve (dashed-dotted line). Obstructive disease (dotted line) elevates both FRC and compliance. (Adapted with permission from Barash PG, Cullen BF, Stoelting RK: *Clinical Anesthesia,* Philadelphia, Lippincott, 1992.)

positive airway pressure (CPAP), or positive end-expiratory pressure (PEEP), expands collapsed alveoli, improving lung compliance and moving the pressure-volume curve to the right. In restrictive diseases due to loss of alveoli, such as pulmonary fibrosis, CPAP may worsen compliance due to overdistension of already open alveoli. In obstructive disease, the pressure-volume curve shifts to the left and the slope increases. Less elastic work is required to inspire, but elastic recoil is reduced significantly and active expiration may become necessary.

On a ventilator, compliance can easily be measured by dividing the tidal volume by the airway pressure. Dynamic compliance refers to the tidal volume divided by the peak airway pressure (minus PEEP), while static compliance refers to the tidal volume divided by the plateau pressure (minus PEEP).

Regional Differences in Ventilation
Dependent or lower regions of the lung ventilate more than upper or nondependent zones. Gravitational forces create lower intrapleural pressures in nondependent areas of the lung than in dependent areas. This difference in intrapleural pressure between the top and bottom of the lung is approximately 7 cmH₂O. At the lung base, the expanding intrapleural pressure is small and there is a small resting volume, which places this portion of the lung on a steeper portion of its regional pressure-volume curve (Fig. 9–5). Because of the improved compliance, a small change in pressure results in a large change in volume. In contrast, the apex of the lung is on a flatter portion of the pressure-volume

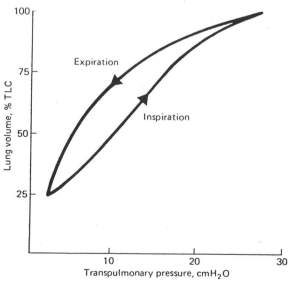

Figure 9–3 Pressure-volume curves during inflation (inspiration) and deflation (expiration) of an excised lung. Note that the inflation and deflation curves are not the same (hysteresis). (With permission from Altose MD: Pulmonary mechanics, in Fishman AP: *Pulmonary Diseases and Disorders,* 2d ed. New York, McGraw-Hill, 1988.)

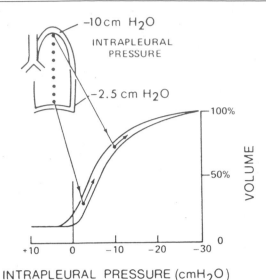

Figure 9-5 Regional differences in lung ventilation. Pleural pressure is less negative at the base; hence, it is relatively compressed at FRC but expands better than the apex with inspiration. (With permission from West JB: Ventilation, Blood Flow and Gas Exchange, 4th ed. Oxford, Blackwell, 1985.)

curve, with a lower compliance. Thus, there is preferential ventilation in the lung base compared to the apex due to regional differences in lung compliance.

It is interesting to note that at very low lung volumes (starting at residual volume), intrapleural pressure at the bases becomes positive (exceeds airway pressure). Under these conditions, the lung at the base is compressed and ventilation is impossible until the intrapleural pressure falls below atmospheric pressure. In contrast, the apex of the lung is at a favorable portion of the pressure-volume curve.

Surface Tension

The surface tension of the liquid film lining the alveoli is a very important factor in the pressure-volume behavior of the lung. Surface tension arises because intramolecular forces between adjacent molecules of a liquid are much stronger than those between the liquid and the surrounding gas. It results in a force acting to collapse the alveoli. The type II alveolar epithelial cells that line the alveoli secrete a lipoprotein material called *surfactant*, which lowers the surface tension of the alveolar lining fluid. Surfactant has several physiologic benefits for the alveoli. First, it increases compliance of the lung and reduces the work of breathing. Second, it helps prevent atelectasis of smaller airways. Third, it prevents transudation of fluid into the alveoli by preventing their collapse.

Airway Resistance   Below critical flow rates, gas flows through a tube in a streamlined fashion parallel to the sides of the tube (laminar flow). Flow rates (V) under laminar conditions can be predicted from Poiseuille's law:

$$\dot{V} = P\pi r^4/8nl \qquad (11)$$

where P is driving pressure, r is radius, n is gas viscosity, and l is tube length. Thus, if tube radius is halved, resistance in-

creases by 16-fold, whereas if tube length is doubled, resistance increases by only 2-fold.

As flow increases, unsteadiness develops, especially at branch points and turns, and departure from streamlined flow occurs as local eddies form. At still higher flow rates, complete disorganization of flow is seen (turbulent flow). The transition from laminar to turbulent flow occurs when the Reynolds number, Re = rvd/n, exceeds 2000. Thus, turbulence is most likely to occur when the flow velocity is high and the tube diameter is large. Low-density and high-viscosity gases also tend to produce less turbulence.

The chief site of airway resistance is the medium-sized bronchi (up to the seventh generation); smaller airways (bronchioles) contribute relatively little to airway resistance because of their large number and cross-sectional area. Increased airway resistance can be secondary to bronchospasm, mucosal edema, mucous plugging, or the presence of a foreign body. Lung volume also contributes to airway resistance. As lung volume is reduced, airways collapse and airway resistance rises. The normal response to increased inspiratory resistance is increased inspiratory muscle effort, with little change in FRC. Accessory muscles of inspiration are brought into play. If airway resistance increases further, the patient will attempt to breathe at higher lung volumes (increased FRC) to reduce airway resistance and improve lung compliance by moving to a more favorable portion of the pressure-volume curve.

On a ventilator, airway resistance is sometimes estimated by determining the difference between peak and plateau airway pressures. Dividing this difference by peak flow rate provides an estimate of total airway resistance. However, this value includes resistance produced by the ventilator circuit and endotracheal tube. Note that peak airway pressure is primarily a reflection of high peak flow through narrow endotracheal tubes, so calculation of airway resistance using this method is of little clinical utility in assessing airway resistance.

CONTROL OF BREATHING

Mechanisms that control ventilation are extremely complex and involve a large network, integrating many parts of the central and peripheral nervous systems. Even with profound variations in CO_2 production and O_2 demand, the respiratory system permits only small fluctuations in P_{O_2} and P_{CO_2}. Respiration is controlled by a central area in the brain stem that integrates neural traffic and results in the periodicity of inspiration and expiration. Several discrete respiratory centers within the pons and medulla control the respiratory motor neurons. The central controller receives input from various receptors throughout the body, all of which affect its output. The cortex can override these centers if voluntary control is desired.

Medullary Center: The Dorsal and Ventral Respiratory Groups   The medulla oblongata contains the most basic inspiratory and expiratory control areas of the brain. Two discrete areas have been identified: the dorsal respiratory group (DRG) and the ventral respiratory group (VRG). The DRG is probably responsible for inspiration and ventilatory rhythmicity. Even in the absence of afferent stimuli, these inspiratory cells generate repetitive contraction of the respiratory muscles. Inhibitory impulses from the pneumotaxic center in the pons (see below) can limit the activity of the DRG.

The VRG is known as the expiratory center. It is unclear whether it is active during normal breathing. Some experts believe that inspiration ceases as a consequence of VRG activity, while others believe the VRG is quiescent during normal breathing and functions only during forceful ventilation. The latter believe that expiration during normal breathing is a completely passive process and requires no neuronal input.

The Pontine Centers: The Apneustic and Pneumotaxic Centers The pontine centers process the information that originates in the medulla. When active, the apneustic center, located in the lower pons, sends impulses to the DRG inspiratory neurons to sustain inspiration. If this center is sectioned in experimental animals, apneustic ventilation (prolonged inspiratory gasps interrupted by expiratory spasms) results. It is not known whether the apneustic center plays a role in normal human respiration.

The pneumotaxic respiratory center, located in the upper pons, stops inspiration. When stimulated, tidal volumes become smaller and ventilatory frequency increases. When the center is sectioned, tidal volumes increase and ventilatory rate decreases.

Chemical Control of Ventilation
Central Chemoreceptors
The most important receptors involved in breath-to-breath control of ventilation are the central chemoreceptors located on the ventral surface of the medulla near the exit of cranial nerves 9 and 10. The chemical chemoreceptors are surrounded by cerebrospinal fluid (CSF) and are exquisitely sensitive to changes in H^+ ion concentration. The H^+ concentration of the CSF is determined by Pa_{CO_2}, which readily diffuses across the blood-brain barrier, where it is converted to carbonic acid. An increase in H^+ concentration stimulates ventilation, while a decrease inhibits it.

For H^+ ions or carbon dioxide to reach these central chemoreceptors, they must pass through the blood-brain barrier. The blood-brain barrier is relatively impermeable to H^+ ions. Thus, metabolic acidosis is not as potent a respiratory stimulus as is hypercarbia. The CSF has minimal buffering capacity, and the CSF H^+ ion concentrations are considerably higher than that found in blood (normal CSF pH = 7.32).

Peripheral Chemoreceptors
The peripheral chemoreceptors include the carotid and aortic bodies. The carotid bodies are located at the bifurcation of the common carotid arteries. They have predominantly ventilatory effects (increased respiratory rate and tidal volume). The aortic bodies are located above and below the aortic arch. They have predominantly circulatory effects (bradycardia and hypertension); their neural output travels to the central respiratory center via the vagus nerve.

Peripheral chemoreceptors rapidly respond to decreases in Pa_{O_2} (not to decreased Sa_{O_2} or Ca_{O_2}) and pH and increases in P_{CO_2}. Only the carotid bodies respond to falls in arterial pH. When PaO_2 falls below 500 mmHg (some investigators say 100 mgHg), neural activity from these receptors increases. When PaO_2 falls to 60 to 65 mmHg neural activity increases enough to substantially augment minute ventilation.

The peripheral chemoreceptors are responsible for increased ventilation associated with hypoxemia. In the absence of these receptors, there would be complete loss of hypoxic ventilatory drive. These peripheral chemoreceptors also respond to changes in Pa_{CO_2} and pH but to a much lesser degree. Only about 20% of the ventilatory response to inhaled CO_2 can be attributed to peripheral chemoreceptors.

Intrapulmonary Receptors
Pulmonary Stretch Receptors
Within the smooth muscle of all airways reside spindle receptors that respond to pressure changes within the airway. In lower-order mammals, the stimulation of these receptors inhibits respiratory activity via vagal afferents (Hering-Breuer reflex or inflation reflex), whereas deflation of the lung stimulates inspiratory activity (deflation reflex). It is unlikely that these reflexes are important in humans; however, stretch receptors probably play a role during exercise when tidal volume exceeds 1 L or when airways are distended in disease states such as pneumonia, pulmonary edema, or atelectasis.

Irritant receptors lie between airway epithelial cells and respond to various noxious inhalants, including cigarette smoke, dust, and cold air. The stimulation of these receptors results in bronchoconstriction and an increase in respiratory rate via the vagal afferents.

J receptors (juxtacapillary receptors) lie in close proximity to the capillaries near the alveolar walls. These receptors are stimulated by interstitial fluid in the alveolar interstitium and engorged capillaries. They may play a role in the increased respiratory rate seen in heart failure and acute respiratory distress syndrome (ARDS). Their afferent impulse also travels via the vagus nerve.

Multiple reflexes are present in the nose, pharynx, larynx, and trachea. Nasal occlusion may promote apnea, especially during sleep. Pharyngeal stimulation from swallowing or vomiting inhibits ventilation. Laryngeal stimulation seen during endotracheal tube placement may lead to laryngeal spasm, and stimulation of the tracheal subepithelium results in coughing.

Impulses from muscle groups are thought to stimulate ventilation during exercise. Studies in animals and humans have shown that passive movements of the limbs stimulate ventilation. The receptors for these reflexes are hypothesized to be located in joints or muscles. These neural pathways may be responsible for the reflexive increase in ventilation during the first few seconds of exercise.

Pain and high temperatures often result in hyperventilation. The increased ventilation secondary to an increase in body temperature may partially explain the increased ventilatory response to exercise.

Integrated Responses

Response to Carbon Dioxide

The most important factor in the control of ventilation under normal conditions is PCO_2 of the arterial blood (Pa_{CO_2}). The stimulus to increase or decrease ventilation (i.e., Pa_{CO_2}) derives mostly from the central chemoreceptors, which respond to increased H^+ ion concentration in the brain extracellular fluid. Approximately 20% of the response to Pa_{CO_2} comes from the peripheral chemoreceptors. The response to changes in Pa_{CO_2} on minute ventilation can be seen in Fig. 9–6 and is referred to as the CO_2 ventilatory response curve. This curve is linear when Pa_{CO_2} is 20 to 80 mmHg, which is most often encountered under normal physiologic conditions. Once the Pa_{CO_2} exceeds 80 mmHg, ventilatory response becomes parabolic, and peak ventilatory response occurs when P_aCO_2 approaches 100 mmHg. Several studies now suggest that, independent of changes in PaO_2 and pH, Pa_{CO_2} does not act as a central nervous system depressant; as such, true CO_2 narcosis may not exist.

The ventilatory response curve is affected by various factors, including PaO_2. When PaO_2 is lowered, ventilation for a given Pa_{CO_2} increases, and the slope becomes steeper (Fig. 9–6). Raising Pa_{O_2} to supranormal levels has little effect on the Pa_{CO_2} curve in normal subjects. The ventilatory response to Pa_{CO_2} is reduced with sleep, increasing age, and central nervous system depressants. Opioids and barbiturates

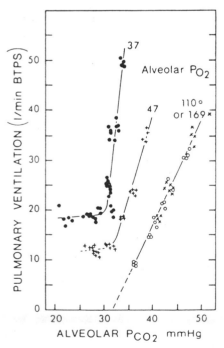

Figure 9–6   Total ventilatory response to changes in PA_{CO_2} varies with Po_2. (With permission from Nielson M, Smith H: *Acta Physiol Scand* 24:293, 1951.)

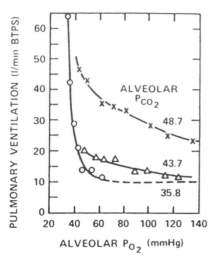

Figure 9–7   Hypoxic response is dependent on P_{CO_2}. Minute ventilation increases to a greater degree for a given P_{CO_2} as the P_{CO_2} increases. (With permission from Loeschke HH, Gertz KH: *Arch Ges Physiol* 267:460, 1958.)

move the CO_2 response curve to the right; low doses cause little change in the slope, whereas large doses depress the slope. Inhaled anesthetic agents also displace the curve to the right and lower the slope. The ventilatory response to Pa_{CO_2} may also be reduced if the work of breathing is increased, as in asthma. Although the neural output from the central and peripheral chemoreceptors are the same, they are not as effective in producing ventilation. The ventilatory response curve to Pa_{CO_2} is enhanced by metabolic acidosis, cirrhosis, anxiety, and various drugs, including aminophylline, salicylates, and norepinephrine. Genetics, race, and personality factors also affect the ventilatory response curve.

Response to Oxygen

Studying the ventilatory response to O_2 is difficult due to large variation between individuals. Ventilatory response to oxygen also varies with Pa_{CO_2} (Fig. 9–7). The role of hypoxic stimulation in minute-by-minute ventilatory control in normal subjects is probably minimal, since the Pa_{O_2} rarely falls below 50 mmHg. However, if the Pa_{CO_2} is elevated, the ventilatory response at any Pa_{O_2} increases. When Pa_{CO_2} is brought to 44 or 49 mmHg, even a Pa_{O_2} below 100 mmHg stimulates ventilation. The combined effects of both stimuli (Pa_{CO_2} and Pa_{O_2}) is greater than the sum of the individual effects.

In some patients with chronic hypercapnic respiratory failure, the hypoxic drive to breath is more important. In these patients, chronically elevated CO_2 levels are compensated for by renal mechanisms, CSF pH is near normal, and consequently there is a much diminished response to Pa_{CO_2}. It is postulated that these patients depend more on Pa_{O_2} for control of ventilation. However, in studies of patients with hypoxemia due to chronic obstructive pulmonary disease (COPD), this is rarely the case. Measures of central respiratory drive, based on the $P_{0.1}$, are high in these patients. Administration of O_2 to these patients results in insignificant reductions in central drive and minimal changes in Pa_{CO_2} (primarily due to alterations in V/Q relationships). Most patients with severe COPD die of hypoxemia, not hypercarbia, which is usually well-tolerated. Thus, maintenance of adequate arterial saturation must be the first aim of therapy in these patients.

Reductions in arterial pH stimulate ventilation, producing hypocapnia and compensatory respiratory alkalosis. This response is most likely due to stimulation of the peripheral chemoreceptors, since the blood-brain barrier is relatively impermeable to H^+ ions.

BLOOD FLOW, VENTILATION-PERFUSION RELATIONSHIPS, AND BLOOD-GAS TRANSPORT

PULMONARY BLOOD FLOW

The Volume of blood passing through the lungs each minute ($\dot{Q}$-pulmonary blood flow) can be calculated using the Fick principle. The Fick principle states that O_2 consumption per minute (V_{O_2}) is equal to the amount of O_2 taken up by the blood in the lungs per minute, or

$$\dot{Q} \times (A - V)_{O_2} \text{ content difference} \qquad (12)$$

Since pulmonary venous O_2 content cannot be readily measured, systemic arterial O_2 content (Ca_{O_2}) is used to estimate the $(A - V)_{O_2}$ content difference, provided a mixed venous measurement is available to calculate venous O_2 content (Cv_{O_2}). Thus,

$$\dot{Q} = \dot{V}_{O_2}/(C_aO_2 - C_vO_2) \qquad (13)$$

$\dot{V}_{O_2}$ can be measured directly by collecting the expired gas in a large spirometer and measuring its O_2 concentration. C_aO_2 and C_vO_2 can be calculated from arterial and mixed venous blood gasses [content $= 1.34 \times$ hemoglobin (gm) $\times$ measured O_2 saturation/100].

Distribution of Blood Flow Blood flow is partly gravity-dependent, and considerable inequality of pulmonary blood flow exists within the lung. To observe this difference, we can inject radioactive xenon dissolved in saline solution into a peripheral vein. When it reaches the pulmonary capillaries, it diffuses into alveoli because of its low blood solubility, and its distribution can be measured. In an upright lung, pulmonary blood flow increases linearly from top to bottom (Fig. 9–8). The uneven distribution of blood flow can be explained by the hydrostatic pressure differences. Like ventilation (see above), blood flow is position-dependent. In the supine position, the distribution of blood flow from apex to base becomes uniform, and blood flow in the dependent posterior regions of the lung is greater than in the anterior regions. As cardiac output increases (e.g., during exercise), blood flow increases throughout and regional differences are minimized.

Based on these varying regional blood flows, West created a lung model that divides the lung into three zones (Fig. 9–9). In zone I, pulmonary artery pressure is less than alveolar pressure, preventing blood flow through alveoli in this region (PA > Pa > Pv) and producing alveolar dead space. This is unlikely to occur under normal conditions because, even in the apices of the lung, pulmonary artery pressure is greater than alveolar pressure. Clinically, zone I may become prominent when alveolar pressure is raised, such as during positive-pressure ventilation or when arterial pressure is reduced, such as in hypovolemic shock. In zone II, pulmonary arterial pressure increases because of the hydrostatic effect and now exceeds alveolar pressure; thus, flow will vary with respiratory swings in alveolar pressure (Pa > PA > Pv). Zone II has well-matched ventilation and perfusion and contains the majority of alveoli. In zone III (Pa > Pv > PA), venous pressure always exceeds alveolar pressure, and blood flow is independent of alveolar pressure. Zone III is found in dependent areas of the lung. In zone III, capillary perfusion is present in excess of ventilation and can contribute to physiologic shunt. The amount of zone III lung increases as pulmonary arterial and venous pressures rise as with congestive heart failure.

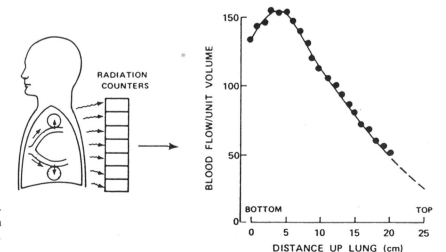

Figure 9–8 Distribution of blood flow in the upright human lung. (Adapted with permission from West JB: *Respiratory Physiology: The Essentials,* 4th ed. Baltimore, Williams & Wilkins, 1990.)

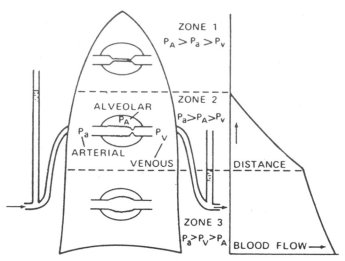

Figure 9–9 West's zones of the lung. P_a = pulmonary arterial pressure; P_A = alveolar presure; P_V = pulmonary venous pressure. (With permission from West JB: *J Appl Physiol* 19:713, 1964.)

VENTILATION-PERFUSION RELATIONSHIPS

The relationship between ventilation and blood flow determines gas exchange. Not all areas of the lung are perfectly matched with respect to ventilation and perfusion. Thus, there are varying ventilation-perfusion (V/Q) ratios throughout the lung. This mismatching of ventilation and blood flow is responsible for most abnormalities of gas exchange in pulmonary disease. The ideal V/Q ratio is 1, and it is thought to occur at the level of the third rib. Above this level the V/Q ratio rises, while below it the V/Q ratio drops.

If a region of lung is ventilated but not perfused (Q = 0), its V/Q ratio approximates infinity. This is physiologic dead space ventilation (see above). Physiologic dead space primarily affects CO_2 elimination. Clinically, CO_2 retention is unlikely if central and peripheral chemoreceptors are functioning to increase ventilation and decrease CO_2. This mechanism explains why patients with a pulmonary embolus rarely have hypercapnia; however, if a patient with a pulmonary embolus is paralyzed on a ventilator and is unable to increase minute ventilation, hypercapnia may develop.

Physiologic Shunt If an area of lung is perfused but not ventilated (V = 0), its V/Q ratio is 0. This phenomenon is referred to as shunt, since the blood is shunted from the pulmonary arterial system to the pulmonary venous system (and systemic circulation) without going through ventilated areas of lung. Some shunt is present in normal individuals; bronchial artery blood is collected by the pulmonary veins, and coronary venous blood drains into the left ventricle (approximately 2 to 5% of total cardiac output). Anatomic shunts of greater magnitude are seen in congenital heart diseases with right-to-left shunting. Arteriovenous malformation seen in certain disease states, including cirrhosis, may also lead to anatomic shunt. The end result of shunt is that poorly

oxygenated blood enters the arterial circulation and lowers arterial O_2 content.

Shunt can be calculated by realizing that the total amount of O_2 carried in the arterial blood equals the sum of O_2 carried in capillary blood and O_2 carried in shunted blood. Using the Fick equation, we have

$$Q_T \times Ca_{O_2} = (Q_S \times Cv_{O_2}) + C_{CO_2}(Q_T - Q_S) \qquad (14)$$

Rearranging and solving gives us

$$Q_S/Q_T = (C_{CO_2} - Ca_{O_2})/(C_{CO_2} - Cv_{O_2}) \qquad (15)$$

where C_{CO_2} is pulmonary capillary O_2 content and Cv_{O_2} is mixed venous O_2 content. Oxygen content is equal to $1.34 \times Sa_{O_2}/100 \times$ hemoglobin (gm). Because hemoglobin concentration is uniform throughout the vascular system, O_2 content in the shunt equation is determined by O_2 saturation. Assuming that end-capillary O_2 saturation is 100% and substituting O_2 saturation for O_2 content, we have

$$Q_S/Q_T = (1 - Sa_{O_2})/(1 - Sv_{O_2}) \qquad (16)$$

This equation reveals that for a given $\dot{V}_{O_2}$ if mixed venous saturation (Sv_{O_2}) is low, shunt is low. If mixed venous saturation increases, then the amount of shunt has increased. Q_S/Q_T measures the shunt fraction. In actuality, there are areas of absolute shunt and areas of "partial" shunt, or V/Q mismatch. Mismatch occurs when alveolar ventilation is deficient in relation to perfusion (V/Q ratio close to 0). Although ventilation to these alveoli is deficient, it is not absent. When supplemental O_2 is given to these patients, Pa_{O_2} increases. This partial shunt, or V/Q inequality, can be seen in pulmonary edema, atelectasis, or COPD. Sometimes patients with V/Q mismatch or partial shunt are not hypoxemic. If there is a fall in mixed venous O_2 saturation from either a drop in O_2 delivery or an increase in O_2 consumption, there will be a concomitant drop in Pa_{O_2} for the same degree of V/Q inequality.

Regional Gas Exchange in the Lung Both ventilation and perfusion increase as we move from the apex down to the base of the lung. Since blood flow increases more than ventilation, the V/Q ratio decreases toward the base of the lung (Fig. 9–10). The ideal V/Q ratio of 1 is seen at about the level of the third rib in the upright lung.

Hypoxic Vasoconstriction and Low-Blood-Flow Bronchiolar Constriction Hypoxic vasoconstriction is a built-in mechanism whereby the lung diminishes areas with abnormally low V/Q ratios or physiologic shunt. When the PA_{O_2} is reduced, smooth muscle in the walls of small arterioles and capillaries constricts, limiting blood flow to the downstream hypoxic region. Marked vasoconstriction does not occur until PA_{O_2} falls to about 70 mmHg. Vasoconstriction redirects blood flow away from the hypoxic regions of the lung. As a corollary to hypoxic vasoconstriction, decreased regional pulmonary blood flow results in bronchiolar constriction, which limits ventilation to these regions.

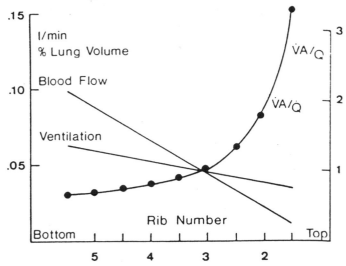

Figure 9–10   Distribution of ventilation and blood flow in the up-right lung. (With permission from West JB: *Ventilation, Blood Flow and Gas Exchange,* 4th ed. Oxford, Blackwell, 1985.)

OXYGEN TRANSPORT

The P_{O_2} falls as gas moves from the atmosphere to the tissues (Fig. 9–11). Air contains approximately 21% O_2, assuming normal barometric pressure (760 mmHg), and body-temperature, inspired $P_{O_2} = 150$ mmHg, [$0.21 \times (760 - 47$ mmHg water vapor pressure)]. The uptake of O_2 at the alveolar-capillary membrane produces an average PA_{O_2} of approximately 100 mmHg. Since complete equilibrium between capillary and alveolus is never reached, capillary P_{O_2} is slightly lower than PA_{O_2}. The Pa_{O_2} is lower than end-capillary P_{O_2} because of normal physiologic shunt and V/Q mismatch.

The gradient between alveolus and alveolar capillary (the A-a gradient) can be calculated from the alveolar gas equation:

$$PA_{O_2} = PI_{O_2} - (Pa_{CO_2}/R) + F \qquad (17)$$

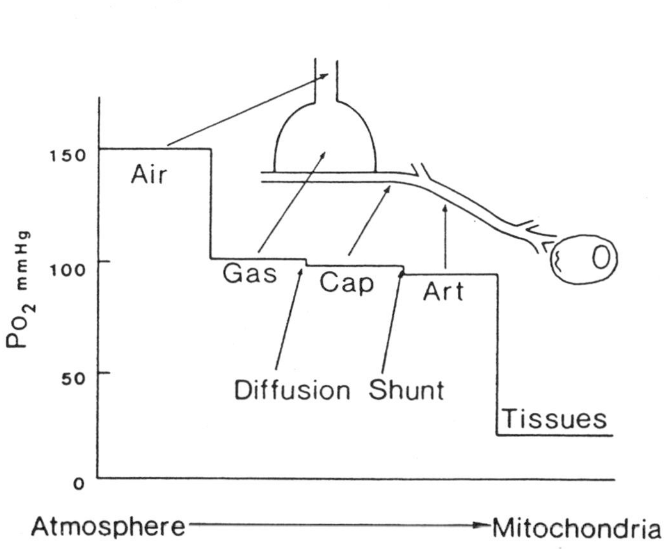

where PA_{O_2} is the alveolar P_{O_2}, PI_{O_2} is the inspired P_{O_2} [$PI_{O_2} = (P_B - P_{WV}) \times FI_{O_2}$)], Pa_{CO_2} is the alveolar or arterial P_{CO_2}, R is the respiratory quotient (V_{CO_2}/V_{O_2}, normally 0.8), and F is a small correction factor that is dependent on the dead space fraction. The normal Aa_{O_2} gradient increases with age but is generally < 20 [or (50 + age)/4] for patients breathing room air. The Aa_{O_2} gradient is a general estimate of V/Q inequality. If the Aa_{O_2} gradient is normal and the patient is hypoxemic, the cause is either alveolar hypoventilation or low fraction of inspired oxygen (FI_{O_2}). All other causes of hypoxemia—shunt, V/Q mismatch, and diffusion impairment—are associated with an elevated Aa_{O_2} gradient. This equation is of particular use for patients breathing room air.

Oxygen Dissociation Curve   Oxygen is carried in the blood in two forms: dissolved and bound to hemoglobin. The amount of dissolved O_2 is proportional to the partial pressure. Under normal conditions, dissolved O_2 is of minimal significance. For each mmHg of P_{O_2} there is 0.003 mL O_2/100 mL blood. If P_{O_2} is 100 mmHg, there is only 0.3 mL O_2/100 mL. Oxygen is most efficiently transported in the blood bound to hemoglobin. Heme is an iron porphyrin compound that is joined to globin. Oxygen forms an easily reversible combination with hemoglobin to give oxyhemoglobin.

Figure 9–12 shows what is known as the O_2 dissociation curve. The curved shape of the O_2 dissociation curve has several teleologic advantages over the linear dissolved O_2 graph. First, the steep portion of the curve, from a P_{O_2} of 20 to 60 mmHg, is where the peripheral tissues remove O_2. A small drop in P_{O_2} results in a large drop in O_2 saturation, allowing peripheral tissues to extract a large fraction of bound O_2. The flat portion of the curve, from a P_{O_2} of 60 to 600 mmHg, in-

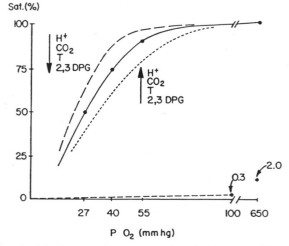

Figure 9–12   Hemoglobin oxygen dissociation curve. The effects of increasing and decreasing concentrations of hydrogen ion (H^+), carbon dioxide, and temperature on oxygen saturation are depicted by the dashed and dotted lines, respectively. (Adapted with permission from Wood LDH: The respiratory system, in Hall JB, Schmidt GA, Wood LDH (eds): *Principles of Critical Care.* New York, McGraw-Hill, 1992.)

Figure 9–11   Depiction of the reduction of P_{O_2} from air through the lung to the tissues. (With permission from West JB: *Ventilation, Blood Flow and Gas Exchange,* 4th ed. Oxford, Blackwell, 1985.)

dicates that a small drop in alveolar P_{O_2} will result in little change in O_2 saturation, which will have little impact on peripheral O_2 delivery. The flat portion of the curve also shows that there will be a large partial pressure difference between alveoli and capillaries, resulting in enhanced diffusion. If diffusion occurred along the steep portion of the curve, incomplete diffusion would result in significant decrease in O_2 uptake in the alveolar capillaries.

The O_2 dissociation curve is shifted to the right by increases in H^+ concentration, P_{CO_2}, temperature, and 2,3-diphosphoglycerate (2,3 = DPG) in the red blood cells. When the curve is shifted to the right, much more oxygen will be unloaded to the tissues. An increase in 2,3-DPG, which is an end-product of red blood cell metabolism, occurs in chronic hypoxia.

The amount of O_2 in the blood is referred to as O_2 content (Ca_{O_2}) and can be calculated from the formula

$$1.34 \times \text{hemoglobin} \times \text{saturation}/100 + 0.003 \times P_{O_2} \quad (18)$$

Since the amount of dissolved O_2 ($0.003 \times P_{O_2}$) is usually minimal (except under hyperbaric conditions), it is usually disregarded. The factor 1.34 comes from the fact that 1 g of pure hemoglobin can combine with 1.34 mL of O_2. Oxygen delivery is simply the O_2 content multiplied by the cardiac output (Q).

Carbon Dioxide Dissociation Curve   The nearly linear relationship between P_{CO_2} and CO_2 concentration is seen in Fig. 9–13. The lower the hemoglobin saturation, the higher the CO_2 concentration for a given P_{CO_2}. Reduced hemoglobin (deoxygenated) is less acidic and therefore facilitates loading of CO_2; in other words, deoxygenated blood carries more CO_2. This is known as the Haldane effect. Conversely, the oxygenation of hemoglobin in the pulmonary capillaries aids unloading of CO_2.

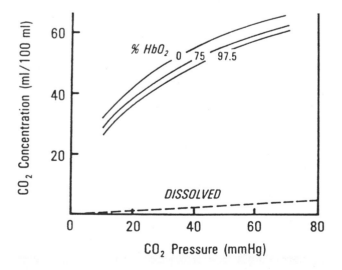

Figure 9–13   Carbon dioxide dissociation curves for various oxygen saturations. (With permission from West JB: *Respiratory Physiology: The Essentials,* 4th ed. Baltimore, Williams & Wilkins, 1990.)

☐ TESTS OF PULMONARY FUNCTION

An important and practical application of respiratory physiology is the testing of pulmonary function. Pulmonary function tests can aid the clinician in a variety of ways: as a diagnostic tool for patients with suspected lung disease, in the management of patients with known lung disease, for the assessment of preoperative risk, and for evaluation of disability. Pulmonary function tests cannot diagnose a disease and do not replace clinical assessment.

STATIC LUNG VOLUMES

In the mid-nineteenth century, Hutchison described a water spirometer to measure pulmonary function and used it to help complement his physical examination. A spirometer measures the volume of inhaled and exhaled gas (Fig. 9–13). Tidal volume is the amount of gas in a normal inspiration, and vital capacity is the maximal volume of gas that can be expelled from the lungs following a maximal inspiration. Functional residual capacity (FRC), residual volume (RV), and total lung capacity (TLC) cannot be measured with a spirometer (see below). The FRC is the amount of gas in the lungs at the end of a normal expiration. The RV is the amount of gas remaining in the lung following maximal exhalation, and TLC is the amount of gas contained in the lung at maximal inspiration.

The FRC, RV, and TLC can be measured by one of two methods: the gas dilution technique and body plethysmography. In the gas dilution technique (Fig. 9–14), the subject breathes a known concentration of helium or other inert gas. Helium is insoluble in blood; thus, after several breaths (to allow equilibration) the concentration of helium can be measured. The degree of dilution is then used to calculate FRC. One drawback of the gas dilution technique is that it measures only the volume of the lung that readily communicates with the airways. In patients with obstructive lung disease or bullae that do not communicate with the airways, the gas dilution technique may underestimate lung volume. A body plethysmograph (or body box) is a large, airtight box in which the subject sits and breathes through a mouthpiece. At the end of a normal expiration, a shutter occludes the mouthpiece, and the subject is asked to make respiratory efforts against this closed mouthpiece. As the subject tries to inhale, he or she expands the gas in the lungs; as lung and chest volume increase, the box pressure rises. Since the box volume is fixed, lung volume can be calculated based on the pressure changes in the box before and after the inspiratory effort using Boyle's law ($P_1V_1 = P_2V_2$). The body plethysmograph measures the total volume of gas in the lung, including any gas that is trapped behind obstructed airways.

In restrictive lung diseases, lung volumes are reduced because of limited lung expansion due to alterations in the lung parenchyma, the pleura, or the chest wall, or to neuromuscular disease. Some causes of a restrictive ventilatory defect are listed in Table 9–1. Restrictive ventilatory defects have been further subdivided by some experts into concentric or non-

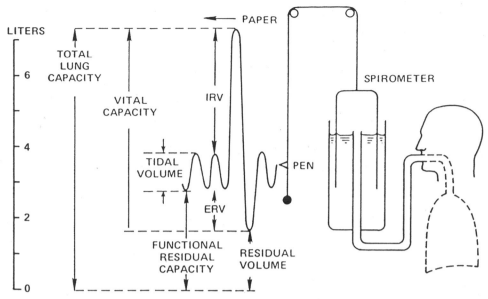

Figure 9–14 Lung volumes and capacities. Note that residual volume cannot be measured with a spirometer. IRV = inspiratory reserve volume; ERV = expiratory reserve volume. (With permission from West JB: Ventilation, blood flow, and gas exchange, in Murray JF, Nadel JA (eds): *Textbook of Respiratory Medicine.* Philadelphia, Saunders, 1994.)

concentric defects. In obstructive lung diseases such as emphysema, the TLC, FRC, and RV are often increased, indicating hyperinflation due to air trapping behind closed airways due to loss of lung elastic recoil. Typically, lung volumes greater than 120% of predicted volume for gender, age, and size are considered hyperinflated.

CLOSING CAPACITY

Closing capacity is a sensitive indicator of early small airways disease and measures the volume at which airways begin to close in dependent portions of the lung. To perform this test, the patient first exhales to residual volume and then, at the beginning of a full inspiration, a bolus of tracer gas (xenon or helium) is injected into the inspired gas. During the initial part of this inhalation from residual volume, the first gas to enter the alveolus is the dead space gas and the tracer bolus; this initial gas enters alveoli already open, presumably in the apices, where compliance is more favorable

and does not enter the bases. As inspiration continues, apical alveoli continue to fill, and then the bases begin to open and fill with gas that does not contain the tracer gas (which has been taken up by apical regions of the lung). When the subject is asked to exhale and the tracer gas is measured, a point is reached where the basilar airways close near end expiration and there is a sudden increase in exhaled tracer gas. The volume of gas remaining in the lung at this point is referred to as the closing capacity. The closing capacity is normally well below FRC but rises with age, obesity, smoking, and supine position. The closing volume refers to the difference between the volume at which the airways close and residual volume (Fig. 9–15). In healthy young patients, the closing volume (CV) is approximately 30% of TLC, whereas FRC is approximately 50% of TLC. Thus, normal tidal ventilation occurs at lung volumes above CV. In a patient whose FRC is low and whose CV is high, atelectasis and arterial hypoxemia result from poor ventilation in areas that are well-perfused. This mechanism is the pathophysiologic basis for postoperative respiratory failure in patients with thoracic and upper abdominal surgery.

FORCED EXPIRATION

Static lung volume measurements provide important physiologic data, but even more useful information can be obtained from dynamic tests of pulmonary function. Total exhaled volume is the forced vital capacity (FVC). The volume exhaled in the first 1 s is referred to as the forced expiratory volume (FEV_1). Figure 9–16 shows a normal tracing. The volume exhaled in 1 s (FEV_1) is 4.0 L, and the total volume exhaled (FVC) is 5.0 L, giving a ratio FEV_1/FVC of 0.80, or 80%. The ratio of FEV_1/FVC has been precisely defined in

Table 9–1
ETIOLOGIES OF RESTRICTIVE VENTILATORY DEFECTS

Interstitial lung disease (idiopathic pulmonary fibrosis, sarcoid, and asbestosis)
Chest wall abnormalities (kyphoscoliosis)
Neuromuscular diseases (amyotrophic lateral sclerosis and muscular dystrophy)
Extrathoracic conditions (obesity and circumferential burns)
Pleural disease (mesothelioma)
Decreased lung compliance (pulmonary edema)

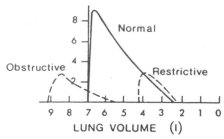

Figure 9–15 Normal, obstructive, and restrictive expiratory loops. (With permission from West JB: *Respiratory Physiology: The Essentials,* 4th ed. Baltimore, Williams & Wilkins, 1990.)

healthy adults and is an important physiologic parameter. This ratio declines with age, varies slightly with gender, and is low in patients with obstructive disease.

In disease states, two general patterns can be distinguished. Figure 9–16 shows measurements of FEV_1 and FVC in a normal patient and in patients with obstructive lung and restrictive lung diseases. In obstructive lung disease, such as asthma or emphysema, the flow of exhaled air is limited by the collapse of small airways, and expiratory time is prolonged. Although FEV_1, FVC, and FEV_1/FVC are all reduced, the FEV_1/FVC has been determined to be the most sensitive marker of obstructive disease. If the FEV_1/FVC is less than 0.80, there is likely to be an obstructive ventilatory defect. If the FEV_1/FVC is less than 0.50 or the FEV_1 is less than 1.0 L, the defect is considered severe.

Figure 9–16 also includes a tracing from a patient with a restrictive lung disease such as pulmonary fibrosis. Here, both FEV_1 and FVC are reduced proportionally, and as such the FEV_1/FVC is normal or increased. These findings are indicative of a restrictive ventilatory defect, which would be confirmed by low lung volumes (TLC, FRC, and RV).

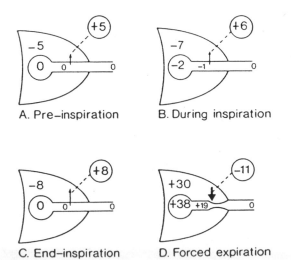

Figure 9–16 Forced expiration is associated with increased pleural pressure which contributes to airway collapse. The resistance distal to the point of collapse determines flow rate. (With permission from West JB: *Respiratory Physiology: The Essentials.* Baltimore, Williams & Wilkins, 1990.)

THE FLOW-VOLUME CURVE

A very useful way of looking at forced expiration is the flow-volume curve. By recording flow rates and volume during maximal inspiration and maximal forced expiration, a flow-volume curve is obtained. Flow rises very rapidly to a high value and then declines linearly over most of expiration. The initial portion of the curve depends on effort. Shortly after development of peak flow, the curve follows a remarkably reproducible path as flow diminishes until RV is reached. At mid- or low volumes, expiratory flow plateaus and cannot be further reduced despite further increases in intrapleural pressure. Flow in this portion of the curve is effort-independent and is due to distal airway collapse. Because the airways collapse, increasing muscular effort cannot increase driving pressure or flow (Fig. 9–17).

When airways collapse during forced expiration, flow rate is determined by the resistance of the airways distal to the point of collapse. Collapse occurs at the point where the pressure inside the airways is equal to interpleural pressure; this is called the equal pressure point, which is in the vicinity of the lobar bronchi early in a forced expiration. As lung volume falls and airways narrow, resistance increases. As a result, pressure is lost more rapidly and the collapse point moves into more distal airways. Thus, late in a forced expiration, flow is principally determined by the properties of small peripheral airways. Figure 9–17 shows the forces acting across an airway within the lung during forced expiration accompanied by their respective flow volume curve. In A, alveolar pressure, which starts at +38 cmH_2O, continues to drop along the airway after flow begins. Eventually, intrapleural pressure rises above alveolar pressure and the airway collapses (the equal pressure point). Once this point is reached, flow becomes effort-independent.

In obstructive lung diseases, TLC is often increased due to hyperinflation and expiration ends early, resulting in an elevated RV. In addition, flow rates are much lower and the curve has a "scooped-out" appearance. This low flow rate in obstructive lung disease is caused by several factors, including airways collapse from acute bronchospasm or from destruction of normal supporting parenchyma; thickened airway walls; increased secretions in the airways; destruction of small airways, including alveoli, by disease process; and reduced static recoil pressure due to destruction of elastic alveolar walls. Patients with obstructive lung disease have lower expiratory flow rates, lower total expiratory volumes, and prolonged expiratory times due to small airways collapse.

In patients with restrictive lung diseases, TLC is reduced, and thus expiration ends in a low lung volume, resulting in a low FRC. Although the maximal flow rate is much lower than normal, if the flow rate is measured in correlation with lung volumes, the flow is greater than normal, especially during the latter part of expiration. This higher flow rate can be explained by the increased lung recoil in patients with restrictive lung diseases. The low lung volumes are due to loss of lung parenchyma and increased lung stiffness, which limits lung expansion.

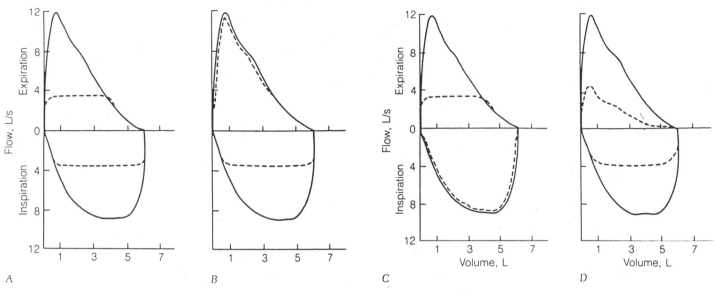

Figure 9–17 Upper airway obstruction. *(A)* Fixed upper airway obstruction. *(B)* Variable extrathoracic obstruction. *(C)* Variable intrathoracic obstruction. *(D)* Chronic obstructive airways disease; note the absence of the plateau seen with variable intrathoracic obstruction. Solid lines denote normal inspiratory and expiratory flow patterns. Note that in all cases peak inspiratory and expiratory flows are reduced. (With permission from Grippi MA, Metzger LF, Krupinski AV, Fishman AP: Pulmonary function testing, in Fishman AP: *Pulmonary Diseases and Disorders,* 2d ed. New York, McGraw-Hill, 1988.)

INSPIRATORY FLOW-VOLUME CURVE

The inspiratory flow-volume curve is useful in detecting airway obstruction outside the thorax (upper airway). A flattening of the inspiratory limb in combination with low inspiratory flows (typically <2 L/min) suggests the presence of a variable extrathoracic upper airway obstruction. This obstruction occurs due to diminution of extrathoracic upper airway caliber due to reduced intraairway pressures during inspiration. The intrathoracic upper airway widens with the negative intrapleural pressures associated with inspiration and narrows with the positive pressures of expiration. Figure 9–17 includes a flow-volume curve of a patient with a variable intrathoracic upper airway obstruction. Instead of the usual rise in expiratory flow rate, there is reduced flow and an expiratory plateau with forced expiration. In contrast, the flow-volume curve from a patient with a variable extrathoracic large airway obstruction typically reveals flattening of the inspiratory limb. Patients with fixed large airway obstructions will demonstrate low flows (typically <2 L/min) with inspiratory and expiratory plateaus.

PEAK EXPIRATORY FLOW RATE

Expiratory flow reaches a transient peak early in the forced expiration maneuver; this is referred to as the peak expiratory flow rate or peak flow. Peak flows can be measured easily with a small, inexpensive device, which makes it ideal for monitoring flows on an ambulatory basis in patients with known chronic lung disease. Measurements of peak flows are becoming routine in emergency rooms and hospital wards as well as on an outpatient basis as a convenient quantitative measure of airway obstruction. Unfortunately, peak flow is effort-dependent and correlates poorly with more objective measures of airflow obstruction, such as FEV_1, that gauge obstruction from the effort-independent portion of the flow-volume curve (see above). Peak flow quantitation is of little clinical benefit unless excellent cooperation can be obtained from the patient, which is unlikely when a patient is dyspneic or has limited communication skills.

MAXIMAL VOLUME VENTILATION

Maximal volume ventilation (MVV) is the maximal volume of air that can be moved by voluntary effort in 1 min. Subjects are asked to breathe rapidly and deeply for 30 s. The maximal volume exhaled over any 15 s is adjusted to liters per minute. The MVV is decreased in patients with airway obstruction and in patients with mild or moderate restrictive defects who are able to compensate for low lung volumes with rapid, shallow breathing. The MVV is also useful in identifying upper airway obstruction, since results of spirometric measurements may be normal but MVV low. The MVV also provides a measure of respiratory muscle endurance, which is useful in diagnosing neuromuscular disease. It is also of prognostic value in preoperative evaluation of patients likely to develop postoperative respiratory failure. In general, the MVV should be 35 to 40 times the FEV_1.

DIFFUSION CAPACITY

Diffusion is the process by which a gas moves across the blood-gas barrier from the alveoli to the capillary. Carbon monoxide (CO) readily crosses the alveoli, and it has a high affinity for hemoglobin, which prevents back-diffusion of

CO into the alveoli. Thus, the uptake of CO provides a ready estimate of the diffusion capacity of the lung. Reductions in the diffusion capacity of CO (D_LCO) suggest the diagnosis of an impaired surface area for the transfer of gases from the alveoli to the pulmonary capillaries. Diffusion capacity is reduced by diseases that increase the thickness of the blood-gas interface, such as in pulmonary fibrosis, or destroy the alveolar capillary, such as emphysema. Conditions associated with increased blood in the lung (e.g., congestive heart failure and pulmonary hemorrhage syndromes) demonstrate increased D_LCO. Diffusion depends not only on the properties of the blood-gas barrier but also on the alveolar volume, capillary blood flow, and concentration of hemoglobin. Diffusion capacity results, then, need to be corrected for lung volume and anemia before any interpretations can be made.

RESPONSE TO BRONCHODILATORS

The response to bronchodilators is often measured in pulmonary function laboratories by performing spirometric tests before and after administration of β agonists. Most experts require a > 15% increase in FEV_1 and an absolute increase in FEV_1 of > 200 mL to suggest a response to inhaled bronchodilators. Although a significant bronchodilator response documents reversibility, the absence of a response does not exclude reversible obstructive lung disease and does not mean that bronchodilators should not be used.

BIBLIOGRAPHY

Barash PG, Cullen BF, Stoelting RK: *Clinical Anesthesia.* Philadelphia, Lippincott, 1992.

Berger AJ, Mitchell RA, Severinghaus JW: Regulation of respiration. *N Engl J Med* 297:92, 138, 194, 1977.

Brown BJ. Asthma and irreversible airflow obstruction. *Thorax* 39:131, 1984.

Burrows B: An overview of obstructive lung diseases. *Med Clin North Am* 65:455, 1981.

CIBA Guest Symposium: Terminology, definitions, and classification of chronic pulmonary emphysema and related conditions. *Thorax* 14:286, 1959.

Crapo RO, Forster RE: Carbon monoxide diffusing capacity. *Clin Chest Med* 10:187, 1989.

Crapo RO, Morris AH, Gardner RM: Reference spirometric values using techniques and equipment that meet ATS recommendations. *Am Rev Respir Dis* 123:659, 1981.

Dantzker DR: Ventilation-perfusion distributions in the adult respiratory distress syndrome. *Am Rev Respir Dis* 120:1039, 1979.

Gardner RM (chairman): ATS statement on standardization of spirometry. *Am Rev Respir Dis* 119:831, 1979.

Gass GD: Preoperative pulmonary function testing to predict postoperative morbidity and mortality. *Chest* 89:127, 1986.

Guz A: Regulation of respiration in man. *Ann Respir Physiol* 37:303, 1975.

Houston JC: A clinical and pathologic study of fatal cases of status asthmaticus. *Thorax* 8:207, 1953.

Huber HL, Koessler KK: The pathology of bronchial asthma. *Arch Intern* Med 30:689, 1922.

Jackson M: Preoperative pulmonary evaluation. *Arch Intern Med* 148:2120, 1988.

Kearney DJ: Assessment of operative risk in patients undergoing lung resection. *Chest* 105:753, 1994.

Kryger M: Diagnosis of obstruction of the upper and central airways. *Am J Med* 61:85, 1976.

Miller RD: *Anesthesia.* New York, Churchill Livingstone, 1990.

Miller RD: Obstructing lesions of the larynx and trachea: clinical and physiologic characteristics. *Mayo Clin Proc* 44:145, 1969.

Miller RD, Hyatt RE: Evaluation of obstructing lesions of the trachea and larynx by flow-volume loops. *Am Rev Respir Dis* 108:475, 1973.

Morgan EG, Mikhail MS: *Clinical Anesthesiology.* Norwalk, CT, Appleton & Lange, 1992.

Pitts RF, Magoun HW, Ranson SW: The origins of respiratory rhythmicity. *Am J Physiol* 127:654, 1939.

Reid L: Chronic bronchitis, asthma, and pulmonary emphysema. *Thorax* 15:763, 1960.

Snider GL, Kleinerman J, Thurlbeck WM, Bengali ZH: The definition of emphysema. *Am Rev Respir Dis* 132:182, 1985.

Weibel ER: Morphometric estimation of pulmonary diffusion capacity. *Respir Physiol* 11:54, 1970.

Weibel ER: *Morphometry of the Human Lung.* New York, Academic Press, 1963.

West JB: *Respiratory Pathophysiology: The Essentials.* 3d ed. Baltimore, Williams & Wilkins, 1989.

West JB: *Respiratory Physiology: The Essentials,* 3d ed. Baltimore, Williams & Wilkins, 1989.

10

Cardiac Physiology

Paul E. Stensrud and Maria DeCastro

The physiologic function of the heart is to ensure the circulation of blood by generating the pressure gradient necessary for blood flow. The activity of individual cardiac myocytes must be tightly coordinated in order for the heart to work effectively. A complex mechanism of intrinsic and extrinsic control mechanisms assures continued blood flow and aids in matching perfusion to metabolic requirements.

☐ CELLULAR CHARACTERISTICS

Cardiac muscle is a syncytium, the cell membranes (sarcolemmas) of individual cardiac myocytes being cross-linked in a complex fashion by permeable intracellular junctions termed intercalated disks. This syncytial arrangement allows communication between cells throughout the myocardium, aiding in coordination of electrical and mechanical activity. The myocytes are surrounded by a supporting lattice of connective tissue. The most common cell type in the heart is the ventricular myocyte, and most descriptions of cardiac cellular morphology refer to the ventricular myocytes. In ventricular cells, the myocardial contractile apparatus is contained within each myocyte as a system of myofibrils made up of bundled protein chains. Complete bundles of myofibrils are referred to as sarcomeres. The contractile proteins are actin and myosin, and the interaction of these two proteins results in progressive shortening of the myofibril (Fig. 10–1). Coordinated shortening of the many myofibrils in a multitude of cardiac myocytes results in myocardial contraction. The troponin-tropomyosin complex is an additional component of the myofibril. In the presence of low cytosolic concentrations of calcium ions, this complex inhibits the interaction of actin and myosin, preventing myofibrillar shortening. In addition to sarcomeres, myocytes also contain other structures necessary for cellular function, including the nucleus, sarcoplasmic reticulum, Golgi apparatus, and mitochondria.

Other cell types exist within the heart. Purkinje cells, forming a portion of the conduction system, are larger than ventricular myocytes and have fewer myofilaments. Their size allows for increased conduction velocity. Sinoatrial nodal cells are much smaller than Purkinje cells, and have different ionic fluxes, as will be discussed later. Atrioventricular nodal cells are structurally similar to Purkinje cells but demonstrate ionic fluxes similar to those of sinoatrial nodal cells. The latter two cell types both have intrinsic "pacemaker" capabilities.

☐ CELLULAR ION PUMPS

Like cell types in other excitable tissues, cardiac myocytes maintain strong electrochemical gradients across the sarcolemma. Ion transport systems ("pumps") allow cells to create ionic gradients with both electrical and concentration components. The most studied ion transport system is the Na^+K^+-ATPase. This system exchanges Na^+ for K^+ using energy derived from adenosine triphosphate (ATP). The exchange appears to be electrogenic, in that the ratio of exchange is not even, producing changes in the resting membrane potential. Conventionally, three Na^+ are considered to be exchanged for two K^+, although this does not seem to be a constant ratio. Pump activity is decreased by hypothermia and digitalis. Activity is increased by increased extracellular K^+ levels.

The other major sarcolemmal ion transporter in cardiac tissue is the Na^+-Ca^{2+} exchanger, in which the Na^+ gradient is used to transport Ca^{2+} extracellularly at a ratio of approximately three Na^+ to one Ca^{2+}. Activity of this system does not seem to be directly linked to high-energy phosphates.

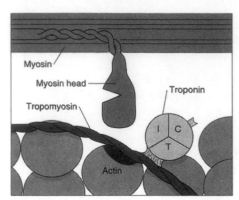
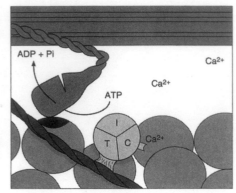

Figure 10–1 Myofibrillar contraction initiated by a rise in cytosolic Ca⁺⁺. Conformational change in tropomyosin allows cross-bridge formation and movement of the heads of myosin molecules, shortening the myofibril. Reprinted with permission from Ganong WF: *Review of Medical Physiology,* 13th ed. Norwalk: Appleton and Lange, 1995, p. 61 (Figure 3-6).

The Ca^{2+}-ATPase, found in high concentrations in the sarcoplasmic reticular membrane, allows for storage of the bulk of the Ca^{2+} required for myofibrillar shortening within the sarcoplasmic reticulum. A transient increase in Ca^{2+} ion permeability at voltage-gated, L-type Ca^{2+} channels within the cardiac cell surface membrane causes a brief increase in cytosolic Ca^{2+} concentration, which in turn triggers release of the large Ca^{2+} stores within the sarcoplasmic reticulum. This "calcium activated calcium release" dramatically increases cytosolic Ca^{2+} concentration, which in turn disinhibits actin-myosin interaction, resulting in myocardial contraction, Fig. 10.1. The Ca-ATPase then utilizes high-energy phosphates to transport cystolic Ca^{2+} into the sarcoplasmic reticulum, replenishing Ca^{2+} stores required for the next cycle of excitation-contraction.

☐ ELECTROCHEMICAL EVENTS

Cardiac ventricular myocytes maintain a resting transmembrane electrical potential (E$_R$) of approximately −90 mV by manipulating ionic gradients via selective ion transport, primarily involving Na$^+$ and K$^+$, but also including Ca^{2+}, H$^+$, and Cl$^-$. By convention, the value of E$_R$ is recorded as the net charge inside the sarcolemma relative to that outside. Thus, a negative E$_R$ indicates net negative charge on the interior of the cell, resulting from net inward movement of negatively charged molecules and/or net outward movement of positively charged ions. The resting membrane potential thus depends on the relative concentrations of ions inside and outside the sarcolemma and the conductance of these ions, as defined by the Goldman-Hodgkin-Katz equation:

$$E_R = \frac{RT}{F} \log_e \frac{P_K[K]_o + P_{Na}[Na]_o + P_{Cl}[Cl]_o + \ldots}{P_K[K]_i + P_{Na}[Na]_i + P_{Cl}[Cl]_i + \ldots} \quad (1)$$

In this equation, P is permeability of the ion involved, the ionic concentrations in the numerator are those on the outside of the cell, and the ionic concentrations in the denominator are those on the inside of the cell. Potassium perme-

ability is the major factor affecting resting E$_R$. Therefore, E$_R$ is close to E$_K$ (−95 mV). Any perturbation of ionic flux must be corrected by opposing fluxes to maintain or restore E$_R$. At rest, concentrations of major ions (in millimoles) are Na$_o$, 150; Na$_i$, 15; K$_o$, 4.5; K$_i$, 172; Ca$_o$, 2; Ca$_i$, 2×10^{-4}; Cl$_o$, 110; and Cl$_i$, 30. As noted, these ionic gradients are maintained primarily by the Na$^+$K$^+$-ATPase and the Na$^+$/Ca^{2+} exchanger, with Cl$^-$ equilibrating passively.

Proper stimulation (local depolarization of the sarcolemma to a threshold potential of approximately −70 mV) results in voltage and time-dependent changes in membrane ionic conductance via specific ionic channels, resulting in temporary depolarization of the membrane (return of the transmembrane potential toward or beyond neutrality) as the resting ionic gradients are altered. This depolarization is the action potential. In ventricular myocytes, the action potential has five major phases, numbered sequentially 0 through 4 (Fig. 10–2). The major ionic currents involved in each phase are: phase 0, sodium entry; phase 1, potassium efflux and chlo-

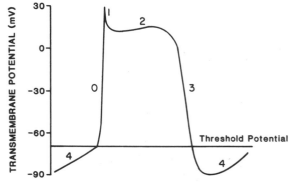

Figure 10–2 The action potential of cardiac myocytes is divided into five phases, 0 through 4. In pacemaker cells, phase 4 is upsloping, demonstrating spontaneous depolarization to threshold potential. In non-pacemaker myocytes, phase 4 is flat. See text for details on ion flux and electrochemical gradients responsible for the action potential. Reproduced with permission from Stoelting RK: *Pharmacology and Physiology in Anesthetic Practice.* Philadelphia, J.B. Lippincott Co., 1987, p. 679 (Figure 47–1).

ride entry; phase 2, calcium entry and continued potassium efflux; phase 3, continued potassium efflux; phase 4, sodium entry. The net current at any point in the action potential is determined by the balance between inward and outward currents (outward currents being defined as positive charges leaving the cell). The major currents involved are I_{Na}, the fast inward Na^+ current; I_{K1}, the K^+ current; I_{X1}, a K^+ with some Na^+ current important in repolarization; and I_{Ca}, also known as I_{SI}, the slow inward Ca^{2+} current.

In ventricular myocytes, phase 0 occurs as the transmembrane potential reaches the threshold potential, causing the membrane Na^+ channels ("fast channels") to open. Na^+ flows into the cell along concentration and electrical gradients, resulting in very rapid depolarization of the cell membrane by I_{Na}. I_{Na} is regenerative, in that the decreasing membrane potential increases Na^+ conductance, speeding depolarization further. During phase 1, early repolarization, I_{Na} slows and ceases as the Na^+ channels are inactivated. Rapid return of the cell to resting potential would ensue, as in skeletal muscle and nerve tissue, but for the activation of I_{Ca}, which partially balances the slowly increasing I_{X1}. This results in phase 2, the plateau phase. As the calcium channels are inactivated, I_{X1} and I_K rapidly return the membrane potential to E_R during phase 3. Phase 4 is a resting phase, during which E_R is maintained, until another stimulus causes repetition of the cycle. Conceptually, the large I_{Na} is primarily responsible for action potential generation and transmission, with the other currents acting to modulate the action potential and "fine tune" myocardial contraction.

Action potential characteristics differ among cell types within the myocardium. Atrial myocytes in the sinoatrial node and myocytes in the atrioventricular node (and other potential cardiac pacemaker cells) demonstrate spontaneous phase 4 depolarization to reach threshold potential as time-dependent decreases in K^+ permeability occur, causing membrane potential to slowly increase. Such spontaneous depolarization, when the threshold potential is reached, causes action potentials in these cells in the absence of outside stimulation, although external factors can alter the rate of spontaneous depolarization. These action potentials are then transmitted to more distal sites within the myocardium, allowing coordination of myocardial contraction and effective myocardial work. In these cells, phase 0 of the action potential is largely due to I_{Ca} rather than to I_{Na}, as in ventricular myocytes.

Action potentials are transmitted along the cell membrane within each cardiac myocyte and on to adjacent myocytes via the intercalated disks. The action potentials are thus distributed throughout the myocardial syncytium and are also more efficiently distributed via specialized conducting tissue (see below). A refractory period, during which membrane depolarization will not trigger membrane depolarization and myofibrillar shortening follows as the ionic gradients are reestablished, preventing retrograde transmission of the action potential. The absolute refractory period is that portion of the refractory period during which no stimulation can result in membrane depolarization. A relative refractory period exists in the later stages of the refractory period, during which supranormal stimulation could result in membrane depolarization. Transmission of the action potential is thus normally a one-way event, with the wave of depolarization proceeding from proximal to distal sites and ceasing once the entire myocardium has undergone myofibrillar shortening.

☐ EXCITATION-CONTRACTION COUPLING

Cardiac myocytes convert electrochemical stimuli into mechanical work (contraction of the myofibrillar network) via a process termed excitation-contraction coupling. Depolarization of the myocyte membrane results in Ca^{2+} entry into the cell via sarcolemmal L-type Ca^{2+} channels. A system of t tubules extending from the sarcolemma throughout the myocyte decreases the distance of the sarcoplasmic reticulum and myofibrillar system to the external environment and decreases the diffusing distance for ions that enter the cell. The increased intracellular Ca^{2+} concentration triggers further Ca^{2+} release from the sarcoplasmic reticulum, a process termed calcium-dependent calcium release. In order to provide sufficient Ca^{2+}, the calcium transporter protein (Ca^{2+}-ATPase) composes up to 90% of the sarcoplasmic reticular protein. The increased cytoplasmic Ca^{2+} diffuses into the myofibrillar bundles, aided by the presence of calmodulin, which binds Ca^{2+} and increases its mobility within the cytoplasm. Ca^{2+} then binds to the troponin C component of the troponin-tropomyosin complex, resulting in a conformational change. This conformational change in tropomyosin disinhibits the interaction of actin and myosin, resulting in repeated sulfhydryl cross-bridge formation between the actin and myosin chains, shortening the myofibril. The shortening of the myofibrils is supported by energy in the form of ATP found on the myosin molecule.

Following the action potential, active reuptake of calcium ions by the sarcoplasmic reticulum reduces the availability of intracellular calcium ions and reinstates troponin-tropomyosin inhibition of actin-myosin interaction, resulting in lengthening of the myofibril and myocardial relaxation. Contraction and relaxation are both active processes requiring high-energy phosphate compounds. Cardiac myocytes are rich in mitochondria, which make up approximately one-third of the cell volume, allowing for continuous synthesis of these high-energy phosphates and sustained contractile activity.

☐ MYOCARDIAL METABOLISM

It is obvious from the foregoing discussion that myocytes must generate a large amount of energy to accomplish many necessary cellular tasks. Furthermore, this energy, in the form of high-energy phosphate compounds, must be generated on a sustained basis, since fatigue of the heart is poorly tolerated by the organism as a whole. Primary substrates used by the heart for generation of high-energy phosphate compounds are fatty acids, glucose, lactate, and amino acids. Fatty acids provide about two-thirds of the myocardial energy needs. Metabolic pathways important in myocardial energy production include glycogen synthesis and glycogenolysis, glycolysis, pyruvate metabolism, and the Krebs tricarboxylic acid cycle. However, direct energy production in the form of high-energy phosphate compounds in these pathways is low. The main source of high-energy phosphates is the respiratory chain, in which products of these metabolic pathways (primarily the energy carriers NADH and FADH$_2$) are used to produce high-energy phosphates by means of oxidative phosphorylation. Anaerobic energy production is thus only a fraction of the capacity of aerobic production (2 ATP molecules per glucose molecule by anaerobic metabolism compared to 36 ATP molecules utilizing aerobic pathways, 32 of which are generated by the respiratory chain). The major storage form for high energy phosphate in the heart is creatine phosphate. This molecule is more rapidly transported through the myocyte than is ATP, which is polar and diffuses poorly. Thus, creatine phosphate is an efficient means of transferring high energy phosphate from its site of synthesis, as ATP in the mitochondria to the intracellular compartments requiring energy. Most ATP produced is therefore converted to creatine phosphate in a reversible reaction catalyzed by creatine kinase:

$$ATP + creatine \xleftrightarrow{CK} creatine\ phosphate + ADP \quad (2)$$

The free energy of hydrolysis of creatine phosphate is greater than that of the terminal phosphate of ATP, and therefore the formation of ATP is favored at sites where it is required (e.g., membrane channels and myofilaments) by the energetics of the reaction. Creatine phosphate thus provides a large store of high-energy phosphate relative to that provided by ATP in the cardiac myocyte. The heart uses about one-third of these high-energy compounds for basal cellular metabolism, about one-half for the contractile process, and about one-sixth for ion pumping.

☐ CARDIAC CONDUCTION SYSTEM

Spontaneous initiation of cardiac action potentials normally occurs only in specialized pacemaker cells, which demonstrate spontaneous phase 4 depolarization to reach the threshold potential. Cells demonstrating spontaneous depolarization are present throughout the myocardium, but the sinoatrial node (SAN), located at the junction of the superior vena cava and right atrium, normally has the most rapid spontaneous depolarization and functions as the primary pacemaker for the heart, the generated action potential stimulating more distal myocytes before spontaneous depolarization can occur (Fig. 10–3). The action potentials generated in the SAN spread locally and are also transmitted via specialized atrial conducting tissue (anatomically ill-defined) to the atrioventricular node (AVN), located posteriorly and inferiorly on the right side of the interatrial septum. In the AVN, the action potential is delayed approximately 0.1 ms before traveling on to the ventricles. This delay is important in the proper coordination of the atrial and ventricular contractions. The action potential is transmitted from the AVN to ventricular tissue via specialized conducting tissue in the bundle of His and the ventricular bundle branches, which further ramify into the Purkinje system of myocardial conduction tissue, terminating in the ventricular myocardium. Proper coordination of myocardial contraction by transmission of the action potential generated in the SAN to the cardiac myocytes in the atria and ventricles results in atrial and ventricular systole and diastole, the alternating phases of contraction and relaxation that make up the cardiac cycle. Pathologic states may slow spontaneous depolarization of more proximal pacemaker cells, in which case more distal cells may assume the primary pacemaker function. Atrial tissue outside the SAN (ectopic atrial pacemakers) may depolarize at a rate close to that of the SAN (60 to 80 times per minute), while more distal pacemaker cells normally depolarize more slowly. The AVN spontaneously depolarizes at a rate of 40 to 50/min,

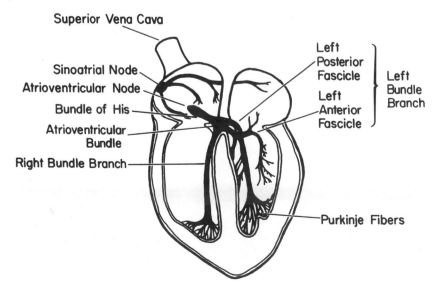

Figure 10–3 Anatomy of the cardiac conduction system. Reproduced with permission from Stoelting RK: *Pharmacology and Physiology in Anesthetic Practice,* 2 ed. Philadelphia, J. B. Lippincott Co., 1991, p. 702 (Figure 47–10).

and distal pacemaker sites in the Purkinje system depolarize at rates of 30 to 40/min. These rates of spontaneous distal depolarization become relevant if conduction is blocked at more proximal sites in the cardiac conduction system, allowing for continued ventricular contraction (ventricular escape), albeit at the expense of heart rate and coordination of atrial and ventricular function, with consequent loss of cardiac efficiency.

☐ THE CARDIAC CYCLE

The repetitive contractile activity of the heart, referred to as the cardiac cycle, is made up of two distinct phases: systole, or contraction, and diastole, or relaxation. The cardiac cycle is conventionally described with reference to the left ventricle (Fig. 10–4). Systole is the phase in which the myocardium contracts, generating increased pressure within the heart. Systole extends from the time just prior to mitral valve opening to the period following aortic valve closure. Systole is, in turn, made up of two subphases: isovolumic contraction and ejection (Fig. 10–5). During isovolumic contraction, the increasing wall tension results in increased intracardiac pressure, causing mitral valve closure. Isovolumic contraction ends when the intracardiac pressure is sufficient to open the aortic valve. Ejection ensues with opening of the aortic valve, as blood exits the heart down the generated pressure gradient, and continues until the intracardiac pressure decreases, resulting in aortic valve closure. Approximately two-thirds of the stroke volume is ejected in a brief period of rapid ejection, followed by the remaining one-third of the stroke volume, which is ejected much more slowly. At normal heart rates, systole normally lasts for one-third of the cardiac cycle. Diastole is the period of myocardial relaxation and filling, preparatory to the next systolic phase. Diastole is an active phase, requiring energy. Conventionally, diastole is regarded as having four subphases: isovolumic relaxation,

rapid filling, diastasis, and atrial systole. Isovolumic relaxation occurs following closure of the aortic valve and before mitral valve opening, when the myocardium relaxes at a fixed volume, since blood cannot transit the closed mitral valve. With opening of the mitral valve, rapid filling of the left ventricle occurs. Eighty percent of left ventricular filling normally occurs at this time. Diastasis, a phase of slow ventricular filling occurring as ventricular pressures approach atrial pressures, follows rapid filling. Finally, atrial systole elevates atrial pressure above ventricular pressure, resulting in a second phase of increased ventricular filling. In the normal heart, atrial systole is responsible for 15 to 20% of ventricular filling. The importance of atrial systole is increased in the presence of increased ventricular stiffness, when loss of the atrial "kick" may result in grave hemodynamic consequences.

☐ MYOCARDIAL FUNCTION IN VITRO

Studies of isolated cardiac muscle provide important data necessary to the understanding of integrated cardiovascular function. Data from such studies has been useful in attempting to understand the behavior of the heart in intact physiologic systems. Contractile characteristics, including resting tension, maximum velocity of shortening (V_{max}), peak tension developed, and time to peak tension can all be measured under varying conditions. Important factors affecting these characteristics of isolated cardiac muscle include preload (the length of the resting fibers prior to stimulation), afterload (the resistance of the fiber to contraction at a fixed resting length), and contractility (the intrinsic strength of the cardiac fibers studied). Although no good single definition of contractility exists, it is generally regarded as an interdependent relationship between force and velocity of contraction at constant preload and afterload. Increases in preload increase resting tension, peak tension, and V_{max} up to the optimal

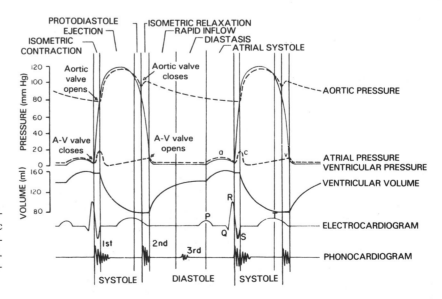

Figure 10–4 The cardiac cycle, with pressure, volume, electrocardiographic, and phonocardiographic changes associated with the various events of the cycle. Reproduced with permission from Guyton AC. *Textbook of Medical Physiology,* 7th ed. Philadelphia, W.B. Saunders, 1986.

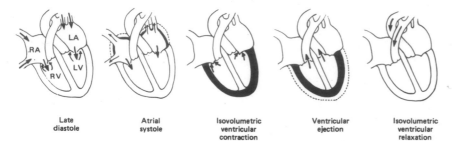

| Late diastole | Atrial systole | Isovolumetric ventricular contraction | Ventricular ejection | Isovolumetric ventricular relaxation |

Figure 10–5 Blood flow during the events of the cardiac cycle. Bold outlined chambers are contracting. Reproduced with permission from Ganong WF: *Review of Medical Physiology,* 13th ed. Norwalk, Appleton and Lange, 1995, p. 514 (Figure 29–1).

length of the muscle strip, at which point these values begin to decrease. Increases in afterload decrease V_{max} and increase peak tension and time to peak tension. An increase in contractility implies increased V_{max} and force of contraction at a given resistance and initial fiber length.

☐ MYOCARDIAL FUNCTION IN VIVO

The physiologic function of the heart is the delivery of blood to organ systems. While studies of isolated cardiac muscle are important, organ perfusion depends on integration of cardiac, vascular, and organ system variables, which are best studied in intact preparations. Work using such preparations has demonstrated four major determinants of cardiac pump function in vivo: preload, afterload, contractility, and heart rate, representing in vivo correlates of the in vitro determinants of myocardial performance noted above.

Left ventricular preload (end-diastolic fiber length) is the most important determinant of cardiac output and is best measured as left ventricular end-diastolic volume (LVEDV). However, it is difficult to conveniently measure LVEDV in the clinical setting, and pressure measurements are often used as correlates of LVEDV. Due to variability in ventricular stiffness, measured changes in pressure do not necessarily result in corresponding changes in ventricular volume, the best analog of preload. Furthermore, since clinical measurement of left ventricular pressure is not routinely performed, especially on a continuous basis, measurement of left atrial, pulmonary artery, or central venous pressure is frequently used to estimate left ventricular end-diastolic pressure and by inference LVEDV. Such estimates require the assumption that cardiac stiffness and cardiac valve function between the point of measurement and the left ventricle are normal or at least constant for trend monitoring. Such an assumption is frequently invalid in critically ill patients, and reliance on absolute values of measured pressures to determine optimum left ventricular preload in a particular patient is dangerous. Measured pressures must be integrated into the entire clinical picture in order for valid conclusions involving ventricular preload to be drawn. Optimization of left ventricular preload is a primary goal in the treatment of critically ill patients, since increasing preload (within physiologic limits) is the most efficient method of increasing cardiac output in terms of the balance between myocardial oxygen demand and supply. Preload is affected by blood volume, body position, in-

trathoracic pressure, intrapericardial pressure, venous tone, skeletal muscle, augmentation of venous return, and the atrial contribution to ventricular filling.

Afterload in vivo is defined as the wall stress across the myocardium during systole. The afterload of any cardiac chamber can be thought of as the impedance to ejection of blood from that chamber. Left ventricular afterload is primarily (93% in the absence of aortic valvular stenosis) dependent on systemic vascular resistance (SVR). Dilation of the left ventricle in response to pathologic states can also result in increased afterload, independent of SVR, according to the law of Laplace:

Tension = (pressure × chamber radius)/(2 × wall thickness) (3)

Increases in afterload result in decreases in the extent and velocity of contraction and stroke volume at a given preload and contractility. Increases in afterload also increase myocardial work and energy demands, while increasing blood pressure for a given cardiac output.

Contractility (also referred to as inotropy) is difficult to measure in intact systems and is usually defined as mechanical work performed by the heart at a constant preload, afterload, and heart rate. In these steady-state conditions, stroke volume and stroke work are functions of contractility. Left ventricular contractility is best determined by plotting stroke work versus fiber length, or LVEDV. However, contractility is often plotted as cardiac output versus pulmonary artery occlusion pressure, since these variables are more readily measured clinically. If curves are plotted as the relationship of cardiac output versus central venous or pulmonary artery pressure measurements, a series of assumptions regarding the relationship of these variables to the actual stroke work and end-diastolic fiber length must be made, as noted previously. Ventricular function curves are not usually plotted in the clinical setting, but an understanding of the concepts underlying their generation aids clinical decisions.

Heart rate has important effects on myocardial performance only at abnormally high or low rates. At constant preload, afterload, and contractility, and in the normal heart rate range, myocardial autoregulatory mechanisms maintain a nearly constant cardiac output by varying the stroke volume. Decreases in heart rate will decrease cardiac output as the limits of increasing stroke volume are reached. Increases in heart rate can decrease ventricular filling as the time spent in diastole decreases relative to that spent in systole, with systole occurring prior to completion of ventricular filling. Decreases in diastolic time can also decrease left ventricular contractile function, as diastolic relaxation may not be complete prior to onset of systole.

☐ DIASTOLIC FUNCTION

Most early studies of cardiac function focused on systolic activity. Diastolic activity was felt to be a relatively minor component of the cardiac cycle. It has now been realized that diastolic function is extremely important. Diastolic dysfunction appears to be the major underlying etiology in up to 40% of patients with congestive heart failure. As stated earlier, the four subphases of diastole are isovolumic relaxation, rapid filling, diastasis, and atrial systole. During isovolumic relaxation, myofibrillar lengthening due to inhibition of actin and myosin interaction by the troponin-tropomyosin complex as Ca^{2+} is removed from the cytoplasm is essentially complete. Further falls in ventricular pressure may occur during the rapid filling phase, but this is due to continued recoil of the ventricular elastic components, which may result in a suction effect and further increase ventricular filling. During diastasis, ventricular filling slows as pressures across the mitral valve equilibrate. As heart rate increases, diastasis is the first component of the cardiac cycle to shorten, as loss of diastasis causes minimal reduction in cardiac efficiency. With onset of atrial systole, a second peak in the ventricular filling rate occurs as the transmitral pressure gradient again increases. Atrial systole normally accounts for 15 to 20% of ventricular filling, but this figure is increased in conditions increasing ventricular stiffness or delaying relaxation. Diastolic function of the heart may be adversely affected by numerous pathologic states, including myocardial ischemia, hypertrophy of cardiac chambers, various cardiomyopathies, atrioventricular valvular stenosis, pericardial disease, aortic or mitral regurgitation, or atriovenous fistula resulting in chronic volume overload.

☐ INTEGRATED VIEW OF MYOCARDIAL FUNCTION

The most frequently used model of myocardial function is the pressure-volume model. Pressure-volume loops plot instantaneous intracardiac pressure versus chamber volume. The resulting plot for the left ventricle (Fig. 10–6) results in a counterclockwise loop that describes ventricular performance through the entire cardiac cycle. In the figure, the portion from point A to point B represents ventricular filling. The portion from point B to point C represents isovolumic contraction. The portion from point C to point D represents ventricular ejection, the period when the aortic valve is open. The portion from point D to point A represents isovolumic relaxation. As can be appreciated from Fig. 10–6, systolic and diastolic dysfunction may produce characteristic changes in the pressure-volume relationship, and both may coexist in a single patient.

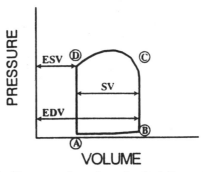

Figure 10–6   Pressure-volume loop for the left ventricle. See text for explanation. Reproduced with permission from Kramer JL, Thomas SJ: Cardiac physiology. In: *Manual of Cardiac Anesthesia,* 2nd ed. Thomas SJ, Kramer JL, eds. New York, Churchill Livingstone, 1993, p. 6 (Figure 1–3).

The pressure-volume relationship is useful in determining many characteristics of cardiac function. The slope of the end-systolic pressure-volume relationship has been useful as a relatively preload-independent analog of contractility. The compliance (stiffness) of a myocardial chamber, defined as the ratio of a change in volume to a change in pressure, can be determined from the pressure-volume curves. Ventricular elastance (the ratio of change in pressure to change in volume) is the inverse of compliance and can be thought of as the snappiness of the myocardium, and ventricular pressure-volume loops are actually plots of the elastance of the ventricle. Such curves were introduced by Suga and Sagawa, and used to describe cardiac mechanics in terms of time-varying elastance, so-called because the elastance of cardiac chambers changes with time during the cardiac cycle (Fig. 10–7). The point of maximum pressure-volume ratio (E_{max}) is defined at end-systole. This value has proven to be an excellent index of myocardial contractility, relatively independent of preload and afterload changes. Since ventricular preload is best defined at end-diastolic volume and end-diastolic pressure measurements are often used as indicators of end-diastolic volume, it must be noted that myocardial elastance strongly influences the relationship of end diastolic pressure and volume. The Frank-Starling law of the heart notes that the cardiac work performed depends on the initial length of the muscle fibers. Understanding of the pressure-volume relationship and the time-varying elastance model of myocardial mechanics aids in interpretation of clinically acquired data, even when formal plots are not generated.

Afterload, while affecting the pressure-volume relationship (although minimally impacting E_{max}), cannot be described in this fashion. Afterload is defined as the systolic wall stress in a cardiac chamber and is dependent on the outflow impedance as well as intrinsic properties of the chamber wall. Left ventricular afterload is dependent on arterial resistance, arterial compliance, and ventricular wall characteristics (e.g., hypertrophy). In normal humans, a large proportion of left ventricular afterload (90%) appears to be due to arterial resistance (systemic vascular resistance, or SVR), and afterload is frequently equated with SVR. Due to the complex

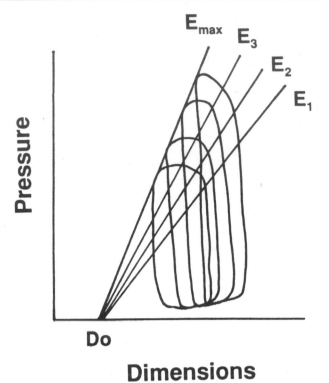

Figure 10-7 Left ventricular pressure-volume relationships at different times during systole, (E1-E3 and Emax). Emax possesses the steepest slope and corresponds to end systole. Do is the common intercept for all lines. Reprinted with permission from Foex, P and Leone, B. Pressure-volume loops: a dynamic approach to the assessment of ventricular function: *J Cardiothoracic Vasc Anesth,* 1994, 8:84-96.

interrelationship of cardiac and vascular factors, the concept of afterload is difficult to use in clinical situations.

MYOCARDIAL WORK AND ENERGETICS

The time-varying elastance concept and the ventricular pressure-volume relationship can be used to determine myocardial work (Fig. 10-8). In the intact organism, these concepts can be correlated with myocardial oxygen demand (V_{O_2}). The area within the pressure-volume loop of the classic cardiac cycle represents external work, or stroke work, performed by the heart. This corresponds to the shaded areas in Figure 10-8. However, in addition to performing external work, oxygen is also consumed by the myocardium in achieving the dimensions necessary for performing this work. The resulting potential energy acquired by this oxygen consumption is analogous to that in a bow drawn before letting the arrow fly, or in a rubber band stretched so it can snap vigorously. It is represented in Fig. 10-8 by the triangular area to the left of the "external work" loop. The total area enclosed, representing the sum of potential energy and external work performed by the heart, comprises the pressure-volume area (PVA). The PVA correlates well with V_{O_2} for a single

contraction. PVA does not vary appreciably with heart rate at rates greater than 80 beats per minute, indicating that myocardial work (hence, V_{O_2}) does not change with higher heart rates on a per-beat basis. V_{O_2} does increase at higher heart rates, but mainly as a result of the greater number of contractions per minute. At heart rates less than 80 beats per minute, the myocardial work performed per beat increases slightly, probably due to the increased contribution of basal metabolic requirements relative to contractile work at these rates. Overall, however, myocardial work and V_{O_2} decrease with decreasing heart rates. Myocardial work and V_{O_2} are dependent on contractile state and increase with increasing E_{max}.

CORONARY CIRCULATORY ANATOMY AND PHYSIOLOGY

The adequacy of coronary blood flow (myocardial oxygen supply) relative to myocardial oxygen demand is an important determinant of myocardial function. The anatomy of the main coronary arteries is illustrated in Fig. 10-9. This system is right-dominant in 50% (more coronary blood flow via the right coronary artery), balanced in 30%, and left-dominant in 20% of patients. In the absence of chronic ischemia, coronary collateral circulation is limited, and stenosis of any of the main coronary arteries will jeopardize perfusion of the area of myocardium perfused by that vessel. The large epicardial vessels illustrated are conductance vessels, responsible for little of the coronary arterial resistance in the absence of stenotic lesions or coronary vasospasm. The main resistance vessels in the normal heart are the penetrating arterioles. Resistance to blood flow in these vessels can be affected by transmural myocardial pressure, and in the left ventricle coronary blood flow occurs primarily during diastole due to the high intramural pressures generated during systole. Thus, the

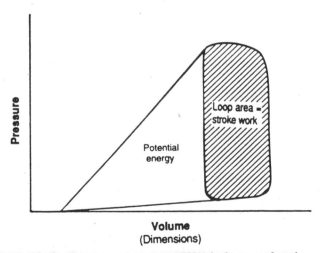

Figure 10-8 Pressure-volume area (PVA) is the sum of stroke, or external, work (shaded area) and cardiac potential energy. PVA is closely related to total myocardial oxygen consumption. Reprinted with permission from Foex, P and Leone, B. Pressure-volume loops: a dynamic approach to the assessment of ventricular function. *J Cardiothoracic Vasc Anesth,* 1994, 8:84-96.

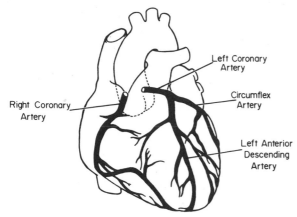

Figure 10–9 Coronary circulatory anatomy. Reprinted with permission from Stoelting RK. *Physiology and Pharmacology in Anesthetic Practice,* 2nd ed. Philadelphia, J.B. Lippincott Co., 1991, p. 697 (Figure 47–5).

endocardium of the left ventricle is the area most vulnerable to ischemia.

Normal coronary blood flow is 75 mL/100 g/min, accounting for approximately 5% of the cardiac output. Due to a high basal myocardial oxygen extraction, the heart accounts for nearly 10% of total body oxygen consumption. The high myocardial oxygen extraction results in a coronary venous oxygen saturation of 30% (normal mixed venous oxygen saturation is 70%, reflecting total body oxygen supply and demand). This degree of oxygen extraction is nearly maximal and requires that coronary blood flow increase in the presence of increased myocardial oxygen demand, as the myocardium is unable to further increase oxygen extraction. Furthermore, the heart has little capacity for anaerobic metabolism. Thus, in the presence of myocardial ischemia, clinical symptoms will develop rapidly.

The heart normally autoregulates the coronary blood flow over a wide range of perfusion pressures, matching myocardial oxygen demand with supply. Autoregulation also occurs in denervated hearts, indicating that local mechanisms are responsible. Myocardial metabolism and oxygen demand are increased in the presence of increases in preload, afterload, contractility, or heart rate. Increases in preload, within physiologic limits, are the most efficient means of increasing cardiac output relative to increasing myocardial oxygen demand. Increases in heart rate result in increased myocardial oxygen demand, while coronary blood flow (oxygen supply) to the left ventricle is decreased by decreasing time spent in diastole. Increases in afterload increase myocardial oxygen demand but may increase coronary blood flow if coronary perfusion pressure (aortic root blood pressure − intramural blood pressure) is increased by increasing systemic blood pressure. In the presence of fixed stenoses (fixed resistance), coronary blood flow to distal regions of the myocardium becomes pressure-dependent, and ischemia may result when myocardial metabolic demands are increased, despite a constant degree of stenosis. Myocardial ischemia may be relieved by decreasing myocardial oxygen demand, increasing

coronary blood flow, or a combination of these two strategies. All current methods of treating myocardial ischemia are based on this principle.

PULMONARY CIRCULATORY PHYSIOLOGY

The pulmonary circulation links the right and left cardiac chambers and regulates the balance between regional pulmonary perfusion and ventilation. The pulmonary circulation is a highly distensible, low-pressure system normally containing 450 mL of blood. This amount may vary with pathologic conditions and with posture (i.e., assumption of supine position increases pulmonary blood volume up to 40%, resulting in orthopnea in the presence of left ventricular failure).

The right ventricle serves as a conduit and assist pump delivering blood via the pulmonary vascular bed to the left heart chambers. Right ventricular function is one determinant of left ventricular preload. As has been demonstrated in animal models and in humans with congenital heart defects resulting in a single ventricle, survival is possible in the absence of the right ventricle, but pulmonary blood flow and left ventricular preload then become more dependent on venous return (right atrial preload) and low pulmonary vascular resistance. Anatomically, the right ventricle is partially wrapped around the left ventricle. Dilation or hypertrophy of the right ventricle, whether due to increased pulmonary artery pressure (primary pulmonary hypertension, mitral valve dysfunction, or impaired left ventricular ejection) or to intrinsic right ventricular dysfunction, may alter left ventricular geometry, diastolic filling, and systolic function.

CARDIOVASCULAR CONTROL SYSTEMS

A number of control mechanisms are responsible for maintaining optimal organ perfusion by coordinating and regulating myocardial and vascular performance.

Arterial baroreceptors are located in the carotid sinus and aortic arch. These are mechanoreceptors that sense mean blood pressure and pulse pressure. Baroreceptor output is inhibitory at the medullary vasomotor center. When blood pressure decreases, inhibition of the vasomotor center is decreased, resulting in increased excitatory outflow and increased cardiac output and blood pressure via sympathetically mediated increases in heart rate and contractility and in systemic vascular resistance. Increases in blood pressure cause the opposite response. These receptors may reset during chronic hypertension.

Cardiopulmonary mechanoreceptors sensing stretch of the atria and pulmonary vasculature also contribute to tonic inhibition of the vasomotor center and cause reflex alterations in cardiovascular function via vagal and sympathetic efferents. Increases in atrial volume (sensed by atrial stretch receptors),

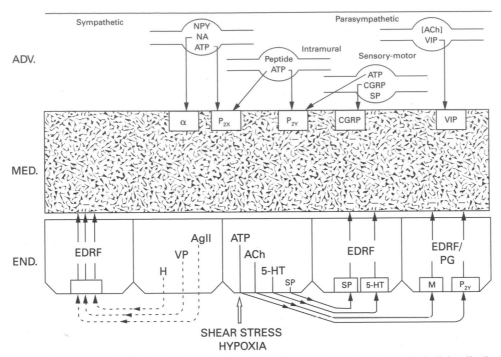

Figure 10-10 Contribution of input from perivascular nerves (above) and endothelial cells (below) to regulation of vascular tone. NPY, neuropeptide Y; NA, norepinephrine; CGRP, calcitonin gene-related peptide; SP, substance P; VIP, vasoactive intestinal peptide; ADV adventitia; MED, media; END, endothelial cells; PG, prostaglandin; AgII, angiotensin II, 5-HT, serotonin; VP, vasopressin; H, histamine; M, muscarinic; pluses indicate vasoconstriction, minuses are vasodilation; boxes are receptors. Reprinted with permission from Burnstock, G. Integration of factors controlling vascular tone. *Anesthesiology*, 1993, 76:1373.

even those not sufficient to cause increases in blood pressure, result in increases in heart rate and decreases in forearm vascular resistance. Such responses serve to maintain constant cardiac volume. In the transition from supine to upright posture, the fall in central blood volume sensed by atrial mechanoreceptors as venous pooling occurs in dependent regions results in reflex constriction of muscle blood vessels, acting to maintain central blood volume. These reflexes may contribute more heavily to basal blood pressure maintenance, with arterial baroreceptors providing fast-response "fine tuning."

Chemoreceptors, located mainly in the carotid bodies, cause reflex increases in ventilation and sympathetic tone in the presence of hypoxia, hypercarbia, and acidosis. The ventilatory responses are instituted to correct the blood gas abnormalities, while the cardiovascular responses divert blood flow to critical organ systems. In the presence of tachycardia and hypertension, the first step is to ensure adequate oxygenation and ventilation.

Skeletal muscle receptors cause reflex increases in blood pressure and heart rate necessary to increase blood flow to muscles during exercise despite the high intravascular pressures present.

The medullary vasomotor center centrally integrates cardiovascular function. This area of the brainstem has many connections to other central nervous system structures, in-

cluding the hypothalamus and higher brain centers. Input from the various mechano- and chemoreceptor systems is integrated with input from higher brain centers and the hypothalamus to determine final central neural cardiovascular regulatory outflow. This system allows coordination of local, neuronal, and hormonal cardiovascular control mechanisms.

Endothelium-dependent vasomotor responses are important in the regulation of vascular tone. Neural-mediated responses act via sympathetic and parasympathetic receptors in the media of blood vessels. Further investigation has shown that many vascular responses are dependent on the presence of intact endothelium rather than mediated by medial receptors. Endothelium-derived relaxing factors (EDRF) and constricting factors (EDCF) act in response to activation of endothelial receptors by shear stress, hypoxia, or any of a number of vasoactive compounds. Nitric oxide (NO) has been identified as an EDRF, and endothelin is considered to be at least one of the compounds acting as an EDCF. Vasomotor responses (either vasoconstriction or vasodilation) are the result of a complex interplay between medial (neural) and endothelial (local and blood-borne) stimuli, as is indicated in Fig. 10-10. Vascular responses are heterogenous, with various vascular beds demonstrating various responses to a single stimulus to the organism. Such heterogeneity is useful in modifying regional blood flow under a variety of conditions to ensure perfusion of key organ systems.

In addition to these cardiovascular control mechanisms, other organs regulating intravascular volume, electrolyte status, and total body metabolic rate are important in determining overall cardiac performance. In this regard, assessment of renal, adrenal, thyroid, and pituitary function is important in the management of the hemodynamically unstable patient. Organ systems do not function in isolation, and the integrated function of multiple organ systems must be simultaneously assessed when one is faced with a critically ill patient.

11 Neurophysiology

J. Michael Jaeger

All the complexities of human behavior have their basis in the structure and function of the neurons and the supporting tissues of the central nervous system (CNS). These behaviors include the perception of sensation, coordinated movement, memory, learning, and emotions. We will focus on the function of the CNS at the cellular level and, whenever possible, relate clinical observations to cellular events. However, human behavior as well as diseases of the CNS cannot necessarily be described solely in terms of isolated cellular events. A detailed knowledge of neuronal networking, complex biochemical interactions, and the simultaneous integration of extensive neuronal activity (information processing) is required. For technical reasons, these areas are not well understood, and, while they are clinically relevant, discussion of them lies beyond the scope of this text.

☐ CELLULAR ORGANIZATION OF THE CENTRAL NERVOUS SYSTEM

The CNS is organized into a vast array of various types of neurons and specialized supporting cells. However, the main features of a "typical" vertebrate neuron are illustrated in Fig. 11–1. The neuron can be divided into functionally distinct regions: (1) the cell body, or soma, which contains the nucleus and the bulk of the components (ribosomes, endoplasmic reticulum, mitochondria, etc.) necessary for the metabolic support of the neuron; (2) the dendrite and the axon, two unique processes that arise from the soma and that function to receive, integrate, and conduct bioelectric nerve impulses; and (3) the axon tip, or presynaptic terminal, which is highly specialized to transmit the nerve impulse to other neurons or excitable tissues by the release of signaling chemicals called neurotransmitters.

The arborization of dendrites from the cell body can be relatively simple, as in the case of an α motor neuron, or extensive, as in the case of a cerebellar Purkinje cell, which can receive as many as 150,000 separate neuronal contacts. A specialized region of the dendritic cell membrane containing aggregations of postsynaptic receptors lies in close proximity to the presynaptic terminus of the apposing neuron. Once bound to a specific neurotransmitter, the neurotransmitter-receptor complex produces electrical excitation or inhibition of the postsynaptic neuron. Dendrites of cells mediating specific sensory modalities, such as vibration, pressure, light or smell, can possess highly specialized regions that transduce their specific mechanical, chemical, or thermodynamic input into an electrical impulse common to all neurons. By virtue of multiple contacts between other neurons and the dendritic tree, excitatory and inhibitory inputs begin to be integrated into a modulated output of the primary neuron.

The axon serves as the main output transmission line for the neuron. An axon can be a simple or complex cylindrical process with a diameter ranging from 0.2 to 20 μm and a length up to 1 m, as in the sciatic nerve α motor neuron. The axon hillock is the initial segment of the axon that normally serves as the point of initiation of the action potential, a transient, self-regenerating electrical impulse that conducts down into the presynaptic terminal virtually without decrement. This region summates the graded intrinsic and extrinsic excitatory and inhibitory inputs and transforms them into a specific pattern of nerve impulses. Branches of the axon may form synapses, or specialized points of contact between the presynaptic terminals and the postsynaptic membranes, of as many as 1000 individual neurons.

Glial cells are actually a family of cells that play an important supporting role within the CNS. To improve nerve impulse conduction velocity, many axons are wrapped at inter-

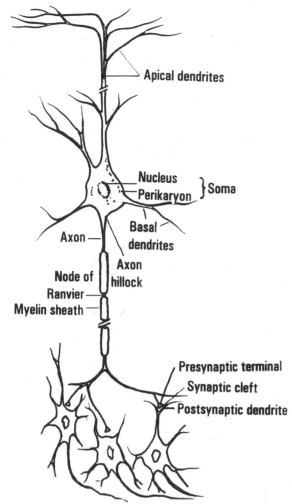

Figure 11–1 This diagram illustrates the typical features of the myelinated neuron. The cell body, or soma, contains the nucleus and perikaryon. Extending from the cell body are two types of processes: apical and basal dendrites and the axon. Nerve impulse initiation occurs at the axon hillock. The myelin sheath, which electrically insulates the axon, is periodically interrupted by nodes of Ranvier. The axon branches terminate in presynaptic terminals, which lie in close proximity to postsynaptic cells at points called synapses. Synapses on the dendrites or soma of postsynaptic neurons enable the transmission of information and subsequent integration of nervous input. (Modified with permission from Kandel, Schwartz, and Jessell, 1991.)

vals in layers of specialized cell membrane called myelin, which, like the insulation around a wire, has a high electrical resistance and a low electrical capacitance improving the transmission of electrical signals. Every millimeter or so, the myelin is interrupted and a few micrometers of axonal membrane are exposed at the nodes of Ranvier. At the nodes of Ranvier, the membrane ion channels responsible for generating the nerve electrical impulse are found in high concentrations and replenish the signal strength. Schwann cells perform this function in individual peripheral myelinated neurons, while the processes of oligodendrocytes are capable of myelinating multiple neurons within the white matter of the CNS.

Astrocytes are very numerous in the CNS, but their role remains unclear. They consist of an irregularly star-shaped cell body with multiple appendages radiating outward with end-feet that make contact with both neurons and capillary blood vessels. While these processes may provide a nutritive or supportive partial sheath around neurons, they also appear to induce the formation of tight junctions between capillary endothelial cells, an essential component of the blood-brain barrier. Astrocytes also sequester neurotransmitters released at synapses, may scavenge neuronal debris following nerve injury, and, because of their high resting permeability to K^+, serve as a sink for extracellular K^+ during periods of increased neuronal activity. Finally, microglia are unique cells that developed from the macrophage line and are phagocytes activated during times of disease and nerve injury.

☐ THE STRUCTURE AND FUNCTION OF THE CELL MEMBRANE

CELL MEMBRANE COMPOSITION

Virtually every aspect of the neuron's function is related to events that occur at the cell membrane. All biological membranes have a common structure consisting of a continuous double layer of lipid molecules approximately 4 to 5 nm thick. The three major classes of component lipids—phospholipids, cholesterol, and glycolipids—are amphipathic, with their hydrophobic tails oriented toward the center and their polar heads toward the aqueous extracellular fluid. The composition of the lipid bilayer imparts a degree of membrane fluidity and stability that is essential for the function of membrane proteins that are embedded within it. Furthermore, membranes provide the cell with the ability to compartmentalize and provide a controlled environment for specific activities.

Membrane-associated proteins are extremely heterogeneous and perform many functions as receptors, ion channels, molecular pumps, reaction catalysts, cytoskeletal anchors, and so on. Certain characteristics appear similar, however. Membrane protein structure and its degree of association with the membrane lipids depends on its amino acid sequence; charged amino acids associate with predominantly aqueous regions (intracellular fluid, extracellular fluid, or pore regions), while the neutral amino acids tend to allow interaction with the lipid region. Within these constraints, membrane proteins are able to twist and migrate within the membrane and to interact with other membrane proteins. The peculiar properties of the cell membrane of excitable tissues allow for the generation of electrical signals that are capable of transmitting information over considerable distances or influencing other tissues by the release of neurosecretions.

CELLULAR ELECTROPHYSIOLOGY OF THE NEURON

The Resting Membrane Potential The plasma membrane, with its associated protein pores, forms the biological counterpart of an electrical capacitor and resistor arranged in parallel. The study of physics teaches us that charged particles, in this case ions in solution, move under the influence of an electrical potential difference (ΔV, volts) or voltage. The rate of charge movement is referred to as current (I, ampere). The ease with which ions move through an ion channel or cytoplasm, for example, is measured in terms of resistance (R, ohms). In biological settings, however, it is often more convenient to use the term conductance (G, siemen), which is the inverse of resistance and given by the rearrangement of Ohm's law:

$$G = I/\Delta V \qquad (1)$$

High membrane conductance generally connotes a large number of open ion channels. Most ion channels have a conductance on the order of 2 to 100×10^{-12} siemens ($10^{-12} = 1$ picosiemens, or pS). Another derived quantity often used is capacitance, a measure of the ability of a device (capacitor) to store an electrical charge. The "membrane capacitor" consists of a thin strip of insulating material, the lipid bilayer, between two conducting plates, the layers of biological salt solution bathing the plasma membrane. The capacitance of biological membranes is about 1 $\mu F/cm^2$.

Several generalizations about the ion content of cells and the extracellular fluid are necessary: (1) K^+ is distributed so that the intracellular concentration (~ 150 mM) is many times greater than extracellular; (2) the intracellular concentration of both Cl^- and Na^+ is always less than that in the extracellular fluid, which can be attributed to the activity of ATP-dependent pumps; and (3) the concentration of positively charged ions equals the concentration of negatively charged ions in the bulk phase (i.e., the extracellular fluid distant from the fixed negative charges on the plasma membrane constituents). Proteins and phosphorylated compounds (e.g., ATP, creatine phosphate, etc.) are responsible for the bulk of the negative charges intracellularly.

Now, consider a mammalian skeletal muscle cell containing a high concentration of K^+, a low concentration of Na^+, and a high concentration of a large anion, A^- (Fig. 11–2). Outside the cell is a high concentration of Na^+ and Cl^- and a low concentration of K^+. If the cell membrane is permeable only to K^+, then the large inward-to-outward concentration gradient will tend to drive K^+ out of the cell. Because electroneutrality must be observed, it is impossible for many K^+ ions to leave the cell or move very far. Thus, it should be noted, K^+ cannot exchange with Na^+, nor can it leave behind an excess of anions. As soon as the first K^+ moves across the membrane, a separation of charge occurs (work is performed by the potential energy stored in the chemical gradient), and an electrical potential difference, or membrane potential, is

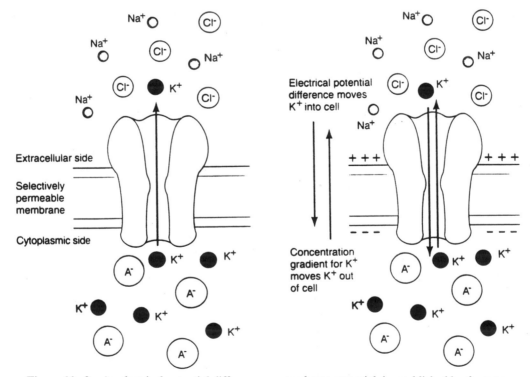

Figure 11–2 An electrical potential difference, or membrane potential, is established by the separation of ionic charges across a selectively permeable membrane. A cell typically contains potassium ions (K^+) and negatively charged proteins (A^-) in high concentrations but sodium ions (Na^+) and chloride ions (Cl^-) in low concentrations intracellularly. Na^+ and Cl^- concentrations are much higher in the extracellular fluid, while K^+ concentration is kept low. Since the cell membrane at rest is relatively permeable to K^+ but not Na^+ or A^-, K^+ moves easily across the membrane via the ionic pores. Because of the electrical attraction to its negatively charged counterpart (A^-), it cannot move very far away. As a result, electrical charge builds up on the membrane (capacitance): the resting membrane potential. (With permission from Kandel, Schwartz, and Jessell, 1991.)

produced, with the inside of the cell negative with respect to the outside. In time, the diffusional force (chemical potential energy) driving K^+ is exactly equal and opposite to the electrical force (electrical potential energy, or membrane potential) that is opposing the outward movement of K^+; the net movement of K^+ will then cease. The movement of ions across the membrane due to diffusion continues, but for each ion these movements are equal and opposite. The K^+ ions (or the anions left behind) do not move very far from the cell but remain in a thin layer adjacent to the plasma membrane, essentially charging the membrane capacitance to a membrane potential that exactly opposes the driving force of the concentration gradient.

It is possible to calculate the membrane potential that exists when electrochemical equilibrium is reached using the Nernst equation:

$$E_{eq} = (RT/zF) \ln\{[K^+]_o/[K^+]_i\} \qquad (2)$$

where R is the universal gas constant, T is the absolute temperature, z is the ion valence, and F is the Faraday constant. The term E_{eq} is referred to as the equilibrium potential of the ion in question. In the situation in which the cell membrane is permselective for K^+, then E_{eq} equals the resting membrane potential.

Since the amount of ion that must move to generate E_{eq} is too small to be measured chemically, no differences in ionic content would be detected if the intracellular and extracellular fluids were to be analyzed. The actual amount of ionic transfer that occurs can be estimated by using the equation for the charge on a capacitor, $Q = CV_m$, where Q is the charge, C is the capacitance of the membrane, and V_m is the measured membrane potential difference. For a typical muscle fiber, $C = 1.6 \times 10^{-8}$ F ($C_m = 10^{-6}$ F/cm^2), $V_m = -90$ mV, and so $Q = 1.4 \times 10^{-9}$ coulombs (C), or only 1.4×10^{-14} molar equivalents, since there are 96,500 C/mol.

Now let us consider a burn patient with a cardiac cell (or any other excitable cell) whose resting membrane potential (-90 mV) is close to the E_{eq} for K^+ (-98 mV, using our sample data). If we inadvertently administer succinylcholine to this patient and drive the serum K^+ concentration to 10 mM, what would happen to the resting membrane potential? Obviously, it will become less, or depolarize, which will lead to arrhythmias and/or cardiac asystole. We can use the Nernst equation to calculate the new membrane potential (use the simplified form, $E_K = 61 \log_{10}\{[K]_o/[K]_i\}$). Note that the Nernst equation can be used to estimate changes in the resting membrane potential of some excitable tissues as long as the concentration gradient is known. In healthy individuals the intracellular $[K^+]$ is probably close to 150 mM. However, in patients with chronic renal failure and persistently elevated extracellular K^+, the intracellular $[K^+]$ is likely to be slightly greater; that is, the concentration gradient, and hence the resting membrane potential, is preserved via Na^+-K^+ pump-mediated redistribution of K^+. Another result of this increase in intracellular K^+ is that it takes a greater change in extracellular K^+ to alter the ratio and produce depolarization.

In reality, if we measure the resting membrane potential as a function of extracellular K^+ concentration, we find that there is a deviation from the anticipated Nernst relationship. There are several reasons for this, but one of the most important is the contribution of other permeant ions to setting the resting membrane potential. The "real" cell membrane is slightly "leaky" to other ions, notably Na^+, Cl^-, and Ca^{2+}. This leak can be via actual ion channels or ion exchange carriers. As the membrane permeability for K^+ drops, the contribution of these leak currents becomes more significant. The Goldman-Hodgkin-Katz equation addresses this situation by summing the E_{eq} for each permeant species and weights their contribution by the relative membrane permeability (P_{ion}) for each ion:

$$E_m = \frac{RT}{zF} \ln \frac{P_K[K]_o + P_{Na}[Na]_o + P_{Cl}[Cl]_o}{P_K[K]_i + P_{Na}[Na]_i + P_{Cl}[Cl]_i} \qquad (3)$$

Since the resting membrane permeability for K^+ is about 10 times higher than that for Na^+, the resting membrane potential is closest to the equilibrium potential for K^+, E_K. The Cl^- is either distributed passively or by ion pumps in such a way that its E_{Cl} is close to the resting potential. Leakage of Ca^{2+} is very small, and that which occurs is readily redistributed via ion pumps or bound by calmodulin, mitochondrion, sarcoplasmic reticulum, and so on. Note that this form of the equation does not take into consideration the contribution of charge transfer by electrogenic ion pumps. (These equations can get very complex!) Furthermore, this relationship can be used intuitively to predict the membrane potential any time changes occur in membrane permeability as long as the ion gradients and permeabilities are known.

Excitation   Nerve impulses are initiated by a variety of external stimuli. Pressure, stretch, chemical neurotransmitters (e.g., acetylcholine, serotonin, glutamate, etc.), and the passage of electrical current across the nerve membrane all can produce nerve activity. In each case, the stimulus produces a change in the membrane potential that can lead to an action potential, a self-regenerative process that allows the spread of excitation to all parts of an excitable cell.

Consider the experiment illustrated in Fig. 11–3, in which a nerve axon is stimulated at one end by the passage of electrical current while the membrane potential is measured at the other by a voltmeter. Figure 11–3 shows the applied current pulses and the associated changes in membrane potential. As the strength of the stimulus (current) increases, the membrane potential is displaced toward zero. The third stimulus was strong enough to cross threshold and elicit a spontaneous abrupt depolarization and subsequent return (repolarization) of the membrane potential to the resting level. Two conditions are crucial to eliciting this all-or-none response with a nerve stimulator. First, the current must be of sufficient magnitude to charge a critical mass of membrane capacitance to a suprathreshold voltage. Second, if the charging of the membrane capacitance occurs too slowly, even if it is sufficiently large, the nerve will fail to initiate an action potential. The reason will become clearer as we discuss the mechanisms underlying the nerve action potential.

A

B

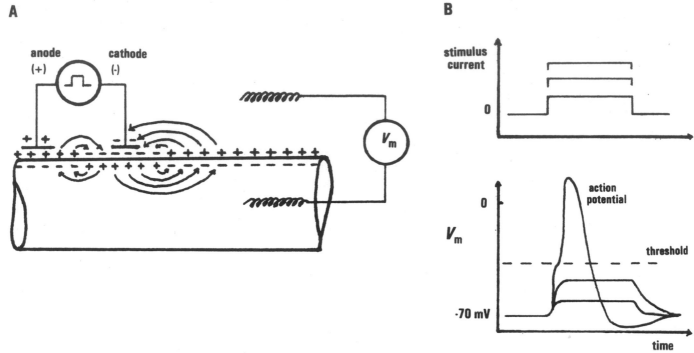

Figure 11–3 (*A*) A nerve axon is stimulated by the passage of extracellular current between two electrodes. Note that the membrane becomes hyperpolarized under the anode and depolarized under the cathode. A voltmeter, V_m, measures the membrane potential some distance away. (*B*) As the magnitude of the stimulus current is increased, the degree of depolarization becomes larger until the threshold for excitation is crossed and a regenerative action potential is triggered.

The Nerve Action Potential The action potential of nerve is produced by ionic current flowing through membrane channels whose conductance displays voltage and time dependence. The prototypical axonal action potential is shown in Fig. 11–4 along with the responsible membrane ionic currents. Starting from the resting potential, a suprathreshold stimulus produces a rapid upstroke (depolarization phase), which actually reverses membrane potential polarity. The membrane potential subsequently falls (repolarization phase) and usually undershoots the resting potential (after-hyperpolarization phase) before resuming the normal resting level. This complicated waveform is generated by a mixture of the inward and outward movements of ions through ion channels and active ion pumps.

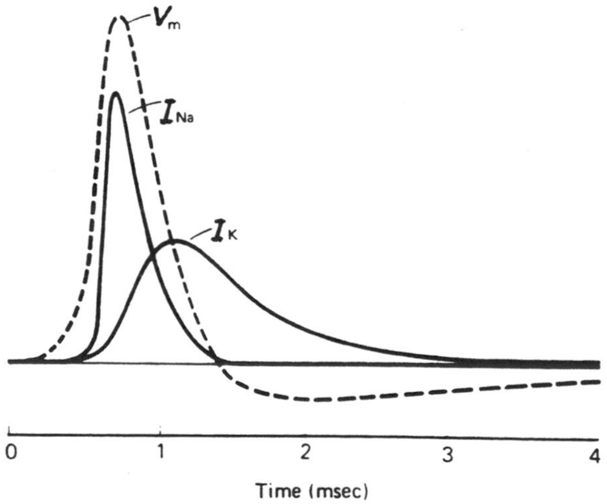

This chapter considers the classical description of the ionic conductance mechanisms underlying the action potential given by Alan Hodgkin and Andrew Huxley in 1952. Although it is not completely accurate, it is conceptually straightforward. The shortcomings of the H-H model are beyond the scope of this text and will not diminish our understanding of nerve electrophysiology from a clinical standpoint.

When a nerve axon is depolarized above threshold, a rapid transient current is produced by the inward movement of Na^+, followed by a more slowly developing and sustained current in the opposite direction, produced by the efflux of K^+. To define the membrane changes that produce these currents, Hodgkin and Huxley used an experimental technique called the voltage clamp on the squid giant axon. This device enables one to measure the membrane potential and control it in a predetermined manner via a series of amplifiers in a feedback circuit. The membrane voltage is "clamped" to a command voltage by the passage of a current through the membrane, which is equal in magnitude but opposite in po-

Figure 11–4 A typical axonal action potential with its rapid upstroke, repolarization, and "undershoot" (hyperpolarization phase) is shown. The time course of the underlying Na^+ and K^+ currents is superimposed. (Modified with permission from Hodgkin AL: *The Conduction of the Nervous Impulse.* Springfield, IL, Charles C. Thomas, p 63, 1964.)

larity to the membrane ionic current flowing in response to the change in membrane potential. By knowing the voltage and the current, Hodgkin and Huxley were able to use Ohm's law to calculate the membrane conductance.

For example, the Na^+ current (I_{Na}) will depend on membrane conductance for Na^+, g_{Na}, and on the difference between the membrane potential during a step depolarization (voltage clamp) and the equilibrium potential for Na^+, E_{Na}:

$$I_{Na} = g_{Na} (V_m - E_{Na}) \qquad (4)$$

A similar equation was written for the K^+ current:

$$I_K = g_K (V_m - E_K) \qquad (5)$$

They observed that, since V_m is held constant during a voltage clamp experiment and E_{Na} and E_K do not change during brief step changes in the membrane potential, then the fact that the currents were a function of time meant that the membrane conductance must be a function of both voltage and time. The voltage and time course of the changes in Na and K conductance were dissected using a variety of methods.

Depolarization produces a transient increase in g_{Na} and a slower and sustained increase in g_K. Immediately after a step depolarization, $g_{Na} >> g_K$, but after the cell has been depolarized for a time, $g_K >> g_{Na}$. In other words, both g_{Na} and g_K are complicated functions of time and voltage.

Hodgkin and Huxley introduced the variables *m*, *h*, and *n* to help them express the time and voltage dependence of the two conductances mathematically. In their nomenclature, *m* represented a Na^+ channel activation parameter, or gate, and *h* a Na^+ channel inactivation parameter. Since the K^+ channel showed only activation in their experiments, it was described by a single parameter, *n*. These parameters actually represent the fraction of the total number of channels available to conduct current or, more accurately, the "probability" that a channel will be in the open state.

They first described the voltage dependence by examining the values reached by *m* and *h* when the membrane potential was held at various values for a long time (i.e., steady-state). It was discovered that at very negative membrane potentials (e.g., the resting potential or greater), the activation gate was closed and the inactivation gate was open. However, as the membrane potential was depolarized with long voltage clamp steps, a larger percentage of the activation gates became opened, and the inactivation gates closed. Therefore, if a nerve cell were partially depolarized to a potential of -60 mV for more than a few milliseconds, as might occur in hyperkalemia, the Na^+ channel will be inactivated by the *h* gate and cannot be opened by further depolarization. A similar relationship for the K^+ channel activation parameter, *n*, as a function of membrane potential can be generated.

Next, Hodgkin and Huxley described the time dependence of *m* and *h*. If the axon is clamped at one voltage for a long time and then quickly changed to a new voltage, *m* and *h* change to new steady-state values at different rates. If substitutions for the permeant ion or selective channel blockers are employed, it is possible to dissect out the Na^+ and K^+ currents (and hence channel conductance time course), as illustrated in Fig. 11–5. The kinetics of the channel gating process are readily apparent when a nerve axon is voltage clamped from -70 to 0 mV instantaneously. The Na^+ channel, or *m* gate, moves the fastest, allowing an influx of Na^+ into the cell. As the *h* gate moves into position, the Na^+ channel shuts down and the Na^+ current tapers off. The K^+ channel, or *n* gate, which has the slowest kinetics of all, opens simultaneously, allowing the efflux of K^+.

From such data, Hodgkin and Huxley, as well as others, were able to produce a model that reproduced much of the behavior of the real squid giant axon action potential. However, investigations in other nerve preparations have revealed that the nerve action potential can be generated by several types of ion channels, including those permeable to Ca^{2+} and Cl^-. This will vary, depending upon the type of nerve, but in all cases, once the membrane threshold is crossed, the summation of voltage- and time-dependent ion currents (although in particular situations Ca^{2+}-activated ion currents may also contribute) produces a brief all-or-none fluctuation in membrane potential that recovers quickly. This important attribute allows the nerve to rapidly recover the ability to generate subsequent action potentials and subserve a role in high-frequency information transmission.

Single-Channel Currents Two German Nobel prize winners (1991), Erwin Neher and Bert Sakmann, have made it possible to record the current flow through individual ion channels by utilizing the patch clamp technique. The technique involves the placement of a micropipette with a fire-polished tip (0.5 to 1 μm diameter) against the membrane. Application of gentle suction in conjunction with the interaction between the negative charge on the membrane phospholipids and the glass wall of the micropipette results in a very high resistance seal (10 to 20 GΩ). This electrically isolates a small area of membrane (~0.8 μm^2) containing one to several ion channels that can be voltage-clamped (Fig. 11–6A).

Typical Na^+ channel recordings are shown in Fig. 11–6B. A step change in membrane potential within the micropipette (trace 1, marked V_p) is produced by the patch clamp amplifier. Each trace in section 3 represents a 60 msec recording of membrane current under the micropipette (I_p). This clearly demonstrates that the opening of a single ion channel (circled events) results in a transient inward jump in current of constant amplitude. This supports the theory that, when a channel transitions to the open state, it has a unit conductance that allows current to be driven by the electrochemical potential across it. The channel remains open for random lengths of time that are exponentially distributed. An open channel can return to one of the closed states (from which reopening is possible) or can enter the inactivated state (whereupon the channel becomes unavailable). Note that the probability of recording an opening event is greater early in the step depolarization and becomes progressively remote with time, presumably because of inactivation. The trace shown in section 2 is the algebraic sum of 300 individual patch recordings

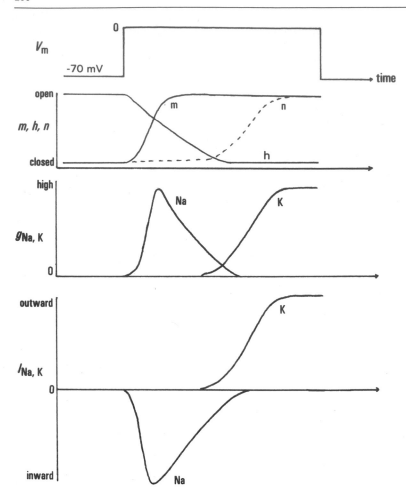

Figure 11–5 The time course of Na$^+$ and K$^+$ currents and their associated membrane conductance changes are shown under voltage clamp conditions. At the top of the figure, a step change in membrane potential from −70 to 0 mV is made. This initiates a sudden increase in Na$^+$-channel conductance as the *m* activation gate opens. Simultaneously but at a slower rate, the *h* inactivation gate closes, shutting off the Na$^+$ channel. The K$^+$ channel is also opening upon depolarization, but the much slower kinetics of the *n* activation gate retard the rate of K$^+$ current development.

made under the conditions that produced the traces in section 3. The summation of multiple single-channel openings recreates the familiar transient inward Na$^+$ current described previously.

The patch clamp has revolutionized the study of both voltage-gated and ligand-gated ion channels by allowing high resolution of channel behavior. Such data will become prevalent in the anesthesiology literature investigating mechanisms of action of anesthetics and other drugs.

Absolute and Relative Refractory Periods Nerve cells are absolutely refractory during most of the action potential; a second stimulus cannot produce another action potential. During this period of time a significant number of Na$^+$ channels are inactivated and unavailable to initiate an action potential. For a short period thereafter, the nerves enter a relative refractory period, whereupon it is possible to elicit a response if the stimulus is larger than normal. This occurs when the Na$^+$ channels are transitioning between the inactivated state and the resting state (without returning through an open state), where they are available to initiate another action potential. However, it requires a critical number of recovered Na$^+$ channels to initiate a propagated action potential. Many factors can retard this recovery process, for example, the presence of channel-blocking drugs such as local anesthetics, inhibitory or excitatory neuronal inputs, general anesthetics,

nerve injury, or low temperature. The latter is commonly seen when cold saline irrigation is used prior to attempts to stimulate exposed nerves during surgical procedures or when attempting to assess the degree of neuromuscular blockade in a cold extremity.

Nerve excitability is also affected by the behavior of K$^+$ channels. The cell cannot fully recover until the K$^+$ channels have returned to their resting state. The reason will become apparent after we discuss the cable properties of nerves and conduction of the nerve impulse. The property of refractoriness places an upper limit on the frequencies at which nerves can conduct electrical impulses.

Conduction of Nerve Impulses A weak current flowing through a nerve may not initiate an action potential; nevertheless, it always produces local changes in the membrane potential. The effects of currents are particularly prominent in nerve and muscle fibers because these fibers are approximately cylindrical and have lengths many thousands of times their diameters. With this geometry, the intracellular plasma offers significant resistance to current flow such that various potentials exist at various distances from a point current source. The combination of this intracellular resistance plus membrane resistance and capacitance accounts for the characteristic attenuation over distance and the retardation in velocity of the effects of a locally applied current on

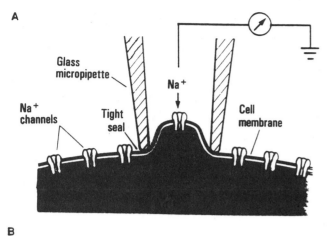

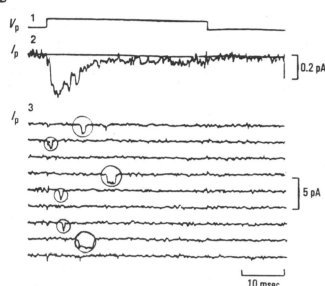

Figure 11-6 (*A*) A small patch of membrane containing a single Na$^+$ channel is electrically isolated by a patch micropipette sealed against the membrane with gentle suction. A special current amplifier measures the single Na$^+$-channel current that flows in response to step changes in membrane potential. (*B*) Recordings of single Na$^+$-channel openings in response to a 10 mV depolarization across the patch membrane are shown. (1) The time course of the step change in patch potential, V_p, is displayed. (2) The patch current, I_p, from the sum of 300 trials of the same step change in membrane potential bears a resemblance to the traces recorded from whole-cell recordings. The whole-cell, or axon, recordings of current represent the openings and closings of thousands of single channels. (3) Nine separate single-channel current traces from the 300 are shown. Individual single-channel openings are circled and are more prevalent at the beginning of voltage step, where the likelihood of inactivation would be less. (Modified with permission from FL Sigworth, E Neher: Single Na channel current observed in cultured rat muscle cells. *Nature* 287: 447-449, 1980.)

membrane potential. These behaviors are referred to as the cable properties of the nerve, after the analogy to the description of signal transmission in trans-Atlantic undersea telegraph cables.

An experiment to study these properties is shown in Fig. 11-7A. Membrane potential is measured simultaneously at several points along the length of a nerve axon. At point V_O a

constant current source injects a subthreshold current pulse via an intracellular microelectrode. The voltmeter at V_O records a large change in membrane potential that rises in a simple exponential manner. At point V_1 the voltmeter records a similar change in membrane potential, although the steady-state magnitude is less than point V_O and it rises more slowly. At point V_2 the membrane potential rises more slowly still and is greatly attenuated. Figure 11-7B illustrates the equivalent electrical circuit used to explain the passive (no action potential) or electrotonic spread of current down the axon. The flow of injected current through the intracellular and extracellular resistances will be proportional to the voltage gradient between points along the axon. As the intracellular current flows along the axon, some of it leaks across the plasma membrane as membrane current and completes the circuit via the extracellular resistor (note $r_a \gg r_e$). It should be apparent that the leakier (or higher the membrane conductance of) the axon, the less current is available to charge membrane capacitance in adjacent patches of membrane "downstream."

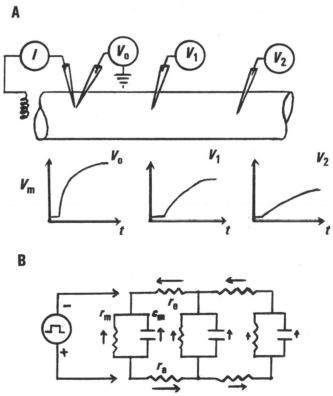

Figure 11-7 An experiment demonstrating the cable properties of neurons. (*A*) A square pulse of current is injected intracellularly at one end of an axon, and the resultant membrane voltage change recorded at several distances away. The change in membrane voltage is fastest and largest near the origin of the current, V_O, and becomes subsequently smaller and slower the farther away V_m is measured (V_1 and V_2). (*B*) The equivalent electrical circuit illustrates the path of current flow down the axon, r_a, to charge the membrane capacitance, c_m, to the new imposed value. However, some current is lost across the membrane resistance, r_m (nongated ionic pores). As more current leaks across the membrane, less is available to charge, c_m, downstream. The current completes its circuit through the extracellular fluid, r_e.

If the nerve relied on the passive spread of an electrical signal, the geometric constraints on the size and shape of the nerve would be enormous and impractical. Fortunately, the nerve is capable of generating an action potential, a self-regenerative process. However, the cable properties of the cell still affect nerve impulse conduction. When a patch of membrane is rapidly depolarized to threshold, Na^+ channels within the activated region allow a large Na^+ current to flow into the cell. This current further depolarizes the membrane potential to positive values. A large membrane potential gradient now exists between the active patch of membrane and adjacent quiescent patches of membrane still at a negative resting potential. The Na^+ current begins to flow into adjacent regions under the influence of this potential gradient and charges the membrane capacitance toward threshold. The rate and the extent to which this occurs will depend upon the cable properties of the cell. The higher the resting membrane resistance (the lower the membrane conductance), the greater will be the amount of current delivered downstream and the faster the adjacent quiescent membrane reaches threshold. This translates into a self-regenerating, rapidly propagating action potential.

A natural example of the application of cable theory is the myelinated axon. In the myelinated peripheral nerve, Schwann cells wrap a thick layer of lipid membrane around the axon, greatly increasing the effective membrane resistance in this region. Between these regions are exposed segments of axon that contain a high density of Na^+ channels, the nodes of Ranvier. An action potential initiated in one node of Ranvier is capable of supplying sufficient excitatory current to the next node of Ranvier, as much as 1 mm away, to bring it to threshold. The process repeats itself as the impulse conducts over long distances very quickly and efficiently. By markedly increasing the membrane resistance with myelin, the intracellular resistance can be greater without decrement in signal transmission. Therefore, myelinated axons are much thinner than their unmyelinated counterparts.

Integration of nervous input within nerve networks such as the ventral horn of the spinal cord also utilizes cable properties. The anatomical arrangement of synaptic inputs to a neuron can markedly influence its output. There are numerous variations of three basic synaptic inputs: axo-dendritic, axo-somatic, and axo-axonic. The axon hillock serves as the trigger zone for action potential generation, and usually numerous excitatory postsynaptic potentials in the dendritic tree must be summated to supply sufficient current to bring it to threshold. Axo-somatic synapses enjoy a strategic advantage in influencing neuronal firing because they can modify the resistance of the cell membrane separating the dendritic tree from the axon hillock. Fortuitously or by design, many inhibitory synapses are found on the soma or proximal dendrites.

In the neuron diagrammed in Fig. 11–8A, excitatory input to the dendritic tree produces small local depolarizations in membrane potential (excitatory postsynaptic potentials, or EPSPs) that set up local circuit currents that spread electro-tonically to the axon hillock. The fact that the membrane resistance of the soma is high and that it is physically large (low intracellular resistance) allows the current to spread with little decrement. Under these conditions, a few EPSPs might be expected to initiate an action potential.

Now, suppose that, after a few moments of nerve activity, a reflex arc is activated downstream. This negative feedback reflex arc activates an inhibitory neuron with its synapse on the soma of our neuron (Fig. 11–8B). It releases gamma aminobutyric acid (GABA), which opens channels permeable to Cl^- and K^+ and produces two major effects. First, it hyperpolarizes the synaptic membrane and tends to have a hyperpolarizing effect some distance away on the axon hillock. Second, by increasing conductance in the somal membrane, it essentially short-circuits the excitatory current coming from the dendritic tree. The combined effect is to prevent the excitatory current from bringing the axon hillock to threshold; thus, the neuron stops firing.

It should be apparent that the interplay among the characteristics of the individual membrane ion channels, the ion concentration gradients, and cell geometry determines the ability to transmit electrical impulses rapidly and repetitively. Numerous clinical examples can be found where these properties are either deliberately modified by pharmacological intervention (e.g., antiarrhythmics, local anesthetics, cardiac glycosides, Ca^{2+}-channel blockers, antiepileptics, etc.) or secondary to pathophysiological conditions (e.g., hyper- and hypokalemia, hyper- and hypomagnesemia, tissue injury, cell edema, toxins, etc.) in nerve, skeletal, cardiac, and smooth muscle.

☐ ION CHANNELS

Ion channels are complex integral membrane glycoproteins that are responsible for the translocation of ions through the cell membrane. So far, we have discussed how these channels function in terms of a model of one of the simplest nerve membranes, the squid giant axon. Most ion channels display more complex behavior. They can be simple ion-selective pores or "gated." Gated channels become permeable only when some specific conditions are met, for example, when a certain voltage exists across the channel or when certain ligands are bound as specific ions, neurotransmitters, or second messenger molecules.

In general, ion channel proteins consist of two or more subunits whose association within the membrane forms a central aqueous pore contiguous with the extracellular fluid and cytoplasm. The genes for seven major classes of ion channels have now been cloned and sequenced, allowing for unprecedented insight into ion channel structure and function. This knowledge will enable the development of drugs designed to modify certain aspects of a particular ion channel or receptor behavior while leaving other aspects unscathed and could lead to a better understanding of those diseases involving defects in ion channel or receptor proteins.

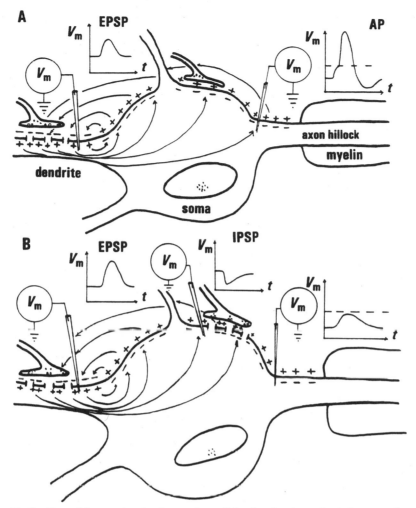

Figure 11–8   Neural integration begins at the cellular level, where the influence of excitatory postsynaptic potentials (EPSPs) and inhibitory postsynaptic potentials (IPSPs) is felt at the axon hillock, the initiation point of the action potential. (*A*) An excitatory input (EPSP) on a dendrite sets up passive, or electrotonic, current flow into adjacent areas of resting membrane. Although the current spreads with decrement owing to the cable properties of the neuron dendrite, soma, and axon, a sufficient amount is able to drive the axon hillock to threshold and an action potential is initiated. (*B*) Simultaneous activation of an inhibitory input (IPSP) on the soma effectively short-circuits the effects of the EPSP by hyperpolarizing the surrounding membrane and by worsening the cable properties (lowering membrane resistance). The net result is the failure of the axon hillock to reach threshold.

VOLTAGE-GATED ION CHANNELS

Neuronal Sodium Channels   The Na$^+$ channel is a prototypical voltage-gated ion channel found in nearly all excitable tissues. At least three subtypes of neuronal Na$^+$ channel have been cloned and sequenced, but all consist of approximately 2000 amino acids, including four highly conserved homologous repeat sequences (Fig. 11–9A). Each internal repeat has five hydrophobic segments (S1, S2, S3, S5, and S6) and one positively charged segment (S4), all spanning the cell membrane. The four repeats (I through IV) associate within the membrane to create an aqueous central pore (Fig. 11–9B). Each segment as well as each repeat sequence is interconnected with the next via cytoplasmic and extracellular loops of amino acids. Each membrane-spanning

segment probably assumes an α-helical structure. Segment S4 may function as the channel voltage sensor, moving outward slightly when the electrical field across the membrane decreases. This realigns the association between the other segments and causes the channel to open. Specific lysine and alanine residues within the core of repeats III and IV function as a highly selective filter, allowing only the passage of Na$^+$. The intracellular linkage connecting repeats III and IV is thought to be crucial for Na$^+$ channel inactivation, a process that closes the channel despite conditions favoring the open state.

Specific mutations in the Na$^+$ channel are thought to underlie certain muscle diseases. Hyperkalemic periodic paralysis is a syndrome manifesting as episodic periods of muscle weakness associated with a rise in serum potassium and oc-

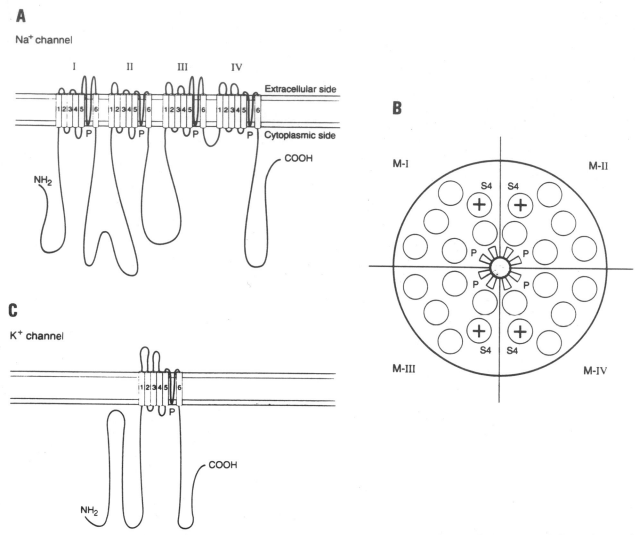

Figure 11–9 Models of the Na⁺ and K⁺ channel structure. (*A*) The amino acid sequence of the Na⁺ channel confers certain associations between the hydrophobic and hydrophilic regions of the chain and membrane. Four homologous repeat sequences (I through IV) span the membrane and are linked by short and long hydrophobic loops. The link between segments 5 and 6, marked with a *P* in each sequence, is felt to form the lining of the ionic pore. The intracellular link connecting repeats III and IV may function as the channel-inactivation gate. (*B*) The four repeat sequences, each with its set of six α helixes, congregate within the membrane to form a central aqueous pore lined by the P region of each repeat. (*C*) The amino acid sequence of the K⁺ channel also consists of six membrane-spanning α helixes linked by hydrophilic loops but has no repeat sequences. Since the formation of a K⁺ selective pore is felt to occur through the same aggregation of four units, it is thought that four similar individual subunits form the K⁺ channel. (Modified with permission from Kendel, Schwartz, and Jerrell, 1991.)

casionally myotonia. The disorder has been linked to a genetic defect of inactivation of skeletal muscle Na⁺ channels. A similar clinical syndrome provoked by cold, paramyotonia congenita, has also been related to a defect in the skeletal muscle Na⁺ channel.

Neuronal Potassium and Chloride Channels The K⁺ channels constitute a large heterogeneous family of membrane proteins that subserve a wide variety of functions. These channels set the resting membrane potential, terminate the action potential, regulate the pattern and rate of repetitive neuronal firing, and terminate bursts of neuronal activity. Despite the much more complex role performed by these chan-

nels, their overall structure seems simple. Similar to the Na⁺ channel architecture described above, the K⁺ channel consists of four polypeptide subunits. Although each subunit contains the familiar six membrane-spanning segments linked by extracellular and cytoplasmic loops of amino acids, unlike the Na⁺ channel, there are no repeat sequences of this sextet (Fig. 11–9C). The K⁺ channel is a tetramer formed by the approximation within the membrane of four distinct subunits or combinations of similar such subunits. The short loop between segments S5 and S6 (P region) dips inward and probably forms the lining of the pore. Analogous to the Na⁺ channel, the S4 transmembrane segment is thought to function as the channel voltage sensor.

Approximately five neuronal K^+ channel subtypes exist. One of the most familiar is the delayed rectifier, which plays a prominent role in the termination of the nerve action potential. The term *delayed rectifier* means that the ionic conductance of the channel increases slowly after depolarization (e.g., the Hodgkin-Huxley axon K^+ channel). This type of channel is predominant in the axon in three varieties, which are voltage-dependent but show various kinetics and pharmacologic sensitivities. The two faster subtypes show inactivation and are sensitive to the K^+-channel blocker 4-aminopyridine.

Neuronal membranes responsible for encoding the summation of input to the dendrites and soma may contain another type of K^+ channel, the A channel. The A channels produce a fast transient outward current that activates upon depolarization *after* a period of hyperpolarization. The channel inactivates rapidly when depolarization is maintained and displays greater sensitivity to 4-aminopyridine than does the delayed rectifier. The voltage dependence of this channel is interesting. It has a very steep voltage-dependent inactivation curve between -80 and -40 mV. This bestows upon the A channel the unique ability to modulate the frequency response (i.e., excitability) of the neuron in the face of a constant, intense stimulus. It does so by activating during the hyperpolarization phase of the preceding action potential caused by the delayed rectifier K^+ current. The additional K^+ current from the A channel suppresses the effect of a constant excitatory stimulus until the channel inactivates itself and the cycle repeats.

Other neurons are spontaneously active. Such "pacemaker" neurons provide a repetitive pattern of nerve impulses essential for timing physiological functions such as respiration. Following a spontaneous burst of nerve activity, intracellular Ca^{2+} rises and opens Ca^{2+}-activated K^+ channels, which hyperpolarizes the membrane and suppresses further neuron firing. As the intracellular Ca^{2+} is sequestered, the channel slowly closes and neuron excitability increases, initiating a new cycle. Two types of channels have been described: one is voltage-dependent, the maxi-K^+ channel (large conductance); and the other is modulated by a neurotransmitter, the SK channel (small conductance). The activity of Ca^{2+}-activated K^+ channels in various cells depends on a complex blend of the kinetics of Ca^{2+} influx, intracellular Ca^{2+} regulation, Ca^{2+} binding to ion channels, and voltage dependence. This channel type has a prevalence in neuronal soma, where it contributes to the slow onset after hyperpolarization and thus influences spike frequency adaptation.

Another class of voltage-dependent K^+ channels is regulated by chemical second messengers. Neurons with this channel subtype show a longlasting depolarization following exposure to acetylcholine or certain peptide hormones, such as luteinizing-hormone-releasing hormone (LHRH) or substance P. This subtype referred to as the M channel (after muscarine, since the acetylcholine effect is blocked by atropine) and is *closed* by these ligands, producing a long (several minutes) depolarization that enhances neuron excitability. The gating of these channels is thought to be mediated either through G proteins directly or indirectly through the production of cAMP.

The role of Cl^- channels in nerve is poorly defined. In other cells, these channels probably function in intracellular pH regulation, cell volume regulation, and the secretion of secretory gland contents. A nongated Cl^- channel contributes a large background permeability in skeletal muscle and probably sets the resting potential. A Ca^{2+}-activated Cl^- channel has been reported in mammalian sensory neurons, but its role is unclear.

Neuronal Calcium Channels Calcium plays an important role in translating electrical signals into a broad range of chemical and mechanical responses. It is essential for excitation-contraction coupling in muscle, synaptic transmission in nerve, and activation and modulation of numerous enzymes and biochemical reactions in addition to excitation-secretion coupling in many tissues.

At least four major types of Ca^{2+} currents have been described. Many subtypes of Ca^{2+} channels are being discovered and classified according to a variety of characteristics (Table 11–1). Some Ca^{2+} channels activate with a low threshold (i.e., small depolarizations from the resting potential turn on these currents), while others require large depolarizations. The Ca^{2+} channels have also been designated according to their kinetics and the size of their conductance. T-type Ca^{2+} channels have *t*iny conductances and produce *t*ransient inactivating currents. L-type channels have *l*arge conductances and produce *l*onglasting currents. It is not surprising that the T-type and L-type channels in one tissue may differ markedly from those in another. A third Ca^{2+}-channel type found extensively in *n*eurons has characteristics intermediate to the T and L types and has been designated the N type for *neither*. Finally, a P-type channel discovered in cerebellar *P*urkinje cells is activated at intermediate thresholds, shows slow inactivation, and has an intermediate-size channel conductance.

These channels can also be distinguished by their sensitivity to Ca^{2+}-channel blockers. Dihydropyridines, such as nifedipine, block L-type channels but not T, N, or P type. The N-type channel can be identified by its relatively selective blockade by ω-conotoxin, a cone shell toxin, while the P type strongly binds the funnel web spider toxin, F toxin.

The Ca^{2+}-channel structure is relatively large, with probably five subunits, denoted $\alpha1$, $\alpha2$, β, γ, and δ. The $\alpha1$ subunit has been studied the most extensively, and variability within this subunit may be responsible for the various characteristics of channel subtypes. The $\alpha1$ subunit of the L-type Ca^{2+} channel consists of the usual four sets of six α-helical transmembrane sequences. Again, the S4 region contains many positively charged amino acids, consistent with a role as an intramembranous voltage sensor. The $\alpha1$ subunit probably folds upon itself within the membrane to form the Ca^{2+}-selective pore in a manner similar to the Na^+ channel. The other subunits, $\alpha2$, β, γ, and δ, are thought to modulate channel kinetics and contain specific binding sites.

Table 11–1
TYPES OF CALCIUM CHANNELS IN NEURONS

	FAST, INACTIVATING		SLOW, PERSISTENT
	T Type	N Type	L Type
Activation range	Positive to -70 mV	Positive to -20 mV	Positive to -10 mV
Inactivation range	-100 to -60 mV	-120 to -30 mV	-60 to -10 mV
Decay rate	$\tau \approx 20$ to 50 ms	$\tau \approx 50$ to 80 ms	$\tau > 500$ ms
Deactivation rate	Rapid	Slow	Rapid
Dihydropyridine sensitivity	Resistant	Resistant	Sensitive

SOURCE: Modified with permission from Table 4.1, Hille, 1992.

LIGAND-GATED ION CHANNELS

Neurotransmitter, or ligand-gated, ion channels are produced from gene superfamilies separate from voltage-gated ion channels. As might be expected, some differences exist between the two types of channels, mostly in their control mechanisms. Ligand-gated channels are either incorporated into a receptor protein or are activated by a second messenger linked to a separate receptor protein. Binding of a ligand like a neurotransmitter usually increases the conductance of the ion channel and results in an ion flux driven by the usual thermodynamic forces described previously. Activation or deactivation of the receptor channel does not typically depend upon membrane voltage, although external influences (e.g., pH, extracellular divalent cation concentrations, and temperature) can modify the kinetics of ligand binding and activation of the channel. Finally, membrane depolarization produced by the activation of a few voltage-gated Na^+ channels can further activate other voltage-gated Na^+ channels, whereas the number of ligand-gated channels activated depends solely on the amount of ligand bound (i.e., it does not produce a regenerative action potential).

Nicotinic Acetylcholine Receptor The nicotinic ACh receptor at the neuromuscular junction is the prototypical ligand-gated ion channel. The transmembrane glycoprotein is so large (molecular weight 275,000) that clustering of ACh receptor channels can be resolved on electron micrographs. The channel pore cross-sectional area is estimated to be more than twice that of the Na^+ channel, allowing both Na^+ and K^+ to pass with nearly equal selectivity. In fact, even Ca^{2+} and small organic cations are permeable. Under physiological conditions, the reversal potential (essentially equivalent to E_m in Eq. 3) for current through this channel is about -5 mV, which is different from the E_{eq} for any of the usual ions. However, it is nearly halfway between the value of E_{Na} and E_K, as might be expected for a channel equally permeable to Na^+ and K^+. Fixed negative charges lining the pore exclude anions regardless of their size.

Five transmembrane polypeptide subunits, designated α, β, δ, and ϵ, comprise the adult nicotinic ACh receptor in the neuromuscular junction (Fig. 11–10A). Only the pair of α subunits are capable of binding ACh, one molecule each. The function of the other subunits is unclear. It is likely that they function in localization of the receptor within the neuromuscular junction and contribute to the gating function of the ion pore. The DNA of all four of the subunits has been cloned and sequenced and shown to be distinct but related genes. Somewhat similar to the structure of the voltage-gated ion channels, each subunit appears to consist of four hydrophobic regions (M1, M2, M3, and M4) containing 20 amino acids forming α helixes that weave back and forth across the membrane. The M2 region with the M2-M3 loop segment probably forms the ion pore lining. Again, the entire aqueous ion channel is formed by the contribution of this region from all five subunits. Neuronal nicotinic ACh receptors have different subunits but retain the pentameric structure with two ACh-binding α subunits.

When both ACh binding sites are occupied, the receptor channel undergoes a conformational change to the open conducting state. With prolonged exposure (seconds versus milliseconds) to ACh or other nicotinic agonists under experimental conditions, the channel can be transformed into a ligand-bound, inactivated state called desensitization. Like Na^+ channel inactivation, the ACh receptor-channel is incapable of being activated until this condition is reversed. This may occur clinically during succinylcholine administration or following inhibition of acetylcholinesterase by organophosphate poisoning. Recovery occurs spontaneously within minutes after the agonist is removed.

The nicotinic ACh receptor described above is the form found in the normal mature neuromuscular junction. However, the muscle fiber produces this junctional type only when there is constant neurotrophic input from an intact functioning α motor neuron. When this influence is interrupted (e.g., due to burns, upper or lower motor neuron lesions, or prolonged immobilization), the muscle fiber will begin to manufacture extrajunctional receptors. This type, which differs only in a substitution of a γ subunit for the ϵ subunit, is not confined to the endplate and can be inserted in large numbers throughout the muscle membrane. Extrajunctional receptors are more sensitive to agonists—both ACh and the muscle relaxant succinylcholine—than are junctional receptors. Extrajunctional ACh receptor channels have smaller single-channel conductances but significantly longer open lifetimes, resulting in a far greater efflux of K^+ from

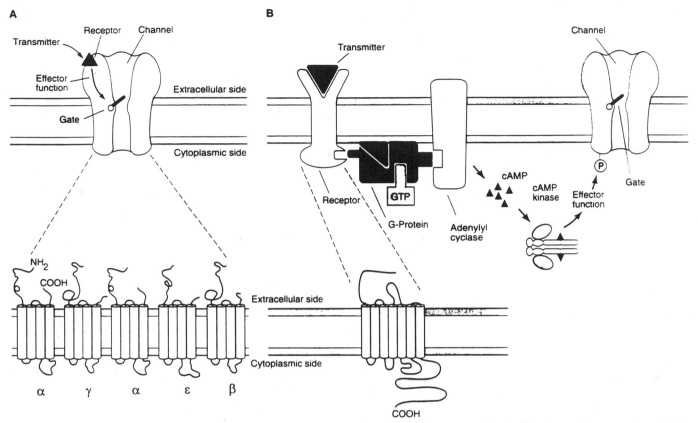

Figure 11–10   Types of receptor channels. (*A*) The junctional nicotinic ACh receptor is an example of a ligand-gated receptor channel. The binding of two molecules of ACh to the α subunits induces a change in the channel structure, allowing Na^+ and K^+ to move through the pore. The three-dimensional structure is similar to that of voltage-gated channels in that five subunits (2α, β,γ, and ε) aggregate to form a pore. (*B*) G-protein-coupled receptors can have widespread effects at a distance. The β-adrenergic receptor is typical, with its seven membrane-spanning α-helical regions. It has no repeat sequences. The α helixes associate in such a way as to create a binding site "pocket" for catecholamines. The third intracellular loop and the *N*-terminal "tail" probably contain binding sites for the heterotrimeric G-protein complex. Activation of the receptor starts a cascade that involves G-protein activation of adenylyl cyclase and then cAMP activation of an effector that can alter Ca^{2+} stores and ion-channel function. (Modified with permission from Kandel, Schwartz, and Jessell, 1991.)

the muscle fiber when activated. Such circumstances can produce dangerous levels of hyperkalemia and have resulted in death from cardiac dysrhythmias.

Gamma-Aminobutyric Acid Receptors   Ligand-gated channels abound in the CNS, where they have evolved into an elaborate system of inhibitory and excitatory mechanisms. One type of particular importance to the anesthesiologist is the inhibitory gamma-aminobutyric acid, or GABA, receptor found throughout the brain and spinal cord. The neurotransmitter GABA actually activates at least two receptors, one that directly gates an ion channel permeable to Cl^-, GABA$_A$, and another, GABA$_B$, which is linked via a G protein to Ca^{2+} and K^+ channels. Because GABA$_A$ is a directly gated channel, its inhibitory current is activated rapidly, in contrast to GABA$_B$, which requires the activation of a cascade of intermediaries.

GABA$_A$ receptors have the familiar pentameric structure, with each subunit possessing four membrane-spanning domains. Molecular biologists have characterized at least 15 GABA$_A$ receptor subunits, designated α_{1-6}, β_{1-3}, γ_{1-3}, δ, ε and ρ. Such diversity of subunits allows the construction of GABA$_A$ receptors with the potential for considerable devel-

opmental plasticity and function. In all cases, the effect of GABA$_A$ activation on the postsynaptic neuron will depend upon E_{Cl}. Since E_{Cl} is generally about ±15 mV around the resting potential, activation of this current will produce inhibition of excitability by stabilizing the membrane voltage at a subthreshold level. Blockade of the channel by picrotoxin, the competitive antagonist bicuculline, and other noncompetitive antagonists produces convulsions.

The GABA$_A$ receptor is the target for several drugs familiar to anesthesiologists. Barbiturates, benzodiazepines, alphaxalone, ethanol, propofol, etomidate, α_2-adrenergic agonists, and even volatile anesthetics have been implicated directly or indirectly in effects on the GABA$_A$ receptor. There seems to be little doubt that specific independent receptor sites exist on the macromolecule for barbiturates, benzodiazepines, and the benzodiazepine antagonists, such as flumazenil. The sedative-hypnotic and anticonvulsant actions of these drugs appear to be linked to their ability to either increase the number of open channels or enhance the total open time of the channel by increasing the duration of bursts of channel openings induced by GABA binding. Finally, there is compelling evidence that GABA$_A$ receptors may play an important role in the mechanism of anesthesia, since such a variety of chemically distinct anesthetic molecules can modulate the function of this receptor.

N-methyl-D-aspartate and Non-NMDA Receptors   The amino acid L-glutamate appears to be the primary excitatory neurotransmitter in the CNS, whereas in the peripheral nervous system ACh predominates. Basically, two broad categories of glutamate-gated ion channels have been described, based on their pharmacology. One important type selectively binds the agonist N-methyl-D-aspartate (NMDA receptor) and has unusual permeability characteristics. Those glutamate receptor channels that are selectively permeable to Na^+ and K^+ are opened by kainate or AMPA (α-amino-3-hydroxy-5-methyl-4-isoxalone propionic acid) and another type sensitive to quisqualate, which activates an unrelated G-protein-coupled receptor, are loosely grouped together as non-NMDA receptors. Most central neurons possess NMDA and non-NMDA receptors, and some actually have both types in the same synapse. Non-NMDA receptors are the sole fast excitatory input to motor neurons of the spinal cord.

The NMDA receptor channels are highly permeable to Ca^{2+}, and increasing intracellular Ca^{2+} levels may be part of their function. Their open-channel burst time is very long, and their affinity for glutamate is high relative to the non-NMDA receptors. However, the most unique characteristic is their voltage dependence. In the presence of glutamate, the channels pass current poorly at the resting membrane potential. However, when the cell is depolarized to -50 mV, channel conductance increases markedly. It is presumed that a voltage-dependent channel blockade by Mg^{2+} is relieved by depolarization, since removal of Mg^{2+} from experimental bathing media eliminates this phenomenon. Activation of this receptor also has an apparent requirement for glycine as a co-agonist. Its functional significance remains unclear.

The NMDA receptors probably play a central role in memory through a process called long-term potentiation. The unique characteristics of this channel enable it to activate in the presence of glutamate only *after* some other intense excitatory input has depolarized the neuron. Thus, it enhances the excitatory signal by increasing Ca^{2+} influx and probably triggers a cascade of intracellular events that lead to a persistent modification of the response of the neuron. In addition, NMDA receptors may function in the anatomical development of neural circuits in response to repeated experiences. Finally, NMDA receptors have been implicated in the phenomenon of excitotoxicity. Neuropathologic processes such as stroke, degenerative diseases, or head trauma may result in excessive excitation of NMDA receptors. High concentrations of intracellular Ca^{2+} may activate Ca^{2+}-dependent proteases and may produce oxygen free radicals that are capable of producing widespread cellular damage.

G-PROTEIN-COUPLED RECEPTORS

The G-protein-coupled receptors utilize an elaborate cascade system to produce widespread cellular effects, with each step allowing considerable amplification and control. This family of receptors includes the α- and β-adrenergic, muscarinic, cholinergic, serotonergic, dopaminergic, histaminergic, purinergic, and opioid as well as receptors for neuropeptides. There may be as many as 16 subtypes of G proteins and 100 receptors coupled to them. The typical receptor molecule is coupled to its effector via a guanosine nucleotide-binding protein, or G protein. Usually, the G protein activates an enzyme (e.g., adenylyl cyclase) that generates many soluble second messengers (e.g., cAMP), which subsequently modify ion-channel behavior, release Ca^{2+} stores, activate or inhibit cellular enzymes, and so on. The action produced by a G-protein-coupled receptor depends upon the type of G protein activated; some produce activation, others inhibition. The main difference between the actions of G-protein-linked receptors and the directly gated receptors is their speed of onset and duration. Whereas directly ligand-gated channels activate with a time course measured in milliseconds, receptors linked to a G protein require hundreds of milliseconds or seconds to produce an effect that can last for seconds or minutes. Such longlasting effects can have marked influences on neuronal information processing.

The β-Adrenergic Receptor and the G-Protein Cell Signaling System   The β-adrenergic receptor was the first to be associated with G proteins and will be used as a model. The entire G-protein-coupled receptor system is complex, employing a receptor macromolecule, a heterotrimeric GTP-binding protein, and adenylyl cyclase. Both β_1 and β_2 receptors are known to be coupled to adenylyl cyclase. The entire system is cell membrane-bound, but the components of the G protein are probably mobile within the membrane and shuttle between receptor and enzyme. The cAMP produced phosphorylates effector proteins via a cAMP-dependent protein kinase such as protein kinase A (PKA).

The mammalian β-receptor is a single-chain glycoprotein (molecular weight 56,000) with N-linked carbohydrates accounting for about one-fourth of its weight. In general, G-protein-coupled receptors have seven hydrophobic domains (amino acids wrapped in α helixes) that are thought to span the membrane and associate to form a cylinder perpendicular to the plane of the membrane (Fig. 11–10B). The amino terminus is extracellular, while the carboxyl terminus is intracellular. Extracellular and intracellular loops of amino acids interconnect the transmembrane segments in a serpentine fashion. Some of these loop segments are quite large and serve as binding sites or phosphorylation sites.

The actual binding site for β-adrenergic agonists and antagonists is not known for certain, but it does not appear to be the extracellular amino terminus. Instead, the protonated amino group on catecholamines interacts with the receptor "pocket" formed by the transmembrane α helixes. Hydrogen bonding with the β-hydroxyl group and the catechol hydroxyl group occurs. Finally, interaction between the receptor and the aromatic portion of the catechol ring may stabilize the "head" of the molecule within the pocket.

The C-terminal portion of the third cytoplasmic loop and

the *N*-terminal portion of the cytoplasmic tail are critical in the formation of the G-protein binding site. Many subtypes of G proteins exist, but the one specific for the β-adrenergic receptor is the *s*timulatory cholera toxin-sensitive G protein, G_s. This protein is a heterotrimeric protein capable of greatly enhancing the activity of adenylyl cyclase. It consists of three subunits, α, β, and γ. The $G_{s\alpha}$ subunit contains the GTP binding site and is responsible for activating the catalytic subunit of adenylyl cyclase. The β-γ subunit of G_s may play a negative feedback role, inhibiting the activation of adenylyl cyclase.

The sequence of events in the G-protein signaling cycle (Fig. 11–11) begins with binding of the G_s heterotrimer to the free β-adrenergic receptor. At this point, GDP is bound to the α subunit. The combination of receptor and G protein markedly increases the affinity of the receptor for its ligand. With ligand binding, a conformational change in the receptor is transmitted to the G-protein trimer. The GDP is released from the $G_{s\alpha}$ subunit and is replaced by GTP. Simultaneously, the α and β-γ subunits dissociate from the receptor and each other. The GTP-$G_{s\alpha}$ subunit diffuses away to interact with its target effector, in this case adenylyl cyclase. The subsequent G-protein-effector interaction has two effects. First, the adenylyl cyclase is activated, and, second, the GTPase activity of $G_{s\alpha}$ is enhanced, leading to hydrolysis of its GTP to GDP. The GDP-$G_{s\alpha}$ is able to combine with another β-γ dimer, and the system is reprimed.

☐ SYNAPTIC TRANSMISSION

Nerve cells are unique in their ability to communicate with one another and other cell types in a rapid and precise manner referred to as synaptic transmission. Intercellular communication may occur via two types of synapses: chemical or electrical. Electrical synapses, or gap junctions, are more prevalent in cardiac and smooth muscle as well as liver epithelial cells. Few exist in the brain. The chemical synapse, with its assortment of neurotransmitters and second messenger linkages, is considerably more versatile and adaptable for subserving such complex roles in the brain as memory and learning. Therefore, we will focus on chemical synaptic transmission.

CHEMICAL NEUROTRANSMISSION

Presynaptic Events The neuromuscular junction, or the pre- and postsynaptic neurons of chemical synapses, are not structurally connected, as in gap junctions, but, rather, are separated by synaptic clefts approximately 20 to 40 nm wide. On either side of the synaptic cleft are highly specialized regions of nerve plasma membrane. The typical presynaptic nerve terminal contains mitochondria, an elaborate cytoskeletal network, numerous small and large synaptic vesicles filled with neurotransmitter, and active zones that are membrane specializations thought to be docking sites for vesicles. Synaptic vesicles are manufactured and filled with a particu-

lar neurotransmitter in the Golgi apparatus of the neuronal soma. The loaded vesicles are transported to the nerve terminal via a unique ATP-driven cytoskeletal transport system. Upon arrival they are released, linked together via actin filaments, and anchored around the active zones that appear as dense bars on electron micrographs. Bordering the active zones on either side are rows of intramembranous particles that are thought to be Ca^{2+} channels of the rapidly inactivating N type.

Depolarization of the nerve terminal by an action potential results in activation of Ca^{2+} channels. The subsequent influx of Ca^{2+} may activate a Ca^{2+}-calmodulin protein kinase, which phosphorylates the protein attachment, synapsin I, of the synaptic vesicles to the actin filaments. Phosphorylation of synapsin I releases the synaptic vesicles, freeing them to move into the active zone. Two low-molecular-weight G proteins may guide the synaptic vesicles into the release site. Although the mechanism is not precisely known, it is thought that vesicle fusion with the active zone induces the formation of a channel or fusion pore that allows the extrusion of vesicle contents into the synaptic cleft by exocytosis. At present, two candidates for the role of fusion pore proteins are synaptophysin and synaptogenin. Synaptophysin, a ubiquitous Ca^{2+}-binding synaptic vesicle membrane protein, is similar in structure to the gap-junction protein and may form a channel for the release of the contents of the vesicle. Synaptogenin, also a synaptic vesicle membrane protein, binds calmodulin and phospholipids, potentially enabling it to bind the synaptic vesicle to the presynaptic membrane in the presence of Ca^{2+}. Once its contents are released, the empty synaptic vesicles are absorbed into the cell membrane only to be retrieved and recycled via incorporation into coated pits at a distant site. The recycled coated vesicle can then be transported back to the nerve soma for degradation or can remain in the nerve terminal for reloading with neurotransmitter. For example, ACh can be synthesized in the nerve terminal from recovered choline and acetyl-CoA.

Postsynaptic Events The response to neurotransmitter release depends upon the postsynaptic cell and the type of ligand-gated receptor. Two types of postsynaptic synapses will be considered: the neuromuscular junction and the central neuronal synapse. The neuromuscular junction is probably the most straightforward example of synaptic transmission and certainly the best documented. It consists of an α motor neuron terminating on a specialized area of the skeletal muscle fiber called the motor endplate. Electron microscopy of this region reveals a depression in the surface of the muscle fiber where the membrane invaginates in a series of deep junctional folds. The surface of these folds is lined by the basement membrane containing several structural proteins and acetylcholinesterase, an enzyme that inactivates acetylcholine (ACh) released by the α motor neuron. At the crest of the junctional folds are clusters of nicotinic ACh receptors ($\sim 10,000/\mu m^2$).

Stimulation of α motor neuron releases about 150 synaptic vesicles in about 1 to 2 msec into the synaptic cleft. This

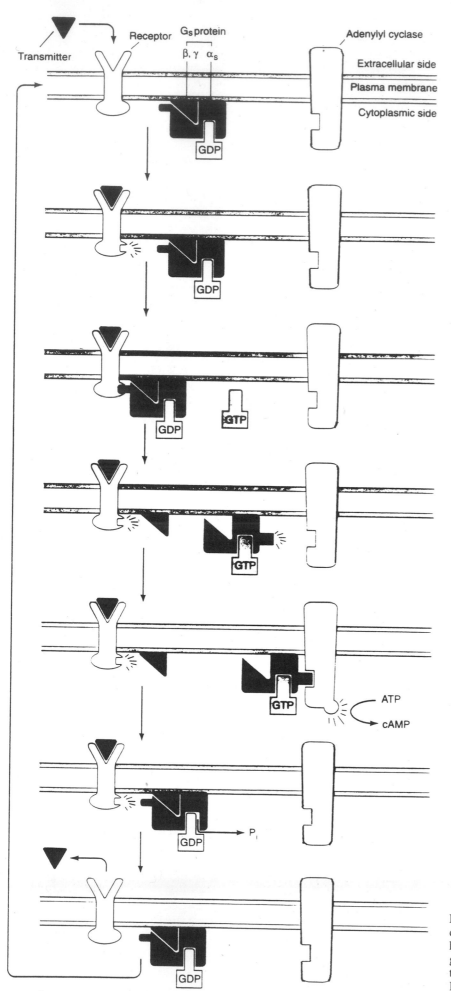

Figure 11–11 The G-protein signaling cascade. Components include a receptor protein, a heterotrimeric G protein (α_s, β, and γ subunits), guanine nucleotide, and adenylyl cyclase. See the text for details. (Modified with permission from Kandel, Schwartz, and Jessell, 1991.)

may represent the release of about 750,000 ACh molecules, which freely diffuse across the cleft to the receptors on the junctional folds. However, perhaps as much as 40 percent of the ACh may be lost by diffusion out of the cleft and the activity of acetylcholinesterase. The remainder binds to the ACh receptor, two molecules per receptor, and opens the channel. The resultant influx of Na^+ and efflux of K^+ depolarizes the endplate membrane potential (EPP), which sets up local circuit currents that depolarize the adjacent skeletal muscle membrane to threshold. The skeletal muscle action potential in turn triggers contraction of the muscle fiber.

The cleft concentration of ACh begins to fall as acetylcholinesterase hydrolyzes ACh into acetate and choline or it diffuses out of the cleft. As ACh comes off the receptors, the ACh channel closes and the endplate current terminates. Choline, which cannot be produced within the neuron, is actively taken up into the nerve terminal to be recycled. The motor nerve replenishes its synaptic vesicles, and the skeletal muscle fiber returns to a quiescent state.

The amount of neurotransmitter released, and therefore the number of receptors that can potentially be activated, can be modified by the influx of Ca^{2+} into the presynaptic terminal. A high-frequency train of nerve action potentials is followed by a period during which individual action potentials will elicit larger than normal EPPs. This high-frequency (50 to 100 Hz), or tetanic, stimulation is thought to increase the influx of Ca^{2+} into the nerve terminal to an extent that transiently saturates the intracellular Ca^{2+} buffering system. The build-up of the free intracellular Ca^{2+} concentration most likely enhances both the release of synaptic vesicles and their mobilization to the active zone. The extra release of neurotransmitter with each subsequent nerve action potential potentiates the size of the endplate potentials, a phenomenon that can last several minutes (posttetanic potentiation). We take advantage of this phenomenon when we use the nerve stimulator to assess the degree of neuromuscular blockade. By testing the response of the muscle twitch to tetanic stimulation, we can assess the balance between the number of available receptors and the ability of the nerve to mobilize and sustain its stores of ACh to effectively compete with residual muscle relaxant.

Synaptic transmission in the central nervous system differs from the neuromuscular junction in utilizing a wide variety of neurotransmitters that produce excitatory or inhibitory effects on the postsynaptic cell. In the CNS, excitatory neurotransmitters such as acetylcholine, glutamate, and aspartate increase the postsynaptic membrane permeability to Na^+ and K^+ or Ca^{2+}, producing excitatory postsynaptic potentials (EPSPs), which result in a heightened state of excitability in the postsynaptic neuron. However, unlike the neuromuscular junction, a single presynaptic neuron is incapable of exciting a postsynaptic cell sufficiently to generate an action potential. A single EPSP is generally too small in amplitude (<1 mV). Therefore, many EPSPs, usually produced by several repetitively firing neurons, are required to bring the postsynaptic neuron to threshold. In fact, while a muscle fiber is usually innervated by only one motor neuron, central neurons may have thousands of synaptic inputs. Inhibitory inputs

mediated by neurotransmitters such as GABA and glycine can increase the postsynaptic membrane permeability to Cl^- or K^+ to generate an inhibitory postsynaptic potential (IPSP). The IPSPs tend to hyperpolarize the postsynaptic membrane and prevent the neuron from reaching threshold. While we commonly think of excitatory and inhibitory inputs as opening ion channels, some types of receptors produce EPSPs or IPSPs of very slow onset by turning *off* either hyperpolarizing or depolarizing currents, respectively, to produce the same response in the postsynaptic nerve cell.

The relative contribution of the inputs at any individual excitatory or inhibitory synapse will depend on its size and location on the dendritic tree or soma and the proximity and strength of other concurrent synergistic or antagonistic synapses. Excitatory glutaminergic synapses tend to occur more often on the dendrites, while inhibitory synapses are found primarily on the cell body. Inhibitory synapses, therefore, enjoy a strategic advantage that enables them to effectively override excitatory inputs. While most integration of neuronal inputs generally occurs at the axon hillock where the action potential threshold is often the lowest, some cortical neurons will possess one or more trigger zones on the dendritic tree that are capable of amplifying weak excitatory inputs. These regions produce nonpropagating, local action potentials generated by the opening of Ca^{2+} channels. The electrotonic spread of current from such regions is then integrated in the soma and axon hillock as before. As described earlier, the cable properties of the cell greatly influences the electrotonic spread of current and has a major impact on the spatial summation of input. The higher the membrane resistance and the lower the intracellular resistance, the farther will be the passive spread of current for a given electrical driving force. Another important property is the time course of the synaptic potential. Obviously, those receptors activating an excitatory or inhibitory current with a slow time course will have a greater impact on the temporal summation of input.

Termination of synaptic transmission by the removal of neurotransmitter can differ, depending upon the type of synapse and the neurotransmitter. Aside from diffusion, which removes a fraction of all neurotransmitter substances from a synaptic cleft, neurotransmitter can be enzymatically degraded or actively recovered by the presynaptic neuron. In the neuromuscular junction and at cholinergic synapses, enzymatic degradation of ACh by acetylcholinesterase removes neurotransmitter rapidly and allows active reuptake of choline for recycling by the neuron. The neuroactive peptides have a long duration of action as a result of their slow rate of metabolism. It is thought that diffusion and proteolysis by extracellular peptidases are the only means of terminating their action. However, most synapses rely on active reuptake of neurotransmitter to terminate transmission. High-affinity cotransporter molecules in the membranes of the presynaptic nerve terminal or surrounding glial cells utilize the energy derived from the movement of ions down their electrochemical gradient and ATP. Norepinephrine, dopamine, serotonin, glutamate, GABA, and glycine are recovered in this manner.

☐ CLINICAL APPLICATIONS

ELECTROENCEPHALOGRAPHY

The electroencephalogram (EEG) is an electrophysiological technique that records the activity of neuronal ensembles, representing thousands of neurons, within the cerebral cortex. Although the various sensory, motor, and cognitive areas of the cerebral cortex differ by their various input and output connections to specific parts of the brain, they all are organized into vertical columns within the cerebral cortex. These columns, which run from the surface of the cortex down to the white matter, contain neurons organized into receptive fields that share similar interconnections and responses. Activity of ensembles is particularly evident in such behavioral states as wakefulness, sleep, and arousal, as well as in disease states such as epilepsy and coma. The EEG has proven to be a clinically useful qualitative tool in monitoring these conditions and in diagnosis.

In contrast to the types of electrophysiological recordings described earlier, the EEG represents an extracellular recording. Comparatively large macroelectrodes are employed to measure the electrical responses of neuronal ensembles either noninvasively by application to the scalp (electroencephalogram) or by placing an array of electrodes directly on the exposed cortical surface intraoperatively (electrocorticogram, or ECoG). This enables the recording of the fluctuations in electrical activity of the large ensembles of neurons directly beneath the arrays of electrodes. The electrical activity that is measured represents the ionic current flowing through the extracellular space surrounding the neurons. This extracellular current originates from the summation of many postsynaptic potentials rather than action potentials.

An understanding of cortical cytoarchitecture is necessary to appreciate the electrophysiological basis of the EEG. Cortical neurons are classified into two major groups. Pyramidal cells are large pyramid-shaped cells that are primarily excitatory and release glutamate as their neurotransmitter. They possess an extensive dendritic tree that enables them to receive many inputs from several layers of cortex, and, in addition, specialized regions of these dendrites are capable of generating localized Ca^{2+}-dependent action potentials that can amplify synaptic currents to increase their effectiveness. Their long axons extend to other parts of the brain and spinal cord, while collateral branches communicate locally with other neuronal ensembles. They are the major projection neurons of the cortex. The nonpyramidal cells have more oval-shaped bodies but are much more heterogeneous than pyramidal cells. Their axons usually do not extend farther than the cerebral cortex and frequently make synaptic contacts only within a cell column or within a restricted group of surrounding columns. Some subtypes, such as basket cells, make extensive synaptic contacts within very localized regions and are thought to produce surround inhibiton to isolate specific columns from the activity of others. These neurons and associated glia are arranged in an elaborate six-layer configuration with pyramidal cells primarily found in layers 4 through 6. The thickness of these layers varies from region to region and relates more to the function and input-output relations of the columns.

The EEG, like the electrocardiogram (ECG), is based on recording the extracellular flow of current from remote sites. Both are based on the theory of volume conduction. Extracellular current flowing between active and inactive or resting areas of excitable membranes produces an electrical potential difference the magnitude of which depends on the distance from the current source, the extracellular resistance (usually quite low), and the magnitude of the current. By convention, the site of current flow into the cell is called the sink, while the site of current flow out of the cell is the source. As depicted in Fig. 11–12A, the flow of synaptic current during an EPSP (I_{EPSP}) completes its circuit by flowing through the axial resistance (R_a), membrane resistance (R_m), and extracellular resistance (R_e). According to Ohm's law, the measured voltage difference (ΔV_e) between an extracellular electrode near the site of the current generator and a remote reference electrode will depend upon I_{EPSP} and R_e:

$$\Delta V_e = I_{EPSP}(R_e) \qquad (6)$$

Since R_e is very small, ΔV_m is small (microvolt range) despite the fact that, in practice, large numbers of EPSPs and IPSPs, not just a single synaptic event, are being summated simultaneously. Also, the recorded signal comes primarily from neurons near the electrode and only to a minor extent from distant neurons. As the exploring electrode is placed farther and farther from the signal generator, the amplitude of the signal becomes attenuated by the square root of the distance.

Direct interpretation of these extracellular recordings in terms of basic cellular events can be misleading. Regional input to the cerebral cortex, either excitatory or inhibitory, frequently occurs in a specific layer. For example, excitatory input from thalamic nuclei may synapse near the cell bodies of pyramidal cells in layer 5, initiating multiple I_{EPSP}s. By convention, scalp recordings of an inward current flow deep in layer 4 or 5 ("sink") with its corresponding outward flow of current in more superficial layers ("source") produces a downward deflection or "positive potential" (Fig. 11–12B). Note that this is different from the convention for intracellular recordings of the same phenomenon. Now, if the excitatory input occurs on the dendrites in the superficial cortical layers, then polarity of the recording will be reversed, since the current sink is close to the electrode and the current source is in the deeper layers. Be aware, however, that the electrode cannot distinguish an inhibitory synaptic current (source) occurring in a superficial layer from an excitatory synaptic current (sink) occurring in a deeper one. Both situations would generate a downward deflection or positive potential on a scalp electrode.

Each recording of an EEG signal requires at least 2 electrodes and as many as 20. One electrode is designated the active, or exploring, electrode and the other, the indifferent, or reference, electrode. The scalp electrodes are typically

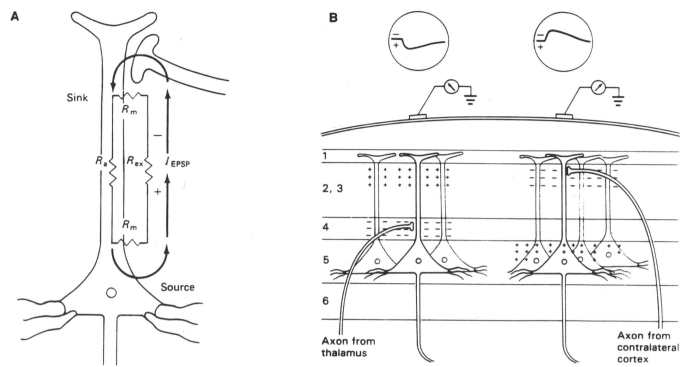

Figure 11–12 Cellular basis of the EEG. (*A*) An EPSP generates passive current (I_{EPSP}) that flows into the synapse (sink), exits the cell through the membrane resistance (R_m, source), and completes the circuit via the extracellular resistance (R_{ex}). The voltage drop across R_{ex} by I_{EPSP} is recorded by surface electrodes. The EEG results from the combined effects of many synaptic events. (*B*) By convention, a downward deflection on a surface EEG is a "positive potential," while an upward deflection is a "negative potential." The difference between the two types of electrical potentials is the location of the source of current. If the source of current is in the superficial cell layers of the cortex, then a positive potential is generated. If the source of current is in the deeper cell layers, then the opposite occurs. (Modified with permission from Kandel, Schwartz, and Jessell, 1991.)

placed over the frontal, parietal, occipital, and temporal lobes according to a standard recording scheme called the "10–20 system". Scalp electrodes are positioned starting at 10 percent of the circumferential distance above the inion, nasion, and external auditory meatus and 20 percent of the circumferential distance apart. Simultaneous recording of many pairs of electrodes allows analysis of the signals in the spatial and frequency domains. The data can be interpreted qualitatively by direct observation of the 16 to 20 channel recording. Alternatively, the raw data can be processed using a fast Fourier analysis to transform the complicated voltage signal into a series of sine wave harmonics that allow interpretation in terms of the power of the signal within specific frequency ranges. This manipulation is used in monitors that display the compressed spectral array (CSA), a three-dimensional display of frequency and power as a function of time, or the density-modulated spectral array (DSA), which presents the same information in a slightly different format.

Most clinical applications describe the EEG in terms of a few dominant frequency bands and amplitudes; β (13 to 30 Hz), α (8 to 13 Hz), θ (4 to 7 Hz), and δ (0.5 to 4 Hz) waves (Fig. 11–13). These frequency bands tend to characterize certain brain activity levels. For example, relaxed wakefulness is typified by α waves, while intense mental activity is associated with low-amplitude β waves. Very large-amplitude, slow θ and δ waves are seen during sleep.

EVOKED POTENTIALS

A currently popular form of intraoperative neurological monitoring, sensory evoked potentials (SEPs), utilizes the electrophysiological response of the nervous system to sensory stimulation as a means to assess functional integrity. Specific sensory stimuli are employed depending on the pathways at risk during surgery, such as a flashing strobe light (visual-evoked potentials), clicking noises (brainstem-auditory-evoked potentials), or electrical stimulation of sensory nerves (somatosensory-evoked potentials). Evoked potentials are frequently of very low amplitude (0.1 to 20 µV), smaller than the spontaneous EEG signal. Therefore, to resolve such small signals from background electrical noise requires filtering and special data processing.

Resolution of the evoked potential signal requires the summation of a consistent response to repetitive stimulation and computer signal averaging. The method is based on the premise that a novel uniform stimulus applied repetitively at a specific frequency elicits a specific CNS response that will appear with the same delay each time. Hundreds or thousands of these responses are recorded, summated, averaged by computer, and then the averaged signal is displayed as a single event. Since all other EEG activity and electrical artifacts are occurring at random times, their contribution to the averaged SEP becomes greatly attenuated, while the SEP sig-

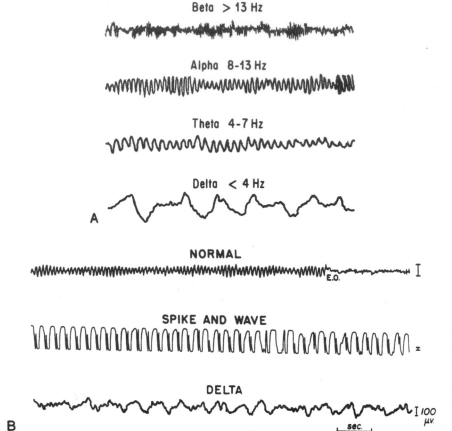

Figure 11-13 Examples of EEG signals. (*A*) Basic waveforms and their wave frequencies. (*B*) Examples of characteristic EEG traces, including a normal EEG with eyes closed and then eyes open (E.O.). (Modified with permission from Cucchiana RF, Michenfelder JD (eds): *Clinical Neuroanesthesia.* New York, Churchill Livingstone p 119, 1990.)

nal becomes enhanced. The SEP waveform is ultimately displayed as voltage as a function of time and can be analyzed according to the poststimulus latency and amplitude of the characteristic positive and negative waves.

The cellular basis for the SEP is presumed to be similar to that of the EEG. Surface electrodes are placed near the synaptic relay stations along the known afferent pathways of the sensory modality of interest. This allows recording of the postsynaptic potentials in a manner identical to the EEG. As with the EEG, the SEP is susceptible to modification by similar environmental conditions and drugs.

PATHOPHYSIOLOGY OF EPILEPTIC SEIZURES

Epileptic seizure activity reflects the abnormal synchronous discharge of large numbers of neuronal ensembles. This recruitment of large populations of neurons from diverse segments of the brain becomes possible because of the extensive networking between the sensory, motor, and associative areas so essential for processing of information.

The synchronous discharge of neurons produces the characteristic paroxysmal involuntary jerking movements and loss of awareness, even convulsions. Seizures can either be focal or generalized. Partial epilepsy is a form of seizure disorder that is limited to a particular region of the brain or subsequently spreads in a limited fashion to adjacent cortex. Manifestations of the seizure reflect the area of cortex involved. Loss of consciousness need not occur. If the limbic

system structures within the temporal lobe and orbital frontal cortex are involved, the seizures are characterized by complicated, semipurposeful movements associated with bizarre sensory phenomenon. Such complex partial seizures are referred to as psychomotor seizures.

Generalized epilepsy differs from focal forms in the extensive involvement of cerebral cortex and subsequent loss of consciousness. There are two primary types of seizures, petit mal and grand mal. In petit mal seizures, cognition, sensory perception, and memory are suddenly and temporarily interrupted but muscle tone remains unaltered. Grand mal seizures begin with loss of postural muscle control and an abrupt loss of consciousness then proceed to characteristic generalized tonic-clonic muscle movements.

The electrophysiological basis of seizures has been studied using an experimental model of focal seizures in animals. Experimental focal epilepsy can be established by the application of convulsant drugs or toxins directly to the surface of the cortex. A seizure focus can also be established by repeated high-frequency stimulation in certain areas of the limbic system. Months later, minimal stimulation of the same area can elicit a focal seizure. This raises the possibility that some forms of epilepsy may be produced by a brief event that induces a series of permanent changes in the properties of neural circuits, a mechanism possibly similar to long-term potentiation.

The initial abnormal electrical event observed on the EEG when a seizure focus becomes active is a series of intermittent high-voltage negative waves called interictal spikes. As their frequency of occurrence rises, they become superimposed on a slower negative wave. Eventually, low-voltage fast waves develop on the crest of the slow negative wave and a full-blown seizure ensues. The interictal spike reflects the synchronous activity of a large neuronal ensemble, possibly numbering in the thousands. The only difference between the EEG during a focal seizure and a grand mal type is that a characteristic spike and wave pattern appears simultaneously over the entire cortex.

Intracellular recordings made in neurons within the seizure focus display a characteristic sudden depolarizing potential referred to as a depolarization shift. This coincides with the initial portion of the interictal spike. A burst of action potentials is triggered during the peak of this depolarization shift, which is thought to be generated by an excitatory postsynaptic potential that is subsequently amplified by voltage-dependent membrane responses (dendritic action potentials). During epilepsy the normal balance between excitatory and inhibitory inputs is disturbed. One mechanism proposed is that cortical GABAergic inhibition is reduced thus removing the constraints (surround inhibition) on one group of neurons that normally would prevent them from exciting their neighbors. Other mechanisms, such as alterations in ion-channel proteins, appearance of novel neuroexcitatory substances, or the destruction of neuroinhibitory ones may ultimately be found.

PHYSIOLOGY OF CEREBROSPINAL FLUID CIRCULATION

The cerebrospinal fluid (CSF) is an aqueous solution of highly regulated constituents that cushions the brain and spinal cord as well as functioning as a chemical buffer between the blood and CNS interstitial fluid. The low specific gravity of CSF (1.007) as compared to the brain (1.040) reduces the effective mass of the brain from about 1400 g to less than 50 g. This greatly assists in reducing the inertial mass of the brain during linear and rotational acceleration movements. Tight regulation of pH, electrolytes, and metabolic substrates ensures greater homeostasis for an organ whose function is exquisitely sensitive to its environment.

About 70 percent of CSF is formed in the choroid plexus, a specialized vascular structure located bilaterally in the lateral ventricles and in the roof of the third and fourth ventricles. The remaining 30 percent is a by-product of utrafiltration of plasma across the ependyma and pia covering the remainder of the brain. The CSF is produced at a rate of approximately 0.4 mL/min, which allows the total adult CSF volume of 100 to 150 mL to be turned over about four times per day.

The choroid plexus consists of tufts of fenestrated (700 Å wide) capillaries separated from the CSF compartment by a single layer of ciliated, interconnected choroidal epithelial cells. The tight junctions connecting the apical portions of the epithelial cells are essential for restricting the passive exchange of solutes with the CSF. This constitutes the blood-CSF barrier at the level of the choroid plexus. CSF production occurs in stages. First, a plasma filtrate is produced by the bulk flow of water, ions, proteins, and other large molecules driven by capillary hydrostatic pressure through the fenestrae into the choroidal stroma. The movement of ions and water into the choroidal epithelial cells from the perivascular space occurs via facilitated ion exchange transporters (Na-H, Na-K, HCO_3-Cl), while essential vitamins, charged amino acids, neutral amino acids, ribonucleosides, and deoxyribonucleosides are transported by active transmembrane carrier proteins (Fig. 11–14). Secretion of CSF on the apical surface requires the active efflux of Na^+ and influx of K^+ under the control of ATP-dependent Na^+-K^+ pumps (Na^+,K^+-ATPase). Simultaneously, facilitated ion exchange produces an efflux of HCO_3^- and an influx of Cl^-, followed by the facilitated efflux of K^+ and Cl^- into the CSF. Intracellular carbonic anhydrase generates the HCO_3 from CO_2 and H_2O that diffuses into the cell or is produced by cellular metabolism. Water follows the osmotic gradient established by the ion fluxes. Essential vitamins, nucleic acids, and so on are secreted by facilitated diffusion into the CSF. Small proteins, Ca^{2+}, and Mg^{2+} gain access to the CSF either through the transcellular movement of pinocytotic vesicles or slip through leaky tight junctions between cells. Normal CSF protein concentration is about 0.5 percent of the plasma concentration.

Glucose transport across the blood-brain barrier is coupled to the movement of Na^+. The rate of glucose transport into CSF is directly related to the plasma glucose concentration although the carrier system does show saturation kinetics. This system appears to be independent of the serum-to-CSF glucose gradient and maintains CSF glucose concentration at about 60 percent of the plasma value.

CSF flows from the lateral ventricles into the third ventricle via the interventricular foramina of Monro. From the third ventricle, CSF passes through the narrow cerebral aqueduct into the fourth ventricle, which lies posterior to the pons and cephalad portion of the medulla. The CSF then enters the subarachnoid space via the median aperature (of Magendie) and the lateral apertures (of Luschka). From the cerebellomedullary cistern the CSF circulates freely through the subarachnoid space and its intercommunicating cisterns, while some passes caudally around the spinal cord as far as the level of the second sacral vertebra.

Most CSF reabsorption occurs within the arachnoid granulations and the villi of the venous sinuses, while approximately 10 percent occurs at the level of the spinal roots. The arachnoid villi are protrusions of the arachnoid membrane into the lumen of the sinuses and are covered with sinus endothelium. The interendothelial clefts act as unidirectional valves allowing CSF to be driven into the venous sinuses by the transvillus pressure gradient. The rate of CSF reabsorption is linearly related to intracranial pressure. At normal steady-state pressure CSF crosses the endothelium by micropinocytotic vesicles and through interendothelial clefts. However, under conditions of sustained elevated intracranial pressure (ICP), CSF reabsorption is enhanced through open

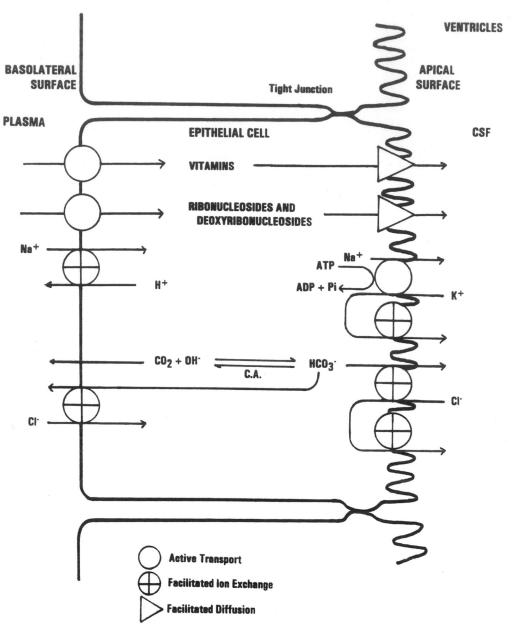

Figure 11–14 Diagram of the choroidal epithelial layer of the brain. A single cell layer of ciliated epithelial cells joined at the apical surface by tight junctions separates the blood plasma (cerebral blood capillaries) from the ventricles containing CSF. The CSF is formed by the translocation of water and numerous ions and large molecular substances by a variety of passive-active transport processes. Ions and some large molecules move across the cell membrane against concentration gradients by the ATP-dependent processes. Others are carried across by the movement of ions down their concentration gradients (facilitated carriers). Sodium bicarbonate is formed by the action of carbonic anhydrase. (Adapted from Spector R, Johnson CE: The mammalian choroid plexus. *Sci Am* 261(5): 68–74, 1989. Copyright 1989 by Scientific American all rights reserved. Fig from pg 72.)

transcellular channels formed by enlarged single vesicles or chains of fused vesicles completely traversing the endothelium.

Production of CSF can be modulated by cerebral perfusion pressure, plasma oncotic pressure, the autonomic nervous system, temperature, and numerous drugs. As anticipated, conditions that decrease cerebral perfusion pressure or blood flow like acute hypocapnia, hypothermia, or metabolic alka-

losis will reduce the production of CSF. It is well-known that acetazolamide, mannitol, and furosemide reduce CSF formation but by different mechanisms. Acetazolamide inhibits choroidal carbonic anhydrase and reduces the flux of HCO_3^-, furosemide inhibits Cl^- and Na^+ transport, while mannitol exerts osmotic effects to reduce the bulk flow of water across the epithelium. Dexamethasone may also inhibit choroidal Na^+,K^+-ATPase. Volatile anesthetics produce myriad effects. Enflurane will increase CSF formation, while halothane can decrease it. However, halothane also appears to reduce the rate of CSF absorption. Isoflurane and N_2O appear to have little influence on CSF formation. Ketamine can elevate ICP by virtue of its ability to increase the resistance to CSF absorption. On the other hand, high-dose etomidate decreases resistance to CSF reabsorption and reduces the rate of formation. The mechanism of action of ketamine and etomidate remains unclear.

INTRACRANIAL HYPERTENSION

One of the long-standing tenets of intracranial physiology has been the relationship between the fixed volume of the intracranial cavity and the incompressible nature of its contents first described by Alexander Munro (1783) and George Kellie (1824). The Monro-Kellie doctrine proposes that addition to or a change in the volume of the intracranial content of blood, CSF, or brain mass can initially be compensated by equivalent volume reductions in the other constituents. Failure to compensate for such additional intracranial mass results in an increase in ICP, referred to as intracranial hypertension. The relationship between changes in intracranial volume (dV) and ICP (dP) is described by the familiar hyperbolic function, which shows complete compensation until a threshold is reached, whereupon small increments in volume produce large increases in ICP. This relationship, dP/dV, is referred to as elastance. In the normal individual, elastance is very low. Note that the more familiar term, compliance, is a misnomer, since it really describes the relationship, dV/dP.

The normal CSF pressure in supine adults should be less than 10 mmHg (1.3 kPa), with the upper limit being 15 mmHg (2 kPa). Note that in an infant the upper limit of normal may be as low as 5 mmHg (0.7 kPa) because of the increased distensibility of an infant's calvarium. In cases of closed head injury, an ICP greater than 20 mmHg (2.7 kPa) produces signs and symptoms of brain dysfunction. However, this can be highly variable and depends upon maintenance of cerebral perfusion pressure. Nonetheless, a sustained ICP of 60 mmHg (8 kPa) is fatal. Normal ICP fluctuates in a cyclic manner as a result of the arterial pressure changes and the intrathoracic pressure changes of respiration. These fluctuations become pronounced in patients with cerebral edema. Brief physiological elevations of ICP occur routinely with coughing, head-down tilt, Valsalva maneuvers, and compression of the jugular veins. These transient rises, as much as 70 mmHg, are tolerated because the pressure is rapidly and equally distributed throughout the craniospinal axis.

The cerebrovascular and CSF circulatory systems are dynamic, and each will influence or be affected by elevated ICP differently. The manner in which ICP rises becomes important. For example, a slow-growing brain tumor might attain a size far exceeding the displaceable fluid volume without producing an increase in resting ICP, while a similar volume added acutely could be devastating. The difference lies in the ability of the intracranial constituents to compensate. Initial

compensation for an intracranial mass includes enhanced reabsorption of CSF and collapse of the dural sinuses and cerebral veins. CSF is also displaced down the craniospinal axis into the more distensible lumbosacral arachnoid space. Gradual changes, such as those encountered with a slow-growing tumor, can produce shifts in interstitial water, compression of nervous tissue, and, eventually, necrosis of the brain.

Pathologic increases in ICP can predispose the brain to two clinically important mechanical effects. First, gross increases can produce herniation of the brain through the foramen magnum or across meningeal-divided compartments. Second, cerebral perfusion (CPP) can be compromised if the mean arterial pressure (MAP) fails to keep pace with the increase in ICP. Cerebral perfusion pressure is related to systemic blood pressure and ICP as follows:

$$CPP = MAP - ICP \qquad (7)$$

As CPP declines, cerebral blood flow and oxygen delivery could diminish if cerebral autoregulatory mechanisms are damaged by drugs or disease processes, or the pressure changes are excessive.

The pathological elevations of ICP have been described and their characteristic waveforms categorized into three classes by Nils Lundberg (1960). The first is the A wave, or plateau wave, which is a sudden elevation of mean ICP to over 50 mmHg (6 kPa) that is maintained for 5 to 20 min before rapidly recovering to near normal levels. They occur at irregular intervals and usually in the presence of an increase in ICP. The ICP pulse pressure increases during the upswing of the pressure to form the plateau as a result of sudden cerebral vasodilatation under conditions of reduced intracranial distensibility. The plateau wave is associated with symptoms of increased ICP, such as headache, nausea, vomiting, and changes in the level of consciousness. Frequent plateau waves carry the most clinical significance and a grave prognosis. B waves are peaked, nonsustained elevations in ICP and occur at a frequency of 1 to 2/min. The ICP undergoes an abrupt upward rise, reaching a peak between 30 and 60 mmHg (4 to 8 kPa) and then immediately descends to normal levels. B waves are frequently seen in patients with severe head injury or disturbances in CSF circulation. They appear to be related to a Cheyne-Stokes type of respiration and are often seen in mechanically ventilated patients. Finally, C waves occur at a frequency of 5 to 6/min and are evident only when the mean ICP is already raised. They may be related to rhythmic oscillations in the systemic arterial pressure (Traube-Hering-Mayer waves). The B and C waves indicate brainstem dysfunction only if persistent for prolonged periods of time.

CELLULAR PATHOPHYSIOLOGY OF BRAIN ISCHEMIA

The maintenance of cellular homeostasis is an expensive energy-dependent process. Proper neuronal function requires continuous synthesis and replacement of damaged or senescent cell membranes, intracellular organelles, and specialized proteins such as receptors, enzymes, ion channels, and the microfilaments and microtubules of the cytoskeleton. The electrophysiological function of the cell is directly dependent upon the maintenance of intracellular Na^+, K^+, Ca^{2+}, Cl^-, and H^+ concentration by several ATP-dependent ion pumps and ion-exchange transporters, a requirement that increases tremendously during times of intense neuronal electrical activity. Axonal transport, which is essential for the delivery of neurotransmitter-laden synaptic vesicles and other proteins to the nerve terminus, is also ATP-driven. In fact, the energy required to sustain electrical activity during peak periods may be more than 50 percent of the total energy production of the cell.

The necessary energy, in the form of ATP, is produced by the usual biochemical pathways (i.e., oxidation of glucose by glycolysis in the cytosol, which itself has an ATP requirement) and the tricarboxylic acid cycle and oxidative phosphorylation within the mitochondria. However, unlike muscle and other tissues, which have a large capacity to store ATP and other high-energy compounds plus glucose or glycogen, the brain has minimal stores of either high-energy phosphates or metabolic substrate. Thus, the maintenance of a high energy consumption by the neuron is exquisitely dependent upon a continuous supply of O_2 and substrate and removal of CO_2 and toxic metabolites via the cerebral circulation. It has been estimated that within 20 s of cardiac arrest, the reserves of O_2 and other metabolic substrate in the brain are depleted. Anaerobic metabolism with ATP supplied by glycolysis continues until the intracellular stores of glucose are exhausted. Unfortunately, anaerobic glycolysis produces a rapid rise in intracellular lactic acid and subsequent acidification of the cell. The ability of the neuron to handle the increased intracellular H^+ load is lost because cellular extrusion requires ATP-dependent transport processes.

Complete global ischemia as produced in cardiac arrest is uniformly fatal to neuronal cells unless it is brief in duration or is preceded by manipulations that markedly reduce cell metabolism (e.g., profound hypothermia). Incomplete ischemia, as might occur with cerebral vessel occlusion but some collateral blood flow, is characterized by a central core of severe ischemia with a peripheral area of ischemic but still potentially viable tissue. This peripheral zone of functionally depressed but possibly salvageable tissue is referred to euphemistically as the ischemic penumbra. It is implied that restoration of blood flow to this region is capable of reversing the cellular changes produced by ischemia. Unfortunately, several detrimental processes can be initiated following the restoration of circulation, so that cell death may be inevitable. These end-stage processes and possible therapeutic interventions are discussed below.

Normal cerebral blood flow (CBF) is about 50 mL/min/ 100 g of brain tissue in the human and is more than adequate to meet the demands of cellular respiration. However, as CBF declines necessary cell functions that are expendable (e.g., synaptic transmission) become inactive in order to preserve those energy-dependent processes essential for the viability of the cell. At a CBF of 22 mL/min/100 g, the EEG, a measure of synaptic transmission activity, begins to slow. The critical cerebral blood flow necessary to maintain neuronal function has been measured to be 15 mL/min/100 g, when the EEG and presumably the cerebral cortex, becomes electrically silent. At this level of cerebral perfusion, synthesis of neurotransmitters ceases and the activity of membrane ion transport systems is slightly curtailed. At the point where structural protein synthesis is compromised, ATP depletion occurs, and consequently total failure of membrane ion transport mechanisms and loss of the ion concentration gradients occurs, the cell damage becomes irreversible. The threshold for membrane failure is about 6 to 8 mL/min/100 g CBF. It should be noted that these values represent critical cerebral cortical blood flows but presumably reflect what occurs in the rest of the brain as well.

Numerous mechanisms have been implicated in producing neuronal damage and cell death. A description of all the proposed mechanisms is beyond the scope of this text. Instead, we shall focus on those pathways that are currently receiving the most attention in the literature. Most investigators would agree that the loss of cellular calcium homeostasis plays an important role in the pathogenesis of ischemic cell damage. The rise in free cytosolic Ca^{2+} concentration depends on both the loss of calcium pump function due to ATP depletion and the rise in membrane permeability to Ca^{2+}.

The loss of Ca^{2+}-transport mechanisms and its consequences are fairly obvious. Major ATP-dependent Ca^{2+} pumps reside within the cell membrane to extrude Ca^{2+} from the neuron and within the endoplasmic reticulum to sequester Ca^{2+} internally. Mitochondria can also sequester Ca^{2+} under situations of calcium overload. However, this mechanism becomes inoperable under conditions of marked intracellular acidosis (pH 6.0 to 6.4), as will be found in ischemic neurons. Furthermore, as cytosolic Ca^{2+} concentration rises, Ca^{2+}-activated degradative enzymes, such as phospholipases and proteases, will destroy both cell and mitochondrial membranes, leading to a marked increase in cell permeability.

At the cell membrane, depolarization of the membrane potential secondary to accumulation of intracellular Na^+ and extracellular K^+ will activate voltage-dependent Ca^{2+} channels. The large influx of Ca^{2+} will strain cellular transport mechanisms further. However, attempts to block this route of Ca^{2+} entry with specific Ca^{2+}-channel blockers such as nifedipine in animal models of focal transient ischemia have not met with great success. It now appears that some of the more important routes of Ca^{2+} entry depend on activation of receptors by glutamate and associated excitatory amino acids released from depolarized presynaptic nerve endings.

Glutamate activates two broad categories of receptor channels, as previously described. The NMDA-type receptor channel is permeable to Ca^{2+} and passes current more easily under depolarized conditions. These conditions are optimized by ischemia. The other type, which binds kainate or AMPA (α-amino-3-hydroxy-5-methyl-4-isoxalone propionic acid), activates a receptor channel permeable to Na^+ and K^+. A third glutamate-sensitive receptor channel is linked via a G protein to phospholipase C. Activation of phospholipase C leads to the formation of the second messengers inositol 1,4,5-triphosphate (IP_3) and diacylglycerol (DAG) from phosphatidylinositol-4,5-biphosphate (PIP_2). The IP_3 mobilizes intracellular stores of Ca^{2+}, while DAG activates protein kinase C. The DAG contains an arachidonic acid skeleton, so its subsequent degradation may produce arachidonic acid, which may initiate additional signaling cascades (prostanoids, leukotrienes, etc.). Various experimental glutamate receptor antagonists or channel modulators have been used with some success in improving the neurological outcome in animal models of focal ischemia. In general, blockade of the Ca^{2+} influx appears to hold the most promise for improving the neurological outcome following ischemia. Unfortunately, those studies that showed the best outcomes administered their channel blockers prior to the period of cerebral ischemia. Therefore, resuscitation following ischemia still lacks a functional approach.

Other recent investigations of the role nitric oxide (NO) might play in mediating neuronal injury have produced mixed results. Nitric oxide mediates a wide variety of functions throughout the body, including regulation of blood vessel diameter, platelet function, possibly neurotransmission, and cytotoxicity. Those studies that have shown the most promise have indicated that inhibition of nitric oxide synthase worsens recovery of cerebral blood flow and subsequent neurological recovery. Interference with other NO-mediated effects in animal models of cerebral ischemia has not been elucidated.

Additional mechanisms of neuronal injury have implicated prostaglandins and oxygen free radicals. Prostaglandins are produced as a by-product of the interaction between free fatty acids and molecular oxygen. Phospholipase A_2, which is activated by Ca^{2+}, converts the abundant free fatty acids releasing arachidonic acid (in ischemic cells). The arachidonic acid follows a variety of pathways, depending on the cell type and available enzymes to produce leukotrienes, endoperoxides (prostaglandin G_2 and prostaglandin H_2, which subsequently form prostacyclin and thromboxane A_2), and the hydroperoxy acids (HPETE). These substances are potent vasoactive substances or platelet aggregators or are damaging to membrane phospholipids by virtue of their potential as free radicals. All of these reactions can alter reperfusion blood flow and the cellular response to reperfusion in many complicated ways. As with the studies of glutamate antagonists, pharmacological interventions that impede these prostaglandin cascades were far more effective if administered prior to the ischemic event.

BIBLIOGRAPHY

Bliss TVP, Collingridge GL: A synaptic model of memory: long-term potentiation in the hippocampus. *Nature* 361:31–39, 1993.

Cooper JR, Bloom FE, Roth RH: *The Biochemical Basis of Neuropharmacology,* 6th ed. New York, Oxford University Press, 1991.

Dichter MA, Ayala GF: Cellular mechanisms of epilepsy: a status report. *Science* 237:157–164, 1987.

Garthwaite J: Glutamate, nitric oxide and cell-cell signaling in the nervous system. *Trends Neurosci* 14:60–67, 1991.

Gjerris F, Borgesen SE: Pathophysiology of the CSF Circulation, in Crockard A, Hayward R, Hoff JT (eds): *Neurosurgery: The Scientific Basis of Clinical Practice,* 2d ed. Boston, Blackwell Scientific, pp 146–175, 1992.

Hille B: *Ionic Channels of Excitable Membranes,* 2d ed. Sunderland, Massachusettes, Sinauer Associates, 1992.

Kandel ER, Schwartz JH, Jessell TM: *Principles of Neural Science,* 3d ed. New York, Elsevier, 1991.

Lynch C, Jaeger JM: The G Protein Cell Signaling System, in Lake CL, Barash PG, Sperry RJ (ed): *Advances in Anesthesia,* vol 11. St. Louis, Mosby-Year Book, pp 65–112, 1994.

Miller JD, Piper IR: Raised Intracranial Pressure and its Effect on Brain Function, in Crockard A, Hatward R, Hoff JT (eds): *Neurosurgery: The Scientific Basis of Clinical Practice,* 2d ed. Boston, Blackwell Scientific, pp 373–390, 1992.

Muzzi DA, Wilson PR, Daube JR, Sharbrough FW: Electrophysiologic Neurologic Monitoring, in Cucchiara RF, Michenfelder JD (eds): *Clinical Neuroanesthesia.* New York, Churchill Livingstone, pp 117–170, 1990.

Siesjo BK: Pathophysiology and treatment of focal cerebral ischemia: Part 1, Pathophysiology. *J Neurosurg* 77:169–184, 1992.

Tanelian DL, Kosek P, Mody I, MacIver MB: The role of the $GABA_A$ receptor/chloride channel complex in anesthesia. *Anesthesiology* 78:757–776, 1993.

12

Hepatic Physiology

Barry Levin and Nancy Burk

A basic understanding of hepatic physiology is crucial to the anesthesiologist. Rarely a day goes by in the operating room that one aspect of hepatic function or physiology does not affect specific management of the patient by the anesthesiologist. This chapter is intended to give an overview of the anatomy, physiology, and basic functions of the liver.

The functions of the liver are many and diverse. Albumin and many plasma proteins, including most coagulation factors, are manufactured solely in the liver. Maintenance of serum glucose levels in the fasting state and synthesis of lipids and plasma lipoproteins are responsibilities of the liver. Many endogenous and exogenous substances, such as drugs, toxins, ammonia, lactic acid, and steroid hormones, undergo extensive metabolism and biotransformation in the liver. The liver is responsible for conjugation and excretion of bilirubin, excretion of bile salts, and storage of vitamins. In addition, the liver is an important component of the reticuloendothelial system.

☐ GROSS ANATOMY AND LIVER BLOOD FLOW

The liver is the largest gland in the human body, weighing over 1500 g in the adult. It resides in the right upper quadrant of the abdominal cavity, extending from the fifth intercostal space to slightly below the costal margin along the midclavicular line. It is divided by the falciform ligament into two unequal halves; the larger right half consists of three lobes, the smaller left half has one lobe. The liver has a dual blood supply; approximately 75% of hepatic blood flow (~1100 mL/min) is via the portal vein and approximately 25% (~350 mL/min) is via the hepatic artery, a branch of the celiac trunk. Total blood flow to the liver represents about 29% of the resting cardiac output. Because the portal vein blood is partially deoxygenated in the preportal viscera (stomach, intestines, spleen, and pancreas), by the time it reaches the liver it supplies only 50% of its oxygen delivery. Because venous blood flow contributes so heavily to hepatic perfusion, liver well-being is highly dependent on an uncompromised cardiac output. This is important clinically. For instance, during anesthesia with an inhalation agent, isoflurane is favored over halothane because this volatile agent reduces cardiac output to a lesser degree. The portal vein, despite being relatively poor in oxygen content, is rich in nutrients and other substances absorbed from the gastrointestinal tract. Normal portal vein pressure is approximately 7 to 10 mmHg. This pressure is determined by portal flow and resistance, which is principally postsinusoidal. Both the portal vein and hepatic artery are ensheathed in connective tissue and enter the liver through the porta hepatis, branching into progressively smaller vessels and pervading the hepatic tissue. Venous drainage of the liver is via the hepatic vein, which empties into the suprahepatic inferior vena cava.

The bile duct, the hepatic artery, and the portal vein constitute the portal triad. Bile from the tiny bile canniculi of the liver flows into progressively larger canals and progresses as follows: canniculi → intrahepatic ductules → interhepatic ducts → right and left hepatic ducts → hepatic duct. The hepatic duct is joined by the cystic duct of the gallbladder to form the common bile duct. The common bile duct is approximately 7 cm in length and empties directly into the duodenum.

Hepatic blood flow is characterized by several unique features. Unlike other vital organs (e.g., the brain and kidney), the liver exhibits no true autoregulation of blood flow over a range of mean arterial blood pressures. Instead, the liver utilizes the "arterial buffer response," which is a phenomenon whereby hepatic arterial vascular tone is influenced by local and intrinsic mechanisms and adjusts hepatic arterial flow to compensate for changes in hepatic portal vein blood flow. Decreases in portal vein blood flow are predictably associated with increases in hepatic arterial flow. This is an apparent attempt to maintain hepatic oxygen supply. The local and intrinsic mechanisms that adjust hepatic arterial tone and hence flow involve neural, myogenic, metabolic factors and portal blood oxygen content as well as the "washout effect." The washout effect refers to the accumulation of a substance, most likely the vasodilator adenosine, which causes hepatic arterial dilatation in the face of diminishing portal vein blood flow. Increasing portal vein blood flow washes out this vasodilator and hence reduces arterial flow.

The liver serves as a substantial reservoir of blood volume. This reservoir function is mediated mainly through the sympathetic nervous system. Stimulation of α adrenoreceptors may cause a release of up to 500 mL of blood into the systemic circulation. In severe acute blood loss, this additional 500 mL of blood may be lifesaving. However, in patients under deep anesthesia (with the resultant decreased sympathetic tone) and in patients with severe liver disease (who are known to have a decreased sensitivity to catecholamines), this mechanism may be attenuated.

☐ HEPATIC MICROANATOMY

The basic histologic or functional unit of the liver has been represented by two different models: the classic lobule and the liver acinus. These two models are not conflicting but, rather, reflect different interpretations of structure and function.

The hepatic lobule is essentially a hexagonal prism of liver tissue, about 0.8 to 2.0 mm in size, with a central vein in the middle and connective tissue with the portal triad (portal vein, hepatic artery, and bile duct) at the corners (Fig. 12-1). The human liver contains approximately 50,000 to 100,000 lobules. The lobule itself consists of many hepatic cellular plates that extend to the periphery of the hexagon, similar to spokes of a wheel (Fig. 12-2).

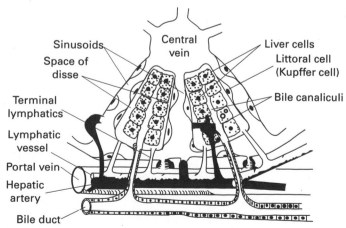

Figure 12-1   Basic structure of the liver lobule. (With permission from Guyton, Taylor, and Granger, 1975.)

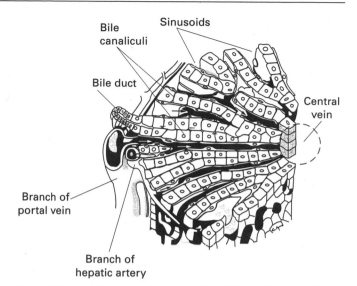

Figure 12-2   Schematic view of the liver lobule. The central vein (CV) lies in the center of the figure, surrounded by anastomosing cords of blocklike hepatocytes. About the periphery of the schema are six portal areas (PA) consisting of branches of the portal vein, the hepatic artery, and the bile duct. (With permission from Jones and Spring-Mills, 1977.)

Between adjacent cells of each hepatic cellular plate lie small bile canaliculi that empty into bile ducts found between individual lobules in the portal triad. Hepatic sinusoids are located between the cellular plates and connect the portal venuoles and arterioles from the periphery of the lobule to the central vein. Two types of cells line the hepatic sinusoid: endothelial cells and large Kupffer cells (tissue macrophages also known as reticuloendothelial cells). Hepatic parenchymal cells, or hepatocytes, lie across the space of Disse on the opposite side of these sinusoidal lining cells. The space of Disse connects with lymphatic vessels in the interlobular septa, enabling excess fluid in these spaces to escape through the lymphatic vessels.

The liver acinus represents a different concept of liver organization. In this model, parenchymal cells are grouped into concentric zones that surround each portal triad (Fig. 12-3). Since zone 1 cells lie closest to the source of oxygen and nutrients they are the least prone to injury. Zone 2 and 3 cells, which are farther from the source of nutrients, are more sensitive to toxins and oxygen deprivation.

Almost 80% of liver parenchymal mass consists of hepatocytes. Hepatocytes are relatively large cells with quite a diverse and complex set of functions. Nutrients (protein, carbohydrate, and lipid) and vitamins originating from splanchnic circulation empty into portal venous blood and are absorbed and subsequently stored by hepatocytes for their final release back into the blood in both bound and unbound forms. Hepatocytes also synthesize plasma proteins, glucose, cholesterol, phospholipids, and fatty acids. In addition, they excrete bile salts, which are required for intestinal fat absorption. Finally, hepatocytes metabolize, detoxify, and inactivate both endogenous (e.g., lactic acid, ammonia, and steroid hormones) and exogenous (e.g., drugs and poisons) substances.

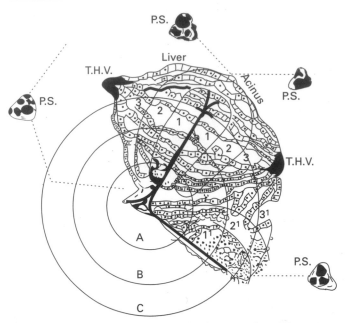

Figure 12–3 Blood supply of the simple liver acinus. The oxygen tension and the nutrient level of the blood in sinusoids decrease from zone 1 through zone 3. Zones 1′, 2′, and 3′ indicate corresponding volumes in a portion of an adjacent acinar unit. Circle A encloses the area commonly designated as periportal; B and C represent the area commonly designated as periportal; B and C represent the areas more peripheral to the portal space (PS) THV, terminal hepatic venules (central veins). (With permission from Rappaport, Borowy, and Lotto WN, 1954.)

Each hepatocyte contains a spectrum of intracellular organelles that carry out the various functions of the cell. Mitochondria are involved in oxidative phosphorylation and oxidation of fatty acids. Lysosomes are involved in digestion and catabolism of exogenous substances. The smooth endoplasmic reticulum is responsible for drug metabolism, while the rough endoplasmic reticulum is involved in protein synthesis. The Golgi complex is involved in very low-density lipoprotein production and albumin and bile salt secretion.

☐ HEPATIC RETICULOENDOTHELIAL SYSTEM

Kupffer cells, the large hepatic macrophages that line the sinusoids, make up the reticuloendothelial system in the liver. Approximately 99% of the bacteria entering the portal vein from the intestines are swallowed by these cells, lodged, and subsequently digested. These phagocytic cells are so efficient that, while results of blood cultures of specimens obtained from the portal system are often positive, systemic blood culture results are almost always negative.

☐ HEPATIC METABOLIC FUNCTIONS

HEMOGLOBIN DEGRADATION, BILIRUBIN CONJUGATION, AND EXCRETION

After roughly 120 days of life, red blood cells lyse and subsequently release free hemoglobin into the circulation. He-

moglobin is phagocytized by tissue macrophages of the reticuloendothelial system (spleen, liver, and bone marrow) and split into globin and heme. Biliverdin is formed from heme and then reduced to free bilirubin and subsequently released into the plasma. Bilirubin binds albumin and is then absorbed by hepatocytes and conjugated primarily with glucoronic acid. Conjugated bilirubin can then be excreted by active transport into the bile.

Intestinal bacteria convert conjugated bilirubin into the very soluble urobilinogen, which is reabsorbed into the blood and mostly reexcreted by the liver into the intestine, with only a small portion (5%) excreted by the kidneys. In urine, urobilinogen becomes oxidized to urobilin. In stool, urobilinogen becomes oxidized to stercobilin.

A thorough understanding of bilirubin metabolism is needed to distinguish the various etiologies of hyperbilirubinemia. Jaundice is defined as a yellowish hue of body tissues usually due to a buildup of bilirubin in the extracellular fluids. When jaundice is due to excessive hemolysis, hematoma absorption, or ineffective erythropoiesis, excessive amounts of indirect or unconjugated bilirubin is noted and accompanied by an increased level of intestinal and serum urobilinogen. When jaundice is caused by obstruction of the bile ducts or damage to the liver cells (e.g., as in hepatitis), increased serum levels of conjugated bilirubin are seen. Also, the presence of clay-colored stools, due to lack of stercobilin and other bile pigment, is noted.

GLUCOSE METABOLISM

One important aspect of hepatic function is its role in the multiple stages of glucose homeostasis. The liver is needed for (1) glycogen storage, (2) conversion of galactose and fructose to glucose, (3) gluconeogenesis, and (4) formation of many intermediate substances from carbohydrate metabolism.

The liver maintains normal blood glucose levels during feeding, after feeding (the postabsorptive state), and during periods of starvation. This maintenance of a relatively narrow range of serum glucose is referred to as the glucose buffer function. During feeding, glycogen stores are built up in the liver, which blunts the rise in serum glucose (glycogenesis). In the postabsorptive state, glycogen is broken down by the enzyme glucose-6-phosphatase to provide glucose for tissues (glycogenolysis). If a fasting state exceeds 48 h, glycogen stores are depleted. Amino acids, lactate, and glycerol are then used as substrates for glucose formation (gluconeogenesis).

In a patient with a poorly functioning liver, immediately after a meal consisting of a high carbohydrate load, serum glucose concentration rises to roughly three times normal. Also, in these patients, a fasting period for a short time (even <48 h) can cause life-threatening hypoglycemia.

PROTEIN METABOLISM

In contrast to its function in glucose and fat metabolism, the liver is indispensable in terms of its protein metabolic functions. Whereas one could sustain life without the glucose-

and fat-metabolizing ability of the liver, one would soon die without its ability to metabolize protein. There are four major functions of the liver in terms of its protein metabolism: (1) synthesis of most plasma proteins, including albumin; (2) conversion of ammonia into urea; (3) deamination of amino acids; and (4) interconversions among the various amino acids.

Hepatocytes are responsible for synthesis of roughly 90% of all plasma proteins. The two major notable exceptions are the procoagulant factor VIII (produced by endothelial cells) and gammaglobulins (produced by plasma cell in lymph tissue). Albumin, a single polypeptide chain containing 584 amino acids, is the major protein secreted by hepatocytes. Because of its relatively long half-life of 21 days, albumin is a poor indicator of liver function in a patient with acute hepatic disease. The daily protein output of the liver is about 50 g, and it can produce up to one-half of the normal total body protein in only 1 to 2 weeks. Even more impressive is the fact that, in the face of severe protein loss (e.g., as in protein-losing enteropathies, nephropathy, or severe burns), liver cells can divide and multiply, increasing the size of the liver and hence protein production.

In addition, the liver is responsible for the urea cycle, the function of which is to convert ammonia (a neurotoxin) into urea (a benign substance), which then can be excreted into the urine. The waste product ammonia is formed by deamination of amino acids as well as by the action of bacteria upon intestinal blood and dietary protein. The liver then needs to convert ammonia to urea, preventing the build-up of ammonia, which can lead to encephalopathy and death. Figure 12-4 is a schematic representation of the urea cycle, which uses a series of enzymes, energy, and water to transform ammonia into urea.

As stated earlier, gluconeogenesis involves the conversion of amino acids into glucose. The liver is the major source of amino acid deamination, which is required for this energy conversion.

Through transamination, the liver is able to synthesize certain amino acids and other important compounds from other amino acids. Some amino acids are referred to as essential (e.g., leucine and glycine) and are required in the diet. In contrast, those produced by the liver are referred to as nonessential amino acids and are therefore not a dietary requirement.

FAT METABOLISM

The liver is responsible for most of the fat metabolism in the human body. It plays a major role in lipoprotein and cholesterol metabolism. Specific functions include (1) β-oxidation of fatty acids into acetylcoenzyme A (acetyl-CoA); (2) formation of cholesterol, lipoproteins, and phospholipids; and (3) conversion of carbohydrates and protein into fat.

Fat is initially split into glycerol and fatty acids. As mentioned previously, gluconeogenesis involves the conversion of glycerol into glucose. Fatty acids are split by β-oxidation and ultimately form acetyl-CoA. Tremendous amounts of energy result from the entrance of acetyl CoA into the Krebs cycle. Leftover acetyl CoA may be condensed from two molecules into acetoacetic acid, which gets released to tissue throughout the body for further energy use.

Roughly 80% of the cholesterol synthesized in the liver is converted into bile salts, which in turn are necessary for cholesterol absorption from the intestine. The remaining 20% of cholesterol synthesized is used as a constituent in tissue cell walls as well as for the production of steroid hormones. Phospholipids, such as cholesterol, are synthesized in liver, transported in lipoproteins, and used as a component of cell membranes.

Most fat synthesized in the body is formed from carbohydrates and protein in the liver and is transported in lipoproteins to adipose tissue, where it is stored. Lipoproteins are divided into four classes: chylomicrons, very low-density lipoproteins (VLDLs), low-density lipoproteins (LDLs), and high-density lipoproteins (HDLs).

☐ THE LIVER AND COAGULATION

The liver produces the majority of procoagulant and coagulation inhibitor factors, with the exception of factor VIII. Vitamin K is required for the synthesis of four procoagulant factors, factors II (prothrombin), VII, IX (Christmas factor), and X; and two anticoagulants factors, protein C and protein S. Vitamin K absorption depends on excretion of bile into the gastrointestinal tract and the absorption of fat. Vitamin K deficiency and its consequent coagulopathy occurs in extrahepatic or intrahepatic cholestasis, malabsorption, antibiotic use, cholestyramine use, and, rarely, in dietary vitamin K deficiency. Prolongation of the prothrombin time (PT) in hepatic disease may be secondary to either vitamin K deficiency, a deficiency of factor production, or an increased level of inhibitors (which are not being metabolized by the liver). Administration of vitamin K will reverse the coagulopathy only from its deficiency and not from the coagulopathy due to liver failure itself. Clinically, when vitamin K replacement does not reverse the increase in the PT, a poor patient prognosis exists because severe deterioration of the liver has already occurred. In addition, administration of exogenous factors (Fresh Frozen Plasma (FFP), etc.) may not correct this coagulopathy because of increased levels of inhibitor factors present in the serum.

THE UREA CYCLE:

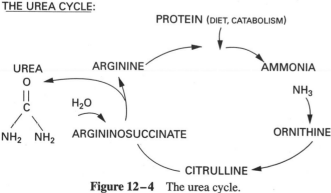

Figure 12-4   The urea cycle.

The half-life of factor VIII (4 to 8 h) is short, therefore, its level decreases early and to a greater extent than other factors during acute hepatic failure. On the other hand, factor I levels are maintained until late in acute liver disease, and it is the last factor compromised. In general, clinical bleeding will not occur until any factor level is reduced to less than 30% of its original level.

VITAMIN AND IRON STORAGE

The liver acts as an excellent storage depot for iron and a variety of vitamins. The vitamins stored in the largest quantity are vitamins A, D, and B_{12}. Vitamin B_{12} can be stored for roughly 2 years. Therefore, a deficiency of this vitamin may not be evident even in a diet lacking it for a prolonged period. Vitamin A can be stored for a 10-month period and vitamin D for 4 months.

Iron is stored in the liver as ferritin. Apoferitin, a protein found in hepatocytes, combines with extra iron in the body to form ferritin. When low serum levels of iron exist, ferritin releases it into the circulation. This system of iron storage and release is referred to as the blood iron buffer system.

FACTORS AFFECTING DRUG METABOLISM

There are two main mechanisms by which the elimination of a drug can be affected: changes in liver blood flow and changes in the ability of hepatocytes to biotransform or excrete a given drug or compound. The second process is called intrinsic clearance. Other mechanisms affecting drug elimination include changes in the ratio of bound to unbound (free) drug and changes in the volume of distribution.

Excretion of an unchanged substance into bile occurs more often with polar, water-soluble compounds or those compounds ionized at physiologic pH. Biotransformation is necessary for nonpolar lipid compounds, which are nonionized at physiologic pH, prior to their excretion and elimination.

Drugs are referred to as having either a high extraction ratio (ER) or a low extraction ratio based on the efficiency of their removal from the liver. Those drugs with a high ER are found in low concentrations in blood leaving the liver in relation to their concentration in blood entering the liver. Drugs with a high ER are more affected by changes in liver blood flow. Two commonly used drugs, lidocaine and propanalol, both with a high ER, have much longer clearance rates when liver blood flow is compromised. Other commonly used drugs, such as sufentinil and midazolam, have a low ER; thus, their clearance is relatively unaffected by alterations in hepatic blood flow.

Volume of distribution (V_d) is defined as the amount of drug administered to give a measured serum concentration of that drug. Elimination half-life ($E_{1/2}$) of a drug has been shown to be directly proportional to V_d and indirectly proportional to clearance (Cl) by the formula $E_{1/2} = 0.693 \times V_d/Cl$. The larger the V_d for a given drug at a set Cl, the greater the $E_{1/2}$. Patients with severe liver disease have an increased V_d due to both a decrease in protein binding and an increase in extracellular water. This contributes to the delayed $E_{1/2}$ of many drugs used in these patients.

DETOXIFICATION AND DRUG BIOTRANSFORMATION

All biochemical reactions responsible for detoxification and biotransformation are divided into two major classes, referred to as phase I and phase II reactions. A phase I reaction involves oxidation, reduction, or hydrolysis and either adds a chemical group to the parent compound or splits the parent compound into two fragments. The goal is to increase the polarity or the water-solubility of the drug to enable it to be excreted into either bile or urine. A phase II reaction (also known as a conjugation reaction) involves a coupling of compounds to a less toxic and more polar group. The substrates for a phase II reaction are frequently, but not always, the products of a previous phase I reaction.

PHASE I REACTIONS

Hydrolysis is the insertion of a molecule of water into a parent compound, forming an unstable intermediate that subsequently splits into more polar fragments. Examples of hydrolysis include metabolism of amide local anesthetics (e.g., lidocaine, bupivicaine, and mepivicaine) as well as metabolism of esters (e.g., succinylcholine). The following equation is an example of a phase I reaction.

$$R-\overset{\overset{\displaystyle O}{\|}}{C}-N-R' \xrightarrow{\text{hepatic esterases}} R-C-O-O-H + R'-N-H2$$

Reductive reactions involve adding electrons to a parent compound. This is the opposite to the process occurring in oxidative reactions, where electrons are removed from a molecule. Reductive biotransformation is inhibited by oxygen, and therefore it is facilitated by tissue hypoxia. This mechanism is responsible for the toxic reactive intermediates produced when halothane undergoes reductive metabolism. This is one proposed mechanism of halothane-induced liver toxicity.

The cytochrome p450 system is a complex of greater than 20 isoenzymes and pigmented hemoproteins responsible for many oxidative and a few reductive biotransformations in the liver. More than half of all drugs metabolized in the liver use this enzyme system. The p450 group of enzymes are formed in the smooth endoplasmic reticulum of hepatocytes. The name is derived from its heme-containing pigment, which, when reduced by carbon monoxide, absorbs light with a peak at the 450 nm wavelength. Many commonly prescribed drugs stimulate and enhance the metabolizing effect of the p450 system. This is referred to as enzyme induction. For instance, when phenobarbital is given as a single, one-time bolus, p450 enzyme activity peaks at 24 h. With continued drug exposure, enzyme activity continues to increase until a new steady state is reached, within 3 to 5 days. Enzyme activity decreases by one-half 24 h after removal of the inducing agent. This suggests that in 4 to 5 days (4 to 5 $t_{1/2}$) p450 enzyme activity returns to baseline. Inhibition of drug metabolism can occur if two drugs compete for the same site on the p450 system. This explains why cimetidine, an H_2 blocker causes increased serum levels of such drugs as meperidine, propanalol, and diazepam. Ranitidine, an H_2 receptor antagonist like cimetidine, has a different structure. It binds the p450 complex at a different site and thus avoids many of these potentially dangerous drug interactions.

PHASE II REACTIONS

Phase II reactions, or conjugation reactions, occur when a parent drug or compound reacts with an endogenous substance (e.g., a carbohydrate or amino acid) to form a water-soluble conjugate. Many drugs that undergo phase II reactions require a suitable functional group as a substrate, which is frequently obtained from a phase I reaction. A minority of drugs, such as morphine, undergo phase II reactions directly. Phase II reactions, like the p450 system, are inducible. Examples of phase II reactions include glucuronidation (the mechanism of bilirubin conjugation), methylation, sulfation, and acetylation. The following reaction (the conjugation of salicylic acid) is an example of a phase II reaction in which hepatic enzymes add a sulfhydryl group to salicylic acid:

$$R{-}C{-}OOH \longrightarrow R{-}\overset{\overset{O}{\|}}{C}{-}S{-}CoA + N{-}H_2{-}CH_2{-}COOH \longrightarrow$$

$$R{-}\overset{\overset{O}{\|}}{C}{-}NHCH2{-}COOH + CoA{-}SH$$

☐ LABORATORY EVALUATION OF LIVER FUNCTION

Elevation in serum transaminases SGOT and SGPT are reflective of hepatocellular injury rather than hepatic function or clinical prognosis. Elevation of these enzymes are fairly sensitive but poorly specific because they are also found in other tissues, such as heart muscle, skeletal muscle, and the kidney. The degree of elevation of these enzymes may reflect the degree of hepatocellular injury; however, a decrease in a previously high concentration may be attributed to decreasing ability to produce the enzyme. This can occur in chronic liver disease and end-stage liver failure, where the SGOT and SGPT may be normal or low.

An elevation in serum alkaline phosphatase occurs in the presence of hepatobiliary disease or obstruction of the biliary ducts. Alkaline phosphatase, like the transaminases, is fairly sensitive but poorly specific because this enzyme is also found in the intestinal tract, bones, and placenta. Hyperbilirubinemia may reflect either decreased hepatic uptake, decreased hepatobiliary excretion, or excessive bilirubin production. As discussed earlier, the amount of conjugated versus unconjugated bilirubin in the serum helps to distinguish hepatocellular dysfunction from cholestatic disease.

The best method of calibrating hepatic function is the measurement of its protein synthesizing ability. Albumin is the major protein synthesized by the liver. In the absence of a protein-losing disease and in the presence of adequate nutrition, low serum albumin levels reflect poor hepatic function. Low serum albumin levels in advanced hepatic disease predict a poor survival rate in patients undergoing surgical procedures. Prolongation of the PT is another indicator of depressed hepatic function because the liver is responsible for production of many coagulation factors (I, II, V, VII, IX, and X). Because only 30% of factor levels are required for a normal PT, an elevation is often a late finding in liver disease. Prolongation of PT is poorly specific. Other reasons for an elevated PT include vitamin K deficiency, poor clearance of coagulation inhibitors, altered plasminogen synthesis, primary fibrinolysis, and disseminated intravascular coagulation (DIC). Prothrombin time serves as an important prognostic indicator. An increase in the PT in the face of acute hepatocellular disease suggests a likely progression to fulminant end-stage hepatic failure. In chronic liver disease, an elevated PT suggests a poor long-term prognosis.

BIBLIOGRAPHY

Barash PG, Cullen BF, Stoelting RK: *Clinical Anesthesia,* 2d ed. Philadelphia, Lippincott, 1993.

Billian TR, Curran RD: Kupffer cell and hepatocyte interactions: a brief overview. *J Parenter Enter Nutr* 15(5): suppl, 1990.

Guyton A: *Textbook of Medical Physiology*, 8th ed. Philadelphia, Saunders, 1991.

Guyton A, Taylor, Granger: *Circulatory Physiology Two: Dynamics and Control of the Body Fluids*. Philadelphia, Saunders, 1975.

Jones AL, Spring-Mills E: In Weiss L, Greep RO (eds): *Histology*, 4th ed. New York, McGraw-Hill, p 702, 1977.

Rappaport AM, Borowy ZJ, Lotto WM: *Anat Rec* 119:11, 1954.

Remmer H: The role of the liver in drug metabolism. *Am J Med* 49:617–626, 1970.

Rogers MC, Tinker JH, Covino BG, Longnecker, DE: *Principles and Practice of Anesthesiology.* St. Louis, Mosby Yearbook, 1993.

Endocrine Physiology and Function

Steven Donatello

The endocrine regulatory and end organs consist primarily of the hypothalamic-pituitary axis, endocrine pancreas, thyroid and parathyroid glands, and adrenal glands. Complex positive and negative feedback loops link the various organs and provide interaction and regulation of hormone secretion. This chapter reviews and discusses the anatomy, regulation, and effects of these organs (with the exception of adrenal physiology, which is discussed elsewhere) and, when applicable, touches upon pathophysiology and its pertinence to the medical care of the patient.

☐ HYPOTHALAMUS-PITUITARY AXIS

The pituitary gland is connected to the hypothalamus via the pituitary stalk, which lies protected within the sella turcica. Physiologically, the pituitary gland lies outside of the blood-brain barrier. Functionally, it can be divided into the adenohypophysis, or anterior pituitary, and the neurohypophysis, or posterior pituitary. The adenohypophysis responds to specific hypothalamic-releasing factors and then secretes adrenocoricotropic hormone (ACTH), gonadotropins, growth hormone (GH), prolactin, and thyroid-stimulating hormone (TSH). It also secretes β-lipotrophin, which is cleaved to amino acid sequences of endorphins which bind to opioid receptors. The neurohypophysis secretes oxytocin and vasopressin in response to end-organ stimulation. These hormones are synthesized in the hypothalamus and transported down the pituitary stalk to the posterior pituitary, where they are stored for future release (Table 13–1).

ANTERIOR PITUITARY GLAND

ACTH is a neuropeptide synthesized in the pituitary gland as part of the large precursor, pro-opiomelanocortin (POMC).

The POMC is cleaved in the anterior pituitary to γ-melanocyte-stimulating hormone (γ-MSH), ACTH, and β-lipotrophin, as illustrated in Figure 13–1. ACTH regulates the secretion of glucocorticoids (primarily cortisol) and mineralocorticoids from the adrenal glands. A natural diurnal variation in the release of ACTH results in elevated morning and decreased evening levels of cortisol. The primary stimulus for increased ACTH release is physiologic stress, and, conversely, elevated cortisol levels have a major suppressive effect on the release of ACTH, as depicted in Figure 13–2.

The administration of exogenous steroids, especially on a chronic basis, may lead to a decrease in the functional integrity of this hypothalamic-pituitary axis. Because of the suppression of the normal feedback mechanisms, the potential for Addisonian crisis exists if steroids are abruptly discontinued. However, despite common medical practice, no controlled data exist to support the routine use of high-dose prophylactic steroids in patients undergoing surgery.

Gonadotropins, namely, follicle-stimulating hormone (FSH) and luteinizing hormone (LH), are synthesized in and released by the anterior pituitary gland. They each consist of two subunits of amino acid sequences that are synthesized independently and subsequently linked by a covalent bond. The α-subunits of the hormones are identical, while the β subunits differ in their amino acid sequences (by approximately 50%). Their primary site of action is the testes or ovaries, with secondary effects on other organs. FSH and LH bind to plasma membrane receptors on target organs (sex organs) and result in increased cyclic AMP (cAMP) formation, with subsequent stimulation and synthesis of various proteins. The end result includes pubertal maturation and the secretion of gonadal sex steroids, which ultimately regulate the development of secondary sexual characteristics.

Table 13–1
HORMONES SECRETED BY THE PITUITARY GLAND

Hormone	Location	Function
Adrenocorticotropic	Anterior pituitary	Stimulates adrenal maturation and secretion
Follicle-stimulating	Anterior pituitary	Stimulates ovarian follicle growth and spermatogenesis
Luteinizing	Anterior pituitary	Stimulates ovulation and testosterone secretion
Growth	Anterior pituitary	Stimulates tissue growth
Prolactin	Anterior pituitary	Stimulates milk secretion and inhibits ovulation
Thyroid-stimulating	Anterior pituitary	Stimulates thyroid growth and secretion
Oxytocin	Posterior pituitary	Stimulates milk release and uterine contraction
Vasopressin	Posterior pituitary	Affects water retention

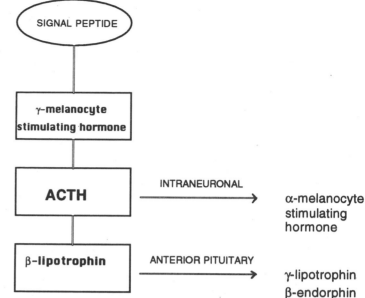

Figure 13–1   POMC structural components.

Growth hormone (GH or HGH) is an α-helical polypeptide chain that has a diurnal variation in secretion with a natural peak occurring at night. In addition, an increased secretion of GH is seen during periods of physiologic stress. GH results in the following effects on all human tissues: (1) stimulation of cell growth and reproduction, (2) an increase in protein synthesis, (3) mobilization of free fatty acids for metabolism, and (4) attenuation of glucose catabolism. The most important effect of GH is on bone metabolism, especially the pronounced growth that occurs at the epiphyseal cartilage of long bones. Thus, excess GH results in giantism prior to, or acromegaly following, epiphyseal closure. GH secretion can be suppressed by the administration of large quantities of exogenous corticosteroids. Metabolically, excess GH leads to glucose intolerance and increased serum glucose level. It is also accompanied by a concomitant increase in the metabolic rate. Other effects of elevated levels of GH may manifest clinically in a variety of pathophysiologic disorders, including cardiomegaly, hypertension, macroglossia, myopathy, neuropathy, and prognathism.

Prolactin (PRL), like GH, is an α-helical polypeptide of just under 200 amino acids. PRL release primarily occurs during pregnancy and results in mammary growth and development. This is in preparation for breastfeeding and increases even further when the infant begins feeding. Prolactin is an inhibitor of ovulation and (secondarily)

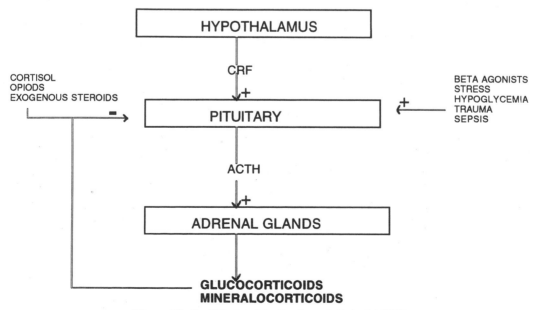

Figure 13–2   Effect and feedback regulation of ACTH.

menstruation. Abnormally elevated prolactin levels due to secretion of the hormone from a pituitary adenoma frequently presents as gynecomastia in males and secondary amenorrhea, galactorrhea, and infertility in females.

TSH consists of two covalantly linked, independently synthesized subunits with an α subunit almost identical to that of FSH and LH. TSH is responsible for the formation of thyroid hormone in the thyroid gland. TSH triggers an increase in circulating thyroid hormone by stimulating proteolytic cleavage of thyroglobulin stores in the gland follicles.

POSTERIOR PITUITARY GLAND

Antidiuretic hormone (ADH or vasopressin) and oxytocin are manufactured in the supraoptic and paraventricular nuclei of the brainstem, respectively. A precursor to vasopressin, prepropressophysin, is synthesized containing the vasopressin molecule bound to a signal peptide, a stabilizing compound called neurophysin II, and a glycopeptide tail. Following transport down the pituitary stalk to the posterior pituitary, the propeptide is cleaved to vasopressin and neurophysin II for storage within granules for future release.

ADH secreted from the posterior pituitary has a role in maintaining volume homeostasis by free-water retention. The release of ADH is stimulated by a host of factors, including hypotension, hypovolemia, increased plasma osmolarity, nausea and/or emesis, pain, and physiologic stress. Following transport in the blood, ADH binds to renal capillary epithelial cell receptors in the distal convoluted tubules and collecting ducts, resulting in the increased formation of cAMP. This causes an opening of pores in the cell membranes, thus providing an increased permeability to extracellular water and therefore free-water resorption. The water-retaining effects of ADH are attenuated by cortisol, fluoride ion (a potentially toxic metabolite of some of the inhalational anesthetics, e.g., enflurane), hypercalcemia, hypokalemia, and lithium. ADH secretion itself is inhibited by α agonists, cortisol, ethanol, and decreased plasma osmolarity. Also, ADH has a direct constrictor effect on arterioles, resulting in increased systemic vascular resistance, which may cause increased blood pressure if cardiac output is maintained.

Excessive release of ADH relative to the patient's volume status is referred to as the syndrome of inappropriate ADH release (SIADH), which can cause severe hyponatremia due to a retention of excess free water. Conversely, inadequate release of ADH in the face of a total body free-water deficit may cause diabetes insipidus (DI). This is sometimes observed with intracranial pathology, such as head trauma, elevated intracranial pressure, or surgical ablation of the pituitary gland. Patients with DI exhibit polydipsia, with the production of large volumes of urine (>250 mL/h) with a low urine specific gravity. This leads to an increase in the serum sodium level and osmolarity. The clinical diagnosis of DI may be confirmed with urine electrolytes (a low urine sodium level) and an increase in the urine osmolarity following the administration of exogenous ADH.

Oxytocin is synthesized, transported, and stored via a mechanism similar to that for vasopressin. Key differences involve the presence of neurophysin I in place of neurophysin II and the absence of a glycopeptide tail. Oxytocin, which is secreted by the neurohypophysis, causes the contraction of myoepithelial cells surrounding the mammary glands, resulting in the release of breast milk. In addition, it decreases the depolarization threshold for some types of smooth muscle (e.g., uterine), thus augmenting myocyte contraction. Clinically, oxytocin release immediately following childbirth causes myometrial contraction, which attenuates uterine blood loss after delivery of the fetus.

☐ PARATHYROID GLAND

Normal calcium homeostasis is mediated by parathyroid hormone (PTH), calcitonin, and vitamin D. Calcium homeostasis relies on a balance between gains from gastrointestinal absorption, losses due to renal excretion, and the balance between bone resorption and deposition. PTH is synthesized as a prohormone, preproPTH. The hydrophobic "pre-" sequence is removed as the peptide enters the endoplasmic reticulum lumen following synthesis. ProPTH, which lacks biologic activity, is proteolytically cleaved in the Golgi apparatus to the highly active hormone. PTH is stored in and secreted by the four parathyroid glands, located in the neck, primarily in response to decreased serum calcium levels. The principle sites of action of PTH are the kidneys and osteoid tissue. In the kidneys, PTH causes an increase in the calcium resorption while concurrently increasing the excretion of bicarbonate, phosphate, potassium, and sodium via transtubular ion transport. In addition, increased renal conversion of 25-hydroxycholecalciferol to 1,25-dihydroxycholecalciferol (the activated form of vitamin D) results in an increased gastrointestinal absorption of dietary calcium. PTH acts synergistically with activated vitamin D to stimulate bone resorption and decrease mineralization of bone collagen stroma. The net effect of PTH secretion, therefore, is an increase in the serum calcium level. Conversely, parathyroid hormone release is inhibited by elevated levels of magnesium and vitamin D. Administration of exogenous steroids, particularly glucocorticoids, may result in decreased serum calcium levels from inhibition of bone resorption and remodeling and thus increased levels of PTH secretion.

The incidence of hyperparathyroidism in the United States is approximately 50,000 patients per year, 50% of whom are asymptomatic and detected on routine laboratory evaluation (elevated serum calcium levels). Benign parathyroid adenomas account for the majority (80%) of these cases, with parathyroid hyperplasia accounting for the remainder. Although rare, neoplastic hyperparathyroidism may be seen in multiple endocrine neoplasia (MEN) type II, usually occurring in conjunction with medullary thyroid carcinoma and pheochromocytoma. Laboratory abnormalities encountered with these conditions include hypercalcemia, calcuria, hypophosphatemia, and decreased serum bicarbonate levels. The signs and symptoms that accompany hyperparathy-

Table 13-2
SIGNS AND SYMPTOMS OF HYPERPARATHYROIDISM

Signs	Symptoms
Cardiac dysrhythmias	Anorexia
Hypertension	Coma
Nephrolithiasis	Constipation
Osteopenia	Depression
Pancreatitis	Mental status changes
Renal tubular dysfunction	Nausea/emesis
Seizures	Weakness

roidism arc listcd in Tablc 13-2. In patients with an increased serum calcium level who undergo general anesthesia, the most frequent problem encountered is cardiac dysrhythmias that may be refractory to the usual medical therapy. Hypoparathyroidism in adults (Table 13-3) is a rare condition and is almost always iatrogenic in nature following surgical thyroidectomy. Hypoparathyroidism in children may be congenital, as is seen in DiGeorge's syndrome.

Calcitonin, which is synthesized in and secreted by the parafollicular C cells of the thyroid gland, is a polypeptide that antagonizes the effect of parathyroid hormone by a minor inhibitory effect on bone resorption and osteoclast activity.

☐ ENDOCRINE PANCREAS

The pancreas is both an endocrine and an exocrine organ; the exocrine portion secretes such enzymes as amylase and lipase to aid in digestive and absorptive functions. This chapter discusses only the endocrine pancreas. The endocrine function is to secrete four hormones: glucagon, insulin, pancreatic peptide, and somatostatin, which work in conjunction to maintain serum glucose homeostasis. All four hormones are synthesized in and secreted by the various cell types found in the islets of Langerhans. The role of pancreatic peptide is currently unknown. Somatostatin provides negative feedback on the islets, thereby decreasing glucagon and insulin secretion. Glucagon is synthesized in α cells, which

Table 13-3
SIGNS AND SYMPTOMS OF HYPOPARATHYROIDISM

Signs	Symptoms
Apnea	Mental status changes
Cardiac dysrhythmias	Paresthesias
Dermal changes	Weakness
Hypotension	
Laryngospasm	
Muscle spasm	
Seizures	
Tetany	

comprise approximately 20% of the mass of the islets of Langerhans. Insulin is synthesized and stored as a propeptide in the β cells, which comprise the remaining 80% of islets cells. Both insulin and glucagon are transported to the systemic circulation after release into the portal venous system.

INSULIN

Insulin is synthesized as preproinsulin, with the hydrophobic "pre-" sequence removed prior to arrival at the Golgi apparatus. Proinsulin is a single-chain polypeptide containing the A and B chains of insulin and a connecting C chain, as shown in Fig. 13-3. The presence of the C peptide chain allows for folding, and therefore correct pairing, of disulfide bridges between the Λ and B chains. Prior to granule secretion, proinsulin is cleaved to yield a double-chain molecule of insulin plus the C peptide.

The primary control of insulin secretion is serum glucose. Maximum stimulation of secretion occurs with glucose levels of 300 mg/dL or greater, whereas levels of 50 mg/dL or less result in cessation of secretion. The autonomic nervous system richly innervates the pancreas and provides insulin release in response to both cholinergic and adrenergic stimulation. Insulin release is further stimulated by growth hormone, corticosteroids, and, to a lesser extent, glucagon. The interaction between steroids and insulin is biphasic. Short-term administration of exogenous corticosteroids initially causes β-cell stimulation; however, following chronic stimulation, β-cell exhaustion and hyperglycemia may occur. Clinically, β blockade (e.g., propranolol) can result in decreased insulin release, which may exacerbate hyperglycemia. Under general anesthesia, the volatile anesthetic agents (to varying degrees) may also cause a decrease in the secretion of insulin, thereby enhancing the hyperglycemia seen during the perioperative period.

Insulin facilitates glucose uptake in hepatocytes by increasing the activity of glucokinase, which phosphorylates glucose intracellularly, resulting in trapping of the molecule.

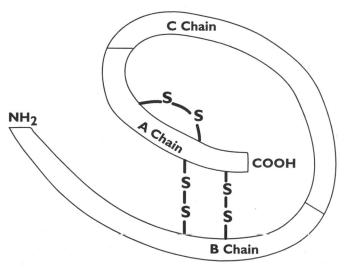

Figure 13-3   The structure of proinsulin.

Insulin also inhibits the phosphorylase enzyme, preventing the intrahepatic degradation of glycogen. Glucose entering muscle tissue under the influence of insulin undergoes a similar fate. Exercise results in an increased permeability of skeletal muscle membrane to glucose; however, the mechanism remains to be elucidated. Neuronal cells are the only human tissue not dependent on the activity of insulin to assist in glucose uptake; they can also utilize other sources of fuel (e.g., amino acids). During a prolonged fast, insulin levels decrease, thereby causing an increase in glucose production by the liver via both gluconeogenesis and glycogenolysis. A concomitant increase in circulating epinephrine and norepinephrine levels (stress mechanism) can further bolster increases in serum glucose levels.

Inadequate insulin levels results in severely depressed transport of glucose into cells, with resultant hyperglycemia. Initially, skeletal muscle is catabolized to provide intracellular substrate, causing an exaggerated elevation of the serum glucose level. Hepatocytes in the absence of insulin are unable to take up circulating glucose and instead catabolize fatty acids, with resulting formation of ketones. They are then released into the bloodstream to provide a usable substrate for cellular energy requirements. If present in high enough quantities, ketones may be excreted into the urine and are easily detected in the laboratory urinalysis. The cellular insulin requirement to prevent lipolysis is significantly lower than that to facilitate glucose uptake; therefore, conditions may occur under which hyperglycemia is present but not accompanied by ketoacidosis. This applies clinically in diabetic patients who are fasting prior to surgery, where low-dose insulin is given to deter the development of ketoacidosis with minimal risk of hypoglycemia.

Diabetes mellitus is a disease process characterized by a failure of cellular glucose uptake secondary to either an absolute or a relative absence of insulin. Type I, or insulin dependent, diabetes mellitus, (IDDM), which usually begins during childhood, is due to an absolute lack of pancreatic insulin production following autoimmune destruction of islet β cells. Patients with type I diabetes are, and remain, insulin-dependent and are therefore prone to the development of ketoacidosis in the absence of exogenous insulin. Type II, or non-insulin dependent diabetes mellitus (NIDDM), which usually has an adult onset, is due to a relative insulin inadequacy either from decreased pancreatic production or from decreased receptor sensitivity on target cells. The serum glucose in these patients can often be managed with oral hypoglycemic agents; in severe cases, such patients require insulin administration. They are not prone to the development of ketoacidosis but may present in hyperosmolar coma, which generally results from dehydration due to an osmoticdiuresis caused by hypercalcemia (Table 13–4).

GLUCAGON

Glucagon is synthesized as a preproglucagon molecule, which is cleaved to the active hormone just prior to release from the pancreas. The secretion of glucagon is triggered by

Table 13–4
CHARACTERISTICS OF DIABETES MELLITUS TYPE I AND TYPE II

Characteristic	Type I	Type II
Onset	Childhood, rapid	Adulthood, gradual
Insulin	Absent	Inadequate
Ketoacidosis	Prone	Uncommon
Hyperosmolar	Rare	Prone
Nutrition	Thin	Obese
Treatment	Exogenous insulin	Variable

serum hypoglycemia. Once glucagon reaches hepatocyte cell membrane receptors, adenylate cyclase is activated, and elevated cAMP results in glycogenolysis and gluconeogenesis, as well as the release of amino and fatty acids to be used as cellular energy substrates. When given in pharmaceutical doses, glucagon enhances myocardial chronotropy and ionotropy and increases mobilization of bile stores from the gallbladder.

☐ THYROID GLAND

The thyroid gland is located in the neck, anterior to the thyroid cartilage, between the larynx and sternal notch and consists of two lobes connected by a vascular isthmus. It is composed of follicles of thyroid cells surrounding a volume of thyroglobulin-bound thyroid hormone termed colloid. Thyroid hormone is an iodinated derivative of thyronine synthesized intracellularly (Fig. 13–4) and secreted into the follicle for storage. When released by the pituitary gland, TSH stimulates protease cleavage of colloid back into thyroxine and thyroglobulin, with the subsequent release of thyroxine into the bloodstream. Thyroxine has a serum half-life of approximately 7 days. Triiodothyronine (T_3), which is 3 to 5 times more potent than triiodothyroxine (T_4), is formed primarily by the hepatic or renal conversion of T_4 (80%) with a small contribution from primary synthesis in the thyroid gland (20%). The peripheral conversion of T_4 to T_3 yields equal amounts of active T_3 and inactive reverse T_3 (rT_3), each with a serum half-life of about 24h. For unknown reasons, physiologic stress may increase preferential formation of T_3. Thyroid hormones are extensively protein-bound in plasma, primarily to thyroxine-binding globulin (TBG) and, to a lesser degree, to prealbumin or albumin. Physiologically active free thyroid hormone accounts for less than 0.5% of the total circulating levels.

There has recently been an explosion of new information on the molecular basis of thyroid hormone action. Once delivered to the surface of a target cell, T_3 enters the cytoplasm and binds to nuclear receptors, resulting in the activation of DNA transcription and subsequent protein formation. Two known genes that code for T_3 receptors are α and β, which are located on chromosomes 17 and 3, respectively. Binding of T_3 to these gene receptors results in the formation of $α_1$,

Colloid

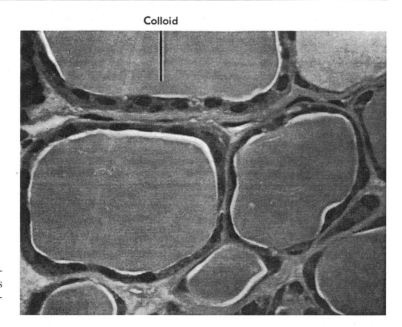

Figure 13–4   Follicles of human thyroid, showing epithelium of various heights and colloid secretion in follicles (×640). (With permission from Bevelander G: *Essentials of Histology*, 8th ed. Mosby-Year Book.)

α_2, β_1, and β_2 receptors. The role of all the receptors has not yet been exactly elucidated; however, it is known that receptor expression is both developmentally and tissue specific.

The end-organ effects of thyroid hormone include increased cellular minute oxygen consumption (except neuronal tissue), stimulation of carbohydrate metabolism, and increased mobilization of free fatty acids. In addition, thyroid hormone is necessary for the normal maturation and function of several tissues, including brain, cardiac, and skeletal muscle. This requirement appears to be mediated by T_3 β-receptor-dependent genes responsible for the formation of normal myelin basic protein, Purkinje cell protein, and TRH. The adrenergic effects of thyroid hormone (e.g. increased heart rate and contractility) are due to indiction of β receptor genes in cardiac muscle. Conversely, down regulation of genes coding for cholinergic receptors by thyroid hormone contributes to tachycardia.

The primary stimulus for thyroid hormone release is TSH, secreted by the pituitary gland in response to hypothalamic release of TRH (see Fig. 13–5). A negative feedback exists in which increased thyroid hormone levels inhibit further pituitary release of TSH, even in the presence of increased TRH.

Multiple laboratory tests can confirm the diagnosis of hyper- or hypothyroidism. Tests used to assess thyroid function frequently measure total T_3 and T_4, often by radioimmunoassay. Because only unbound hormone is able to exert a physiologic effect, the levels of circulating TBG must also be known. Alternatively, free T_3 can be measured by the T_3 resin uptake test, which provides an estimate of the unoccupied TBG sites. Free T_4 index (an estimate of unbound T_4) is the product of T_3 resin uptake and total T_4. Measurement of TSH levels can be useful in a variety of clinical settings, including differentiating primary hyperthyroidism (elevated thyroid hormone and decreased TSH) from secondary hyperthyroidism (elevated thyroid hormone and elevated TSH) and

hypothyroidism (elevated TSH and low thyroxine). Hypothyroidism may be either primary (elevated TSH and low thyroxine) or secondary (low TSH and low thyroxine).

THYROID DISORDERS

Hyperthyroidism   The clinical manifestations of hyperthyroidism may range from no apparent abnormalities to frank thyroid storm, with a majority of patients presenting somewhere in between. Clinical signs of the hyperthyroid state include atrial fibrillation, exophthalmos, goiter, hyperkinesis, and tachycardia. Clinical symptoms include diarrhea, dyspnea, fatigue, heat intolerance, palpitations, psychomotor agitation, sweating, and weight change. Secondary hyperthyroidism may be caused by the presence of an immunoglobu-

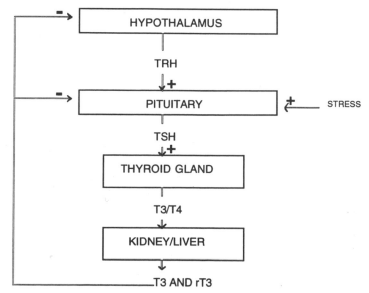

Figure 13–5   Regulation of thyroid hormone secretion.

lin A, which binds to the TSH receptors on thyroid cells, resulting in stimulation of synthesis and release of thyroid hormone.

The cardiopulmonary effects of hyperthyroidism are multiple. Baseline increases in cardiac rate and stroke volume occur, resulting in augmentation of cardiac output. A concurrent increase in myocardial oxygen consumption is present, which may be detrimental in patients with poor myocardial reserve (coronary artery disease). Arrhythmias, including atrial fibrillation and premature ventricular contractions, are common. Although a high incidence of congestive heart failure is seen in elderly patients, the mechanism of cause and effect remains to be determined. Cardiac death in hyperthyroid patients most frequently occurs with poor myocardial reserve and is secondary to myocardial infarction, myocarditis, or atrial thrombus formation. Respiratory complications due to excess protein catabolism and muscle wasting, resulting in muscle weakness, can significantly decrease vital capacity. If a resulting decreased minute ventilation is superimposed on the increased metabolic production of carbon dioxide, severe hypercarbia results and mechanical ventilation may become necessary.

Thyroid storm is a clinical diagnosis made by the existence of exaggerated symptoms of the cardiovascular and gastrointestinal systems. Frequent manifestations include nausea and emesis, tachycardia, pulmonary edema, pain, and frank cardiac failure (high output). Hyperpyrexia may or may not be seen. The mortality rate for untreated thyroid storm exceeds 80%; with proper, timely intervention, the mortality rate is less than 10%.

Hypothyroidism The clinical severity of hypothyroidism may, as with hyperthyroidism, not correlate well with the absolute laboratory values of thyroid hormone. Some signs of hypothyroidism include alopecia, thinning of the eyebrows, and bradycardia. Symptoms may include amenorrhea, anorexia, cold intolerance, constipation, depression, dyspnea, fatigue, impaired central nervous system function, myalgias, and voice changes. In severe hypothyroidism, patients often present with muscle weakness secondary to myxedematous infiltration, which causes elevated Creapine phosphokinase (CPK) levels. However, CPK values may be elevated even in the absence of gross muscle weakness. Hypothyroidism may lead to decreased myocardial contractility; paroxysmal angina can occur, with a proposed mechanism of increased end-diastolic wall tension. Despite a decrease in cardiac output, heart failure is unlikely because of a decreased total metabolic rate and decreased overall oxygen consumption. It remains unclear whether hypothyroidism is a risk factor for the development of coronary atherosclerotic disease.

The respiratory effect of hypothyroidism manifests as a decreased responsiveness of minute ventilation to hypoxia and hypercarbia. In addition, severe cases of hypothyroidism may involve myxedematous infiltration of the respiratory muscles, resulting in a decreased ventilatory reserve. Various other effects of hypothyroidism include hypoglycemia, hypothermia, and SIADH, causing hyponatremia. Myxedema coma, which is most often seen in elderly females, may manifest as hypercarbia, gastrointestinal bleeding, marked hyponatremia, hypotension, and coma. Although rare, this disease state has a mortality rate approaching 80%.

BIBLIOGRAPHY

Brent GA: The molecular basis of thyroid hormone action. *N Engl J Med* 331:847–853, 1994.

Guyton A: *Textbook of Medical Physiology,* 8th ed. Philadelphia, Saunders, 1991.

Katzung BG: *Basic and Clinical Pharmacology,* Los Altos CA, 1982.

Pattens HD, Fuchs AF, Hiller B, Scher AM, Steiner R: *Textbook of Physiology,* 21st ed, vol 2. Philadelphia, Saunders, 1992.

Wilson JD, Foster DW: *Williams Textbook of Endocrinology,* 8th ed. Philadelphia, Saunders, 1992.

Renal and Acid-Base Physiology

Timothy P. Staudacher, James Lash and Nancy Burk

The anesthesiologist is responsible for the intraoperative monitoring and maintenance of renal function of surgical patients. Therefore, a thorough understanding of renal physiology and the mechanisms for maintaining electrolyte and acid-base homeostasis is mandatory. The kidney plays a crucial role in many physiologic functions, including control of fluid homeostasis via the regulation of sodium and water absorption and excretion, regulation of acid-base homeostasis, regulation of blood pressure (via neurohumoral and vascular mechanisms), metabolic and hormonal regulation, and excretion of waste products (e.g., urea) from the plasma into the urine. In addition, the kidney regulates other physiologic functions, such as the production of red blood cells (through the synthesis of erythropoietin) and the activation of vitamin D. This chapter summarizes the complex physiologic processes of the renal system, with clinical examples where relevant.

☐ ANATOMY, BLOOD SUPPLY, AND INNERVATION

The kidneys are paired, bean-shaped organs that weigh about 125 to 150 g each and are located in the retroperitoneal space caudad to the diaphragm. The center of each kidney rests approximately at the level of the second lumbar vertebra, although the left kidney is usually slightly more cephalad. The final position of the kidney is dependent on their cephalad migration during embryologic development.

Blood reaches the kidney via the renal arteries, which arise from the descending abdominal aorta. Each kidney has a single renal artery (occasionally anamolies occur in which multiple renal arteries exist), which divides into interlobar, arcuate, and in-

terlobular arteries. The interlobular arteries branch further into afferent arterioles, which carry blood to the glomerular capillaries. The anatomic organization of the blood flow through the glomerulus is unique in that it interposes a capillary network between two sets of arterioles. Blood leaving the nephron travels via interlobular, arcuate, and interlobar veins, which progressively increase in caliber. These veins empty into the renal veins, which ultimately continues into the inferior vena cava.

The glomerular capillary wall is composed of highly differentiated endothelial and epithelial cells resting on a semipermeable basement membrane that acts as a filtration barrier in the renal corpuscle. It is composed of three distinct layers: the capillary endothelium, the glomelular basement membrane, and the capillary epithelium.

Efferent arterioles carry blood from the glomerulus into peritubular venous capillaries. These capillaries, called vasa recta, descend in the juxtamedullary region with the thin loops of Henle into the renal medulla. Medullary blood flow is only a fraction of that of the renal cortex, and only 1 to 2% of total renal blood flow (RBF) passes through the vasa recta. The vasa recta capillaries control the rate of solute removal from the interstitium and therefore are a critical component of the countercurrent mechanism. They also provide most of the oxygen supply to the loop of Henle.

The glomerular capillaries lie within Bowman's capsule, a dilated blind end of the renal tubule. Glomerular ultrafiltrate is formed here and passes into the proximal convoluted tubule, the loop of Henle, the distal convoluted tubule, and eventually the collecting ducts, which deliver fluid from several nephrons into the renal pelvis. From there the urine is delivered by means of peristaltic waves in the ureter to the urinary bladder. Schematic diagrams of the kidney are shown in Figs. 14–1 and 14–2.

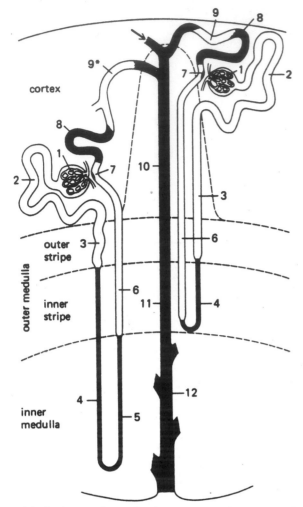

Figure 14–1 Nomenclature for the structures of the kidney from the 1988 Commission of the International Union of Physiological Science, numbered per protocol: 1) renal corpuscle which includes Bowman's capsule and glomerulus, 2) proximal convoluted tubule, 3) proximal straight tubule, 4) descending thin limb of the loop of Henle, 5) ascending thin limb, 6) thick ascending limb, 7) macula densa, 8) distal convoluted tubule, 9) connecting tubule of the juxtamedullary nephron, 10) cortical collecting duct, 11) outer medullary collecting duct, 12) inner medullary collecting duct. Reproduced with permission from W Kriz and L Bankir, *Am J Physiol* 1988; 25:F1-F8.

Autonomic nervous system innervation to the kidneys is from the splanchnic nerves, which arise from the vagus nerve via the celiac axis (Fig. 14–3). Vasomotor and pain fibers originate from spinal levels T4 through T12. The secretion of the hormone renin is mediated by the juxtaglomerular apparatus, a group of tubular and vascular cells located at the angle of the afferent and efferent arterioles close to the distal convoluted tubule. The macula densa is a cluster of specialized columnar-type epithelial cells in the distal tubule close to the vascular pole of the glomerulus. A group of tightly packed cells called the extraglomerular mesangium underlies the macula densa.

☐ PHYSIOLOGY

GLOMERULAR FILTRATION

The formation of urine is a complex process that involves three basic components: glomerular filtration, tubular secretion, and tubular reabsorption. These processes are depicted in Fig. 14–4. Renal function depends largely on RBF, normally 20 to 25% of the cardiac output, or approximately 1250 mL/min in the average adult. The glomerulus filters 10% of RBF, or 125 mL/min on average. Net filtration depends on hydrostatic versus osmotic pressures according to the following formula:

$$NFP = (PGC + P_iBC) - (PBC + P_iGC) \qquad (1)$$

where NPF is net filtration pressure, PGC, glomerular capillary hydrostatic pressure; P_iBC, oncotic pressure of fluid in Bowman's capsule; PBC, hydrostatic pressure in Bowman's capsule; and P_iGC, plasma oncotic pressure in glomerular capillary. Because there is virtually no protein in Bowman's capsule, (Fig. 14–5) the equation simplifies to

$$NFP = PGC - PBC - P_iGC \qquad (2)$$

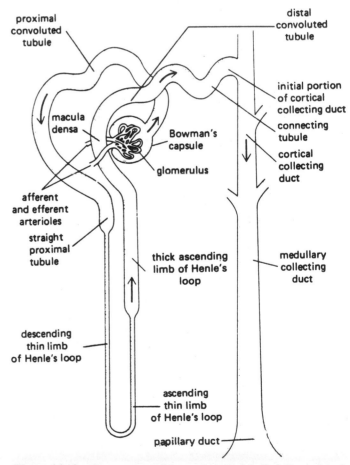

Figure 14–2 Components of the nephron as labelled. Reproduced with permission from Vander A, *Renal Physiology,* 4th ed. New York, McGraw-Hill, 1990.

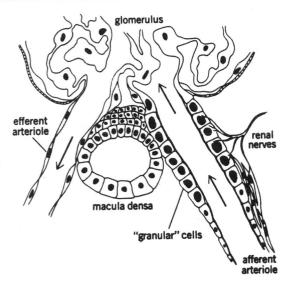

Figure 14–3   Schematic diagram of the glomerulus showing the JGA (juxtaglomerular apparatus). The granular cells help control systemic blood pressure via secretion of renin and functioning as baroreceptors. Adapted with permission from JO Davis, *Am J Med* 1973; 55:333.

Changes in the glomerular filtration rate (GFR), or the net filtration pressure, most commonly result from changes in hydrostatic pressure. Such changes are achieved by either constriction of afferent versus efferent arterioles (mediated by angiotensin II) or vasodilation (mediated by adenosine or prostaglandins).

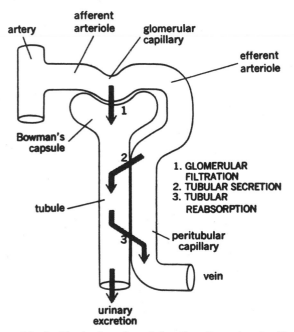

Figure 14–4   The basics of renal function. Reproduced with permission from Vander A, *Renal Physiology,* 4th ed. New York, McGraw-Hill, 1990.

TUBULAR TRANSPORT

After glomerular filtrate is formed, the final composition of the urine is altered by two steps: tubular secretion and tubular reabsorption. When the direction of flow is from the tubular lumen to plasma, it is called tubular reabsorption; flow that travels in the opposite direction is termed tubular secretion.

Approximately 65% of the filtered sodium, chloride, and water is reabsorbed via the proximal convoluted tubule into the peritubular capillaries. Most renal oxygen consumption is due to obligatory sodium reabsorption, which occurs against a concentration gradient. Water and chloride absorption is passive and requires no energy input. Glucose absorption in the proximal tubule is an active process, which therefore requires energy. The maximum transfer rate at which glucose can be absorbed is 180 g/dL; at higher levels, glycosuria develops. In poorly controlled diabetics with plasma glucose levels above 180 g/dL, glycosuria may result in an osmotic diuresis that can lead to intravascular volume depletion.

Sodium and water absorption continues to occur throughout the loop of Henle, and ultimately 25% of total filtered sodium is reabsorbed. Countercurrent concentration of tubular fluid occurs in the loop of Henle of the juxtamedullary nephron as it descends into the renal medulla (Fig. 14–6). Since sodium is actively reabsorbed in the proximal tubule and water passively diffuses from the tubule, the tubular fluid osmolarity approximates that of plasma. Concentration gradients in the hypertonic renal medulla favor passive diffusion of water out of the tubule into peritubular capillaries and of sodium into the tubule. Thus, the osmolarity of the tubular fluid progressively increases as it travels down the descending limb of the loop of Henle.

In the ascending limb of the loop of Henle and in the outer medullary portion of the distal tubule, sodium is actively transported out of the tubule. Since this portion of the nephron is relatively impermeable to water, the osmolarity of the tubular fluid progressively decreases as it passes from the loop of Henle into the cortical portion of the distal tubule. This is schematically represented in Figure 14–7.

Reabsorption of sodium, chloride, and water takes place in the distal convoluted tubule under the influence of aldosterone. Only about 1% of the originally filtered sodium is excreted in the urine. Secretion of hydrogen ion, potassium, and ammonia also occurs in the distal tubule. Secretion of H^+ facilitates elimination of acid metabolites. Secretion of ammonia, which combines with H^+ to form ammonium, allows further H^+ elimination. Systemic acidosis results in preferential excretion of H^+ over K^+; alternatively, alkalosis favors excretion of K^+. The permeability of the distal tubule and collecting ducts to water is regulated by the antidiuretic hormone (ADH), which is secreted by the posterior pituitary gland. Volume depletion and surgical stress enhance the release of ADH; conversely, decreases in plasma osmolality and hypervolemia inhibit its release.

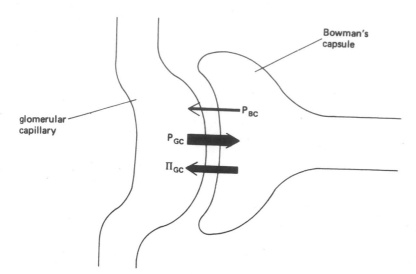

Figure 14–5 The determinants of the net filtration pressure as discussed in the text. Reproduced with permission from Vander A, *Renal Physiology,* 4th ed. New York, McGraw-Hill, 1990.

AUTOREGULATION

Autoregulation is a physiologic mechanism whereby RBF is maintained over a wide range of systemic arterial blood pressures. The kidney is able to autoregulate RBF and GFR between mean arterial pressures (MAP) of 60 and 160 torr (Fig. 14–8). Autoregulation is thought to occur mainly by two intrinsic intrarenal mechanisms: a tubuloglomerular feedback response and a myogenic mechanism. Tubuloglomerular feedback is a complex process whereby the regulation of GFR is primary and the maintenance of RBF secondary. A schematically depicted theory of the tubuloglomerular feedback response is shown in Fig. 14–9. The physiology of the myogenic mechanism is similar to that seen in other autoreg-

ulating beds. Vascular smooth muscle has local stretch receptors that, when stimulated, cause the vessel to contract. This increased arteriolar pressure then distends the arteriolar wall and increases its passive tension. The vascular smooth muscle then contracts, increasing the resistance offered by the vessel, and hence maintains RBF.

Many other factors may also be active in the maintenance of autoregulation and hence RBF. The endogenous chemical transmitter adenosine has multiple functions in the renal vascular bed. It constricts afferent arterioles, dilates efferent arterioles, and decreases the release of renin from the juxtaglomerular (JGA). Adenosine also modulates tubular function and may be active in tubuloglomerular feedback. In addition, it is likely that prostaglandins may somehow participate in the autoregulation process, and inhibitors of these substances (e.g., non-steroidal anti-inflammatory drugs like ibuprofen) may be deleterious, in that they might inhibit this vital mechanism.

The value of autoregulation of the renal system is twofold. Most important, as in any other vital organ, it helps prevent major blood flow changes despite changes in arterial pressure, thereby preserving organ function during periods of hypotension. Moreover, it also modulates large changes in solute and water excretion that occur because of large changes in GFR when MAP is altered. However, autoregulation of RBF is not wholly protective of the kidneys, and alterations of RBF and GFR can occur via other mechanisms, including the sympathetic nervous system and the renin-angiotensin-aldosterone axis.

Sympathetic stimulation causes constriction of the afferent arterioles, which reduces glomerular capillary blood flow and, to a lesser extent, GFR. This is independent of autoregulatory mechanisms and probably results from direct release of catecholamines from renal sympathetic nerves rather than from the effects of circulating catecholamines (from the adrenal medulla). Both α- and β-adrenergic receptors are found in the kidney. There are

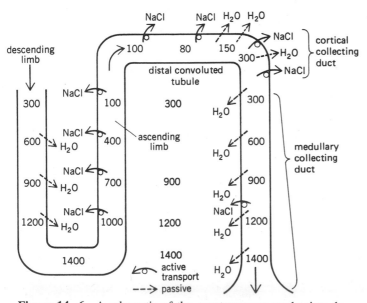

Figure 14–6 A schematic of the countercurrent mechanism depicting the increases in urine osmolality along the loop of Henle and collecting duct. Reproduced with permission from Vander A, *Renal Physiology,* 4th ed. New York, McGraw-Hill, 1990.

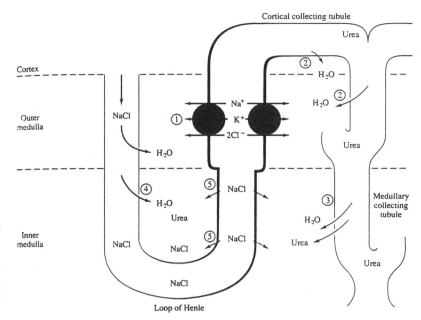

Figure 14–7 The steps involved in countercurrent multiplication in which a concentration gradient is established by passive NaCl reabsorption in the thin ascending limb in the inner medulla. The bold lines represent water impermeability. From Jamison, RL, Maffly, RH, *N Engl J Med,* 295:1059, 1976. Reproduced with permission of the Massachusetts Medical Society.

more α receptors than β receptors, and both catecholamines epinephrine and norepinephrine will produce renal vasoconstriction. Dopamine, on the other hand, has a dual action that is dose-dependent. At low doses, dopamine produces vasodilation of renal arterioles via specific dopamine receptors located in the renal vasculature, but at higher doses it produces vasoconstriction via α receptors. Clinically, this phenomenon is often demonstrated in hypotensive patients who are started on exogenous vasopressors (e.g., epinephrine) to increase their blood pressure. Despite increases in the patient's MAP, the expected increase in urine output (renal perfusion) does not occur. That is why clinicians who are concerned with renal preservation in hypotensive patients often begin an infusion of low-dose dopamine to try to utilize its vasodilating effect.

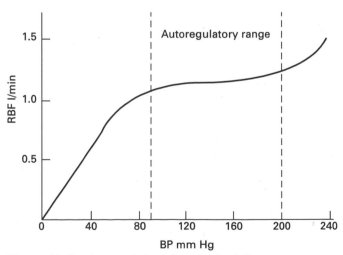

Figure 14–8 Autoregulation of renal blood flow occurs over a range of systemic mean arterial pressure as depicted. Reproduced with permission from Vander A, *Renal Physiology,* 4th ed. New York, McGraw-Hill, 1990.

☐ RENAL HOMEOSTATIC FUNCTIONS

EXTRACELLULAR FLUID REGULATION

The kidney is responsible for the regulation of the volume status, which it does primarily by manipulating the extracellular fluid (ECF), which allows for indirect control of intracellular fluid (ICF). The human body is composed of approximately 50 to 70% water by weight; of this, one-third is ECF and the remainder is ICF. Intravascular fluid is the most important compartment for the clinician in the operating room and accounts for 25% of ECF, or just one-twelfth of the total body water. The distribution of free water in the body is primarily determined by osmotically active solutes (mainly Na^+ and Cl^-) distributed throughout the various compartments. The most important of these is NaCl, since the ECF approximates normal saline solution in composition, and 90% of the solutes in ECF are sodium salts.

OSMOLAR REGULATION

Water moves freely across cell membranes, and the kidneys are able to regulate total body water by manipulating ECF water balance. The kidney is able to do this as long as the portion of the nephron proximal to the collecting ducts is functioning normally. Plasma concentration of solutes is used as an indicator of total body water balance. Minor changes (as little as 1 to 2%) in the osmolality of the blood are sensed in the internal carotid circulation by the osmoreceptors located in the wall of the third cerebral ventricle. An increase in serum osmolality stimulates ADH secretion by the posterior pituitary gland and also simultaneously increases thirst sensation. ADH then increases the permeability of the renal collecting ducts to water and facilitates free-water retention. The osmoreceptor mechanism is very sensitive; even small

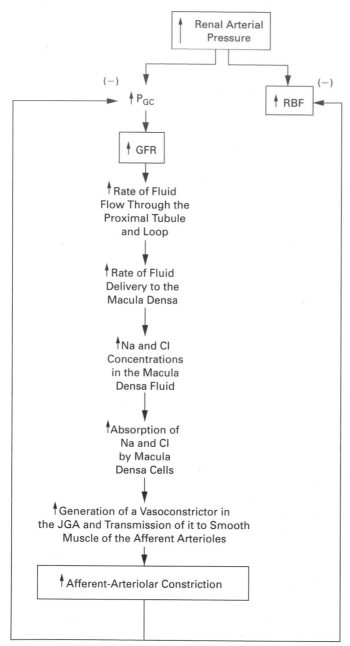

Figure 14–9 A schematic depiction of the contribution of tubuloglomerular feedback. Reproduced with permission from Vander A, *Renal Physiology,* 4th ed. New York, McGraw-Hill, 1990.

changes in NaCl concentration are countered by increased water resorption. Alternatively, when total body water is in excess and serum osmolality is decreased, the opposite mechanism occurs; thirst and ADH secretion are suppressed, and water is excreted. Atrial natriuretic peptide (ANP) also probably participates in a negative feedback loop, further suppressing the release of ADH. The ANP is released following stretch of the atrium and binds to a biologic receptor, which forms cyclic GMP. This cGMP then causes a series of effects, including vasodilation of the renal vasculature, glomerular hyperfiltration, and inhibition of sodium transport in the inner medullary collecting duct.

In addition, arterial baroreceptors (which are pressure-sensitive) can stimulate ADH release irrespective of blood osmolality if ECF volume decreases by 10% or more. This occurs via neuronal pathways and constitutes an "overriding" of the osmoreceptor mechanism. Angiotensin II serves to stimulate thirst in this scenario.

WASTE, TOXIN, AND DRUG EXCRETION

The kidneys play a vital role in the elimination of metabolic wastes and toxins. The first step in elimination of toxins by the kidney is via glomerular filtration. Glomerular filtration is the bulk flow of protein-free plasma (containing the toxin or waste product) from the glomerular capillaries into Bowman's capsule, forming the ultrafiltrate that will eventually be urine. The end products of metabolism and exogenous toxins are necessarily kept at low concentrations in the plasma to minimize toxicity. This means, however, that the kidneys must process large volumes of plasma to rid the body of significant amounts of toxin. Indeed, normal ultrafiltrate volume is 180 L/day, of which 99% of the bulk volume is reabsorbed. The second mechanism of renal elimination is via tubular secretion. Tubular secretion occurs when the toxin is "secreted" from the peritubular glomerular capillaries (plasma) into the tubular lumen. This mechanism serves to eliminate toxins that are highly protein-bound (and therefore do not undergo glomerular filtration to an appreciable amount) with a low free fraction in plasma. Substances eliminated by this route include organic acids, such as urate, citrate, and lactate, and organic bases, such as creatinine. Some drugs, such as certain antibiotics and diuretics, are also eliminated in this way.

BLOOD PRESSURE REGULATION

The kidney also influences blood pressure by exerting control over ECF volume (Fig. 14–10). In clinical practice, one of the mainstays of therapy for hypertension is diuretics, which respond to changes in ECF volume. Hypertension may involve impaired ECF volume control and a "resetting" of MAP to a higher level. The kidneys also release vasoactive substances that directly or indirectly influence blood pressure. Renin is a proteolytic enzyme synthesized and stored in the juxtaglomerular cells. There are three major triggers of renin release: an increase in the sodium concentration of tubular fluid, a fall in renal perfusion pressure, or direct stimulation of renal sympathetic nerves. Renin is also released in response to decreased MAP, which is sensed either at central vascular baroreceptors or at the efferent arterioles. Renin enzymatically converts angiotensinogen, which is synthesized in the liver, to the prohormone angiotensin I. Angiotensin I is converted by angiotensin-converting enzyme (ACE) in the lungs to angiotensin II. Angiotensin II is an extremely potent vasoconstrictor that increases systemic vascular resistance, is critical for renal autoregulation and blood pressure, and stimulates aldosterone secretion. Aldosterone causes sodium conservation and water retention and facilitates the excretion of potassium and hydrogen ions.

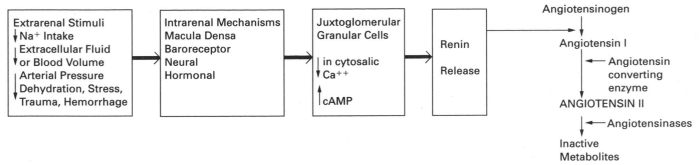

Figure 14–10 The renin-angiotensin system.

The kidneys also release vasodilating substances, renal prostaglandins and kinins, that are intrarenal vasodilators and probably do not act systemically. Nitric oxide is an endogenous compound formed in the endothelium of most vascular beds. It acts primarily as a vasodilating substance, and its effect on the kidney has been the subject of much recent investigation. In addition to its vasodilating properties, possible roles of nitric oxide in renal function include the regulation of RBF, inhibition of renin release, and pressure natriuresis. It may also play a role in changes in sodium excretion in response to the changes in sodium dietary intake and probably inhibits contraction and proliferation of mesangial cells. How nitric oxide works in conjunction with all the other known factors to alter and modulate renal function remains to be clearly elucidated.

MINERAL REGULATION/IONS

Potassium is freely filtered at the glomerulus and is almost completely reabsorbed along the length of the proximal convoluted tubule and then secreted in the distal tubule. Potassium secretion occurs in response to the hormone aldosterone, which is the primary mechanism for the control of plasma concentrations of K^+. Small changes in plasma K^+ concentration result in large changes in aldosterone secretion and plasma concentration. In addition, K^+ secretion also increases with increasing rates of fluid flow, which is coupled with increasing sodium delivery to the distal nephron. Despite serum hypokalemia, the kidney has a limited ability to conserve K^+ (obligatory loss), even in states of severe depletion of the ion. The normal minimal urinary concentration of K^+ is 10 to 12 mEq/L, which is reduced only in states of severe total body K^+ depletion.

Calcium is also freely filtered at the glomerulus and, like sodium, 60% is reabsorbed in the proximal tubule. In the distal tubule, however, it does not parallel the handling of sodium. Distal tubule reabsorption of calcium is governed by parathyroid hormone (PTH), whose release is sensitive to changes in serum calcium. In states of hypocalcemia, PTH increases calcium reabsorption and efficiently corrects the calcium depletion. The kidney, however, is less efficient at controlling hypercalcemia. When plasma calcium levels are high, the filtration rate for calcium increases. Usually, however, hypercalcemic states are accompanied by reduced in-

travascular volume, which increases sodium reabsorption and results in further increases in plasma calcium. With profound hypercalcemia (12 to 15 mg/dL), RBF and glomerular filtration rates may be decreased, and calcium filtration also decreases. Reabsorption of filtered phosphate is also under parathyroid control. Parathyroid hormone decreases phosphate reabsorption and facilitates its excretion.

Magnesium is also absorbed in the proximal tubule, but at a much slower rate than sodium. Most of its reabsorption occurs in the loop of Henle. Magnesium reabsorption is decreased (i.e., excretion is increased) by decreases in the fractional proximal tubular reabsorption, as occurs in states of increased ECF volume. The Mg^{2+} excretion can also be increased by a decrease in the absorption of NaCl in the loop of Henle, as occurs with diuretic use. Renal losses are a common cause of hypomagnesemia, and, conversely, increases in plasma levels of Mg^{2+} are almost always due to renal insufficiency with reduced GFR.

METABOLIC AND HORMONAL REGULATION

The kidney also has a number of other physiologic functions concerning the regulation and metabolism of specific hormones. The kidney degrades metabolically important peptides such as the pituitary hormones, glucagon, and insulin. About one-fourth of insulin is usually degraded by the kidney, and this metabolism decreases with progressive decline in renal function. Such decreases are often seen clinically in diabetic patients who develop renal insufficiency because of their disease. Insulin may have a prolonged duration, and therefore requirements for exogenous insulin can be decreased dramatically. Also, the activation of vitamin D (cholecalciferol), which regulates intestinal calcium reabsorption, is under the control of the kidney in specific situations. Normally, the molecule initially undergoes hydroxylation in the liver. However, in the face of low serum ionized calcium levels, elevated PTH levels, and lowered cellular phosphorus levels, renal tubular cells may add a second hydroxyl group to the molecule, yielding the potent hormonal form of the vitamin. This allows for further actions of vitamin D.

The kidney also has important synthetic functions. The most important substance produced by the kidney is probably erythropoietin. Erythropoietin is a protein (molecular weight

39 kilodaltons) that acts in erythroid-producing tissue both as a differentiating factor that promotes the transition to the pro-erythroblast stage and as a growth factor that promotes mitosis in the series of cells leading to the mature erythrocyte. In general, erythropoietin production increases in states of decreased tissue oxygen delivery, such as with chronic hypoxemia and anemia. Since the kidney makes most of the erythropoietin, patients with chronic renal insufficiency have decreased erythropoietin levels due to decreased nephron mass, and anephric individuals rely solely on erythropoietin produced elsewhere (in the liver 10 to 15% of total). Clinically, this is observed in the severe anemia seen in patients with end-stage renal disease.

☐ RENAL FUNCTION TESTS

ASSESSMENT OF GLOMERULAR FUNCTION

The measurement of GFR would ideally be performed by measuring a substance that is completely filtered by the glomerulus but neither secreted nor reabsorbed by the renal tubules and is at a stable level in the serum. Several chemical markers, namely, serum creatinine and blood urea nitrogen (BUN), are utilized clinically with this goal in mind, both with some limitations in accuracy. The most clinically useful and sensitive marker of renal function is serum creatinine. It is a metabolite of creatine, which undergoes constant release from muscle tissue. Creatinine is almost completely eliminated by glomerular filtration, and its measurement is a fair clinical indicator of glomerular function. Daily production remains relatively constant in a given individual but depends on muscle mass. Absolute values may therefore differ between individuals with different muscle masses. This is especially true in elderly and female patients, whose muscle mass is significantly less than in males. Factors that significantly increase the serum creatinine level, and therefore cause underestimation of true renal function, include rhabdomyolysis (muscle destruction) and intake of the dietary proteins. Conversely, compounds that decrease creatinine excretion, such as the drugs cimetidine and trimethoprim, may cause underestimation of the true GFR.

BUN is a measure of serum urea, a product of protein catabolism. Urea is filtered by the glomerulus but reabsorbed to varying degrees in the renal tubules. Its reabsorption is enhanced in hypernatremic states and with decreased GFR; therefore, measurement of BUN does not accurately reflect glomerular function, since it can be affected by serum sodium levels and ECF volume. The normal BUN-creatinine ratio is approximately $10:1$; if the ratio exceeds $20:1$, other causes for alteration of these serum metabolites (e.g., dehydration or gastrointestinal blood loss) should be suspected. The clearance of a substance is the volume of plasma from which that substance is completely cleared by the kidneys over a specific time interval. The measurement of creatinine clearance involves a timed collection of urine from which the urine creatinine concentration is measured. The following formula yields creatinine clearance:

$$GFR = U \times V/P \tag{3}$$

where U is urine creatinine concentration; V, urine volume in milliliters per minute; and P, plasma creatinine concentration in milligrams per deciliter. Because it measures both the urine volume and the plasma concentration, creatinine clearance is a more accurate representation of glomerular function than are the measurements of BUN or creatinine alone. However, since creatinine is secreted by the renal tubules to a small degree, creatinine clearance causes a slight overestimation of GFR. In the absence of a 24h collection of urine, GFR can be estimated by the following formula:

$$GFR = \frac{(140 \times age) \times lean\ body\ mass\ (kg)}{P_{Cr} \times 72} \tag{4}$$

Because of the decreased muscle mass in women, this number needs to be multiplied by 0.85, or it will overestimate the GFR. Again, several limitations should be considered, including an unusually large muscle mass (e.g., in weightlifters) or, more frequently, an unusually low muscle mass, common in elderly, alcoholic, and severely deconditioned patients.

In addition to the measurement of the GFR, clinical assessment of tubular function may also be necessary. This is important in some forms of acute renal failure, in which the cause of renal failure is a pathologic condition in the tubules, as opposed to the glomerulus. In these instances, urinalysis is performed to check for tubular casts, which imply damage to the kidneys at that level. Urinalysis is also helpful in looking for infection (pyelonephritis), when white cell casts can be observed.

☐ ACID-BASE DISORDERS

An acid is any compound that tends to lose hydrogen ions (H^+), and a base is any compound that tends to gain H^+. Acids and bases usually exist as pairs, with the acid giving up protons, which are accepted by a corresponding base. The normal plasma concentration of H^+ is 40 nEq/L. In an exponential form, this is 40×10^{-9}. In 1909, Sorenson proposed using the pH scale, which is equivalent to the negative logarithm of H^+ concentration. A normal blood H^+ concentration corresponds to a pH of 7.40. Under normal conditions, arterial pH is maintained within a narrow range, between 7.35 and 7.43. Three mechanisms are important in the regulation of pH: extracellular and intracellular buffering, pulmonary ventilatory exchange, and renal H^+ excretion. Bone, proteins, hemoglobin, and the bicarbonate-carbonic acid ($HCO_3^- - H_2CO_3$) system are important elements in the buffer system. The importance of both the renal and respiratory components is seen in the Henderson-Hasselbalch equation:

$$pH = 6.10 + \log[HCO_3^-] - \\ 0.03 \times P_{CO_2} \tag{5}$$

Table 14–1
SIMPLE ACID-BASE DISORDERS

Acid-Base Disturbance	Primary Disorder	Compensatory Response	pH	Predicted Compensation	Limits of Compensation
Metabolic acidosis	$\downarrow HCO_3^-$	$\downarrow P_{CO_2}$	$\downarrow$	$\Delta P_{CO_2} = 1.0-1.5 \times \Delta HCO_3^-$	10 mmHg
Metabolic alkalosis	$\uparrow HCO_3^-$	$\uparrow P_{CO_2}$	$\uparrow$	$\Delta P_{CO_2} = 0.5-1.0 \times \Delta HCO_3^-$	60–70 mmHg
Respiratory acidosis	$\uparrow P_{CO_2}$	$\uparrow HCO_3^-$	$\downarrow$	Acute: $\Delta HCO_3^- = 0.1 \times \Delta P_{CO_2}$	32 mEq/L
				Chronic: $\Delta HCO_3^- = 0.4 \times \Delta P_{CO_2}$	45 mEq/L
Respiratory alkalosis	$\downarrow P_{CO_2}$	$\downarrow HCO_3^-$	$\uparrow$	Acute: $\Delta HCO_3^- = 0.2 \times \Delta P_{CO_2}$	18–20 mEq/L
				Chronic: $\Delta HCO_3^- = 0.5 \times \Delta P_{CO_2}$	12–15 mEq/L

SOURCE: Modified with permission from Saxton CR, Seldin DW: Clinical Interpretation of Laboratory Values, in Kokko JP, Tannen RL (eds): *Fluids and Electrolytes.* Philadelphia, Saunders, 1986.

Primary changes in HCO_3^- are seen with metabolic disorders, whereas primary changes in P_{CO_2} are seen with respiratory disorders. Changes in HCO_3^- and P_{CO_2} may also reflect compensatory responses. It is important for the clinician to predict the expected magnitude of compensation for a given acid-base disorder (Table 14–1). When the observed response differs from what is predicted, a mixed acid-base disorder is present.

METABOLIC ACIDOSIS

Metabolic acidosis is characterized by a primary decrement in HCO_3^-. Metabolic acidosis can be categorized according to the anion gap (Table 14–2). The anion gap is calculated as follows:

$$Anion\ gap = [Na^+] - [Cl^- + CO_2] \qquad (6)$$

The gap is made up of anions that are not routinely measured, such as proteins, phosphate, sulfate, and organic acids. An elevated anion gap is associated with acidosis due to the acid gain, whereas a normal anion gap is seen with acidosis

Table 14–2
CAUSES OF ANION GAP AND NONGAP ACIDOSIS

High Anion Gap	Low or Nongap
Uremia	Gastrointestinal HCO_3^- loss
Ketoacidosis	Renal HCO_3^- loss (RTA)
Lactic acidosis	Gain of HCl
Salicylate toxicity	
Methanol toxicity	
Ethylene glycol toxicity	
Paraldehyde toxicity	

due to HCO_3^- loss. Common causes of high anion gap acidosis include lactic acidosis, ketoacidosis, renal failure, and certain toxic ingestions. Lactic acidosis is a common problem in the critically ill. Lactic acidosis occurs as a result of the overproduction or impaired metabolism of lactate. The overproduction of lactate is usually due to inadequate oxygen delivery, as occurs with shock (septic, hypovolemic, or cardiogenic). Impaired lactate metabolism is usually due to hepatic failure. In shock states, both overproduction and impaired metabolism are important in the genesis of lactic acidosis. Lactic acidosis is associated with a grim prognosis. The underlying cause of the lactic acidosis must be identified and corrected whenever possible.

Ketoacidosis may be seen in the settings of diabetic ketoacidosis (DKA), alcoholic ketoacidosis, and starvation ketoacidosis. When the GFR falls below 25% of normal, net acid excretion can no longer be maintained and, as a result, acidosis develops. The anion gap is elevated due to the retention of phosphoric and sulfuric acids, which are the products of protein metabolism. Earlier in renal failure, a normal anion gap may be present. Finally, salicylate overdose and the ingestion of toxic alcohols (methanol and ethylene glycol) can cause an elevated anion gap acidosis. Ethanol is useful in the treatment of toxic alcohol ingestion because it is a substrate for alcohol dehydrogenase and thus competitively inhibits the formation of toxic intermediates responsible for causing acidosis and other problems.

Normal anion gap or hyperchloremic metabolic acidosis may be due to the gain of hydrochloric acid (HCl) or the loss of bicarbonate. The two most common causes of hyperchloremic acidosis are diarrhea and renal tubular acidosis.

Bicarbonate therapy should be administered if acidosis is severe (pH < 7.1). In the operating room, a measurement of arterial blood gas can provide a determination of the "base excess." The base excess is a derived value obtained by multiplying the deviation of bicarbonate from normal by an empiric factor. The base excess will be negative in the setting of acidosis. The amount of bicarbonate (milliequivalents) to be administered is usually calculated as follows:

$$\text{Body weight (kg)} \times 0.2 \times \text{base excess}$$

Half of this value is administered, and the arterial blood gas measurement is repeated to further determine therapy. Complications of bicarbonate therapy include fluid overload; hypertonicity; and, during overshoot, alkalosis. In some cases, bicarbonate therapy may also be associated with an increase in lactate production since it results in an increase in CO_2 production and may worsen intracellular acidosis.

METABOLIC ALKALOSIS

Metabolic alkalosis is characterized by a primary incremental increase in the serum HCO_3^-. Many factors are responsible for the generation and maintenance of metabolic alkalosis. Metabolic alkalosis can be generated by either bicarbonate gain or HCl loss. Once metabolic alkalosis is generated, it is often maintained by the presence of volume depletion and/or hypokalemia. Both of these factors may exacerbate the alkalosis because of a decrease in the GFR which may limit bicarbonate excretion.

The kidney has an extraordinary capacity to excrete bicarbonate so that metabolic alkalosis due to bicarbonate administration is relatively uncommon, but can occur when there is a limitation in the renal excratory ability (for example when bicarbonate is administered to a patient with renal insufficiency or when it is given during CPR). Metabolic alkalosis is usually generated by loss of bicarbonate from the gastrointestinal (GI) tract or in the urine. Vomiting and nasogastric (NG) suction are the most common causes of GI HCl loss. Exogenous diuretics are the most common cause of metabolic alkalosis due to renal losses of HCl. This occurs because diuretics increase distal Na^+ delivery and can lead to secondary hyperaldosteronism (by inducing volume depletion). The combination of these two factors results in an increased distal H^+ secretion.

In the evaluation of metabolic alkalosis, it is useful to measure the urine chloride concentration. Metabolic alkalosis with a low urine chloride concentration (< 15 meq/L) is associated with volume contraction and is usually due to vomiting, NG suction, or diuretics. This type of alkalosis is called "chloride-responsive" because volume repletion with sodium chloride is an essential part of therapy. Metabolic alkalosis with a high urine chloride is usually due to mineralocorticoid excess (primary or secondary). This alkalosis is called "chloride resistant" because the alkalosis can not be corrected with sodium chloride.

Treatment must be directed toward the correction of factors responsible for the generation of the alkalosis (e.g., discontinuing diuretics or removal of an adrenal adenoma). Therapy must also be directed toward the correction of factors responsible for the maintenance of the alkalosis (e.g., volume and potassium repletion).

RESPIRATORY ACIDOSIS

Respiratory acidosis is characterized by a primary rise in P_{CO_2} due to alveolar hypoventilation. This disorder can be due to diseases that effect the respiratory center, the lung tissue, or the chest wall muscles. In the operating room, the most common cause is relative hypoventilation of a paralyzed patient or oversedation of an awake patient (e.g., during administration of a spinal anesthetic). Intracellular buffering constitutes the initial compensatory response. After several days, renal net acid excretion rises, and compensation is more complete (see Table 14–1). The treatment of respiratory acidosis must be directed at the underlying cause of hypoventilation and must include correcting hypoxia and improving pulmonary function.

RESPIRATORY ALKALOSIS

Respiratory alkalosis is characterized by primary fall in the P_{CO_2} due alveolar hyperventilation. This disorder can be due to stimulation of the central respiratory center or peripheral and intrathoracic chemoreceptors. During anesthesia, a patient who is hyperventilated will also develop a respiratory alkalosis. Compensatory responses to acute and chronic respiratory alkalosis are as listed in Table 14–1. Again, treatment must be directed at the underlying cause.

☐ PATHOPHYSIOLOGY

ACUTE RENAL FAILURE

Acute renal failure occurs when there is an acute deterioration of renal function to the point where dialysis is required. It may be caused by a variety of insults, and categories of acute renal failure are described based on the etiology of the dysfunction. Oliguria is defined as urine output of less than 0.5 mL/kg/h (or < 500 mL/day) and can result from many kinds of disease processes. Prerenal oliguria implies acute reductions in GFR that may be due to decreased perfusion of the kidney from either a low cardiac output state or hypovolemia. Acute increases in water reabsorption, salt reabsorption, or both may also cause a prerenal picture. Renal (or intrarenal) oliguria implies a malfunction in glomerular filtration, tubular reabsorption, or both. It is caused by nephrotoxins, severe renal hypoperfusion, or a combination of the two. The renal tubules are particularly prone to ischemic injury because of their relatively high oxygen consumption, needed for the active transport of solutes. Postrenal oliguria denotes obstructive uropathy, which, in the perioperative period, may be iatrogenic (e.g., a kink in the Foley catheter). Laboratory tests (BUN-Cr ratio, urinalysis, etc.) can be used to aid the clinician in distinguishing prerenal from renal oliguria and to direct treatment accordingly.

CHRONIC RENAL FAILURE

Patients with chronic renal failure have a progressive loss of renal reserve capacity accompanied by a decreased GFR and progressive loss of nephron function. Patients often remain asymptomatic with as few as 40% of their nephrons functioning normally. Renal insufficiency (defined as serum Cr > 1.5) occurs with 10 to 40% of nephrons functioning, and, even though the kidneys are able to excrete toxins, their reserve capacity is nonexistent. Patients with such a condition are therefore more prone to develop renal failure with any added degree of stress or insult to the kidneys. Polyuria and nocturia reflect diminished urine-concentrating ability. With further loss of nephrons, uremia results.

There are many causes of chronic renal failure. Chronic glomerulonephritis occurs with deposition of precipitated antigen-antibody complexes in the glomerular capillary membrane. The resulting inflammation leads to progressive thickening of the basement membrane and subsequent fibrosis and nephron loss. An infectious or inflammatory process like pyelonephritis may cause renal failure. It can start in the renal pelvis as an ascending urinary tract infection and extend into the renal parenchyma, where the damage occurs. The renal medulla is usually affected to a greater degree than the cortex, and urine-concentrating ability is usually impaired. Enteric bacteria (e.g., *Escherichia coli*) from the colon are the most common causative organisms.

NEPHROTIC SYNDROME

Another common pathologic condition of the kidneys that can be acute or chronic in nature is the nephrotic syndrome. The nephrotic syndrome results in increased permeability of the glomerular capillary membrane, resulting in loss of large amounts of protein (up to 30 g/day) into the urine. This decreases the serum colloid oncotic pressure and results in generalized edema and ascites. Effusions in the pleura, pericardium, and joints may also occur. Causes include acute glomerulonephritis, amyloidosis, and lipoid nephrosis. Patients with nephrotic syndrome may have a variable degree of renal insufficiency and for a prolonged period of time have normal renal function, except for their severe loss of protein and its attendant sequelae, as described. Glucocorticoids can be used to treat lipid nephrosis but are usually ineffective in treating the other causes of the nephrotic syndrome. Many of these patients will develop end-stage renal disease and ultimately require nephrectomy to control the severe protein loss.

BIBLIOGRAPHY

Guyton A: *Textbook of Medical Physiology,* 8th ed. Philadelphia, Saunders, 1991.

Rogers MC, Tinker JH, Covino BG, Longnecker DE: Principles and *Practice of Anesthesthesiology.* St. Louis, Mosby Yarbook, 1993

Rose BD: *Clinical Physiology of Acid-Base and Electrolyte Disorders.* New York, McGraw Hill, 1984.

Rose BD: *Renal Physiology: The Essentials.* Baltimore, Williams & Wilkins, 1994.

Schrier R: *Renal and Electrolyte Disorders.* Boston, Little, Brown, 1992.

Stoelting RK: *Pharmacology and Physiology in Anesthetic Practice,* 2d ed. Philadelphia, Lippincott, 1991.

Vander A: *Renal Physiology,* 4th ed. New York, McGraw Hill, 1991.

Coagulation: Components and Functional Interactions in Hemostasis

Juan Chediak and Sabet Siddiqui

The human body possesses a remarkably intricate hemostatic system designed to keep the circulating blood clot-free under physiological conditions and yet respond to vascular injury by closing the site of damage and preventing further blood loss. With a complex array of both formed and soluble elements, injuries to the vascular tree are effectively plugged in a timely manner, while the entire hemostatic process is localized to the site of injury.

Ongoing research has immensely increased our understanding of the coagulation process. With better delineation of soluble coagulation factors, we have gained new insights into factor activation and inhibition. The active roles played by both platelets and vascular endothelium have also assumed major importance. Similarly, we have just begun to appreciate the myriad interactions between the coagulation and the fibrinolytic systems. The purpose of this chapter is to review recent advances on the structure and function of the components of the hemostatic system and their interactions.

☐ OVERVIEW: FUNCTIONAL INTERACTIONS IN HEMOSTASIS

Following a vascular injury, hemostasis can be considered to occur in two interrelated stages. Primary hemostasis represents the initial generation of a platelet plug as platelets adhere and aggregate on the damaged subendothelium, with soluble von Willebrand factor (vWF) serving as bridge in between. Tests of bleeding time give an estimation of the adequacy of the primary hemostatic elements: platelets, vWF, and blood vessel wall. This platelet plug is labile to the shear forces of the circulating blood and is susceptible to disruption. Secondary hemostasis is said to occur as fibrin deposition on the platelet aggregate cements this primary plug to

form the secondary plug, which is now able to resist the shear effects of blood flow. Finally, endothelial cells release tissue plasminogen activator, which facilitates the conversion of plasminogen to plasmin. Plasmin binds to the clot and lyses it, thus restoring blood circulation. Let us now examine in greater depth the various interactions occurring during clot formation and clot lysis.

PLATELET PLUG FORMATION

The endothelium serves as a barrier separating the intravascular coagulation factors from the highly thrombogenic substances located in the subendothelium. With injury to the blood vessel wall, circulating platelets become exposed to subendothelial collagen, proteoglycans, and other thrombogenic substances. Platelets then become activated and undergo three important reactions: adhesion and cellular shape change, secretion of granular contents (release reaction), and aggregation.

Upon contact with subendothelium, platelets spread broadly by extending long pseudopods and, with vWF serving as a molecular ligand, become tightly adherent to the exposed collagen. A metabolic activation process then occurs and induces platelets to externalize a phospholipid complex on the platelet surface by an unknown mechanism.[2] As shall be seen, this phospholipid layer serves as a surface template for soluble coagulation factors to bind and interact freely.

Platelet adhesion and subsequent activation result in the release reaction and platelet aggregation. Several substances metabolized or released by platelets participate in platelet aggregation. Functionally, the most important species are adenosine diphosphate (ADP) released from platelet granules and thromboxane A_2, a product of arachidonic acid stimulation. Thrombin, generated by a simultaneous activation of the coagulation cascade, also plays a powerful role in platelet aggregation. Together, these three substances are powerful platelet aggregators and thus increase the size of the platelet plug. Platelets then bind to each other using fibrinogen molecules as a link in between. The receptor for fibrinogen binding is the glycoprotein heterodimer GPIIb/IIIa on the platelet surface.

FIBRIN FORMATION

The second phase leading to the development of a hemostatic plug is the formation and deposition of a tenacious fibrin meshwork at the site of injury. Historically, the "cascade" or the "waterfall" hypothesis proposed in 1964 was in vogue until recently, when the revised coagulation pathway was proposed. The cascade is a series of reactions of zymogens that undergo cleavage of one or more peptide bonds and become activated, finally culminating in the generation of fibrin. As mentioned, activated platelets present a phospholipid surface layer, providing the template for the zymogen reactions. Tissue factor is the key trigger for the coagulation sequence. As injured endothelium releases tissue factor, it complexes with and activates factor VII, leading to the formation of tissue factor VIIa complex. In turn, this complex activates both factor X and factor IX (the activated moieties being denoted by factor Xa and IXa). It is envisioned that the factors bind to the phospholipid membranes and freely migrate about on the membrane, reacting to form the "prothrombinase" complex (factor Xa-Va complex), which converts prothrombin to thrombin. The small amounts of thrombin thus formed activate factor XI, factor VIII, and factor V. This activation rejuvenates the formation of factor Xa, and thus more thrombin is generated. Though the tissue factor VIIa complex is a powerful activator of factor X, it is inhibited by the recently described "tissue factor pathway inhibitor." Thus, the maintenance of adequate levels of thrombin is provided by the activation of factor X by the factors VIII and IX. In the absence of this positive feedback mechanism, factor VIII- or factor IX-deficient patients (i.e., those with hemophilias A or B) bleed severely.

The endpoint of clot formation is the cleavage of fibrinogen to fibrin by thrombin. Fibrin monomers then rapidly polymerize to form a tight meshwork. Factor XIII also undergoes thrombin activation; its function is to retract and further stabilize the resultant clot by transaminating the fibrin polymers.

CLOT DISSOLUTION

Thrombin, generated by the activation of various coagulation factors, plays a central role in clot dissolution, since it also activates the fibrinolytic system. A simplified view of this system includes the conversion of plasminogen into plasmin by the presence of several tissue activators or proactivators. Plasmin is a powerful enzyme that primarily digests fibrin; however, it also has proteolytic effects on fibrinogen, factor V, and factor VIII. Plasmin activation is attenuated in the presence of inhibitors or neutralized by the presence of antiplasmins.

☐ COMPONENTS OF HEMOSTASIS

Figure 15-1 shows a simplified view of the interaction of several components of the hemostatic system. In order to better understand their relationships, we will describe these components as separate entities, with the understanding that during physiological or pathological situations they interact at various levels. Table 15-1 summarizes the main components of several systems.

ENDOTHELIUM

The endothelium plays a primary role in the regulation of hemostasis. Besides being a barrier that separates the intravascular elements from the highly thrombogenic subendothelium, endothelial cells provide anticoagulant and procoagulant components (Table 15-2). In addition, the endothelium participates in the elaboration of a number of vasoactive compounds, including endothelins (endogenous vasoconstrictors) and endothelially derived relaxing factor (EDRF), now known to be nitric oxide.

Following a variety of tissue insults, endothelial cell sloughing has been observed to occur. In the perioperative arena, this would most likely be due to direct vascular injury; however, other conditions producing similar sloughing include acidosis, hypoxia, and endotoxin exposure. With subendothelial contact, platelet-mediated events unfold as described elsewhere in this chapter.

In the uninjured state, endothelial cell function tends to favor those factors inhibiting thrombosis. Following vessel injury, the balance of endothelial effects sways to promote hemostasis and limitation of blood loss. Local vasoconstriction at the site of injury serves to limit hemorrhage. This vasoconstriction is the result of multiple factors, the most important being vasoactive humoral substances released from platelets. Platelet compounds influencing vessel tone include epinephrine, norepinephrine, ADP, thromboxanes, and kinins. An appropriate balance of vasodilation and vasoconstriction is teleologically important, since excessive or prolonged vasoconstriction predisposes to tissue ischemia. Following the formation of the hemostatic plug, reparation of the breached vessel occurs in the form of cellular migration and repopulation from adjacent vessel walls. At the conclusion of the reparative process, endothelium is reconstituted as migrating cells traverse the internal elastic lamina and redifferentiate into new nonthrombogenic endothelial cells.

In summary, uninjured endothelial cells serve to inhibit platelet adherence and initiation of clotting. Upon injury, endothelial cells manifest both prothrombotic and antithrombotic properties, the balance normally favoring localized thrombosis. It is the overall combination of these factors that maintains hemostasis under normal conditions.

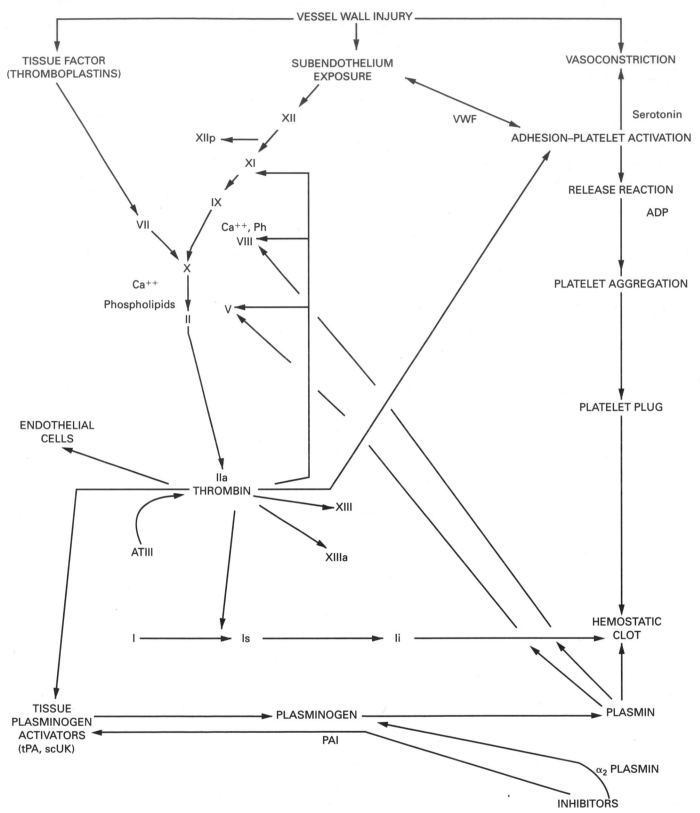

Figure 15–1   A simplified view of the interactions of coagulation, fibrinolysis, and platelet components in response to tissue injury.

Table 15–1
COMPONENTS OF HEMOSTASIS

Endothelial Cell	Platelet Components	Coagulation Factors and Cofactors	Fibrinolytic System	Coagulation Inhibitors
Von Willebrand Factor Prostacyclin (PGI$_2$) Tissue plasminogen activators (PAI-1 and PAI-2) Heparinlike substances Thrombomodulin	Membrane receptors: GPI, GPIIb/GPIIIa, and GPIX Platelet membrane phospholipids Prostaglandin products: thromboxane A$_2$ Granular components: dense bodies (nucleotides and serotonin), α granules (factors I, V, vWF, PDGF, PF-4, and thrombospondin), mitochondrias (ATP production), lysozomes (hydrolases and proteases)	Factors I, II, V, VII, VIII, IX, X, XI, XII, and XIII Von Willebrand factor (vWF) Proteins C and S	Plasminogen and plasmin Activators and inhibitors	Antithrombin III α$_2$ plasmin α$_2$ macroglobulin Activated proteins C and S

PLATELET STRUCTURE

These tiny membrane-bound structures are amazingly versatile, circulating in a tireless search for damaged endothelium. Morphologically, platelets can be considered to be made up of three somewhat arbitrary regions: the peripheral region, consisting of the plasma membrane and its appendages; a sol-gel region containing microtubules, microfilaments, and the contractile protein thrombosthenin; and a cytoplasmic zone containing mitochondria and secretory granules. A glycocalyx surrounds the platelets as the outermost layer of a typical plasma membrane. Various glycoproteins present in the glycocalyx serve as receptors and impart to platelets blood group specificity and antigenicity. Plasma membrane glycoprotein Ib (GPIb) appears to be the receptor for vWF, and glycoproteins IIb and IIIa (GPIIb and GPIIIa) function as receptors for fibrinogen and fibronectin. The membrane has also binding sites for the coagulation factors, ADP, thrombin, and other vasoactive amines.

Table 15–2
MAIN ENDOTHELIAL CELL PRODUCTS WITH COAGULANT OR ANTICOAGULANT PROPERTIES

Anticoagulant	Procoagulant
Heparin-like molecules augment the action of antithrombin III.	Tissue factor initiates the extrinsic pathway of coagulation.
Thrombomodulin activates protein C with the help of thrombin.	Von Willebrand factor (vWF) binds to platelets and to the subendothelium, and serves as a vital element of the primary platelet plug.
Nitric oxide and prostacyclin (PGI$_2$) oppose platelet aggregation and are powerful vasodilators.	Synthesize platelet activating factor, which plays a role in platelet aggregation.
Tissue plasminogen activator (tPA) converts plasminogen to plasmin.	Synthesize plasminogen activator inhibitors include PAI-1, PAI-2, and others.

In the gel-sol matrix of platelets are found microtubules and microfilaments, forming the cytoskeleton of the platelets. These structures participate in the shape change of platelets that occurs during platelet activation. In the cytoplasm are dispersed three types of storage granules: dense bodies, α granules, and liposomal inclusions. Dense bodies are electron-dense organelles and are saturated with Ca^{2+}, ADP, and ATP. These bodies have been designated the storage pools of adenine nucleotides. The α granules contain several proteins whose role has not been clearly defined. Platelet agonists, such as collagen, thrombin, thromboxane A$_2$, ADP, and epinephrine induce the secretion of dense bodies and/or α granule contents.

Table 15–3 summarizes the platelet components and their functions.

PLASMA COAGULATION FACTORS AND COFACTORS

The ultimate substrate for clot formation is fibrinogen, which is converted to fibrin by the fast-acting enzyme thrombin.

Fibrinogen, recognized as factor I, is produced by the liver as a duplicate of three chains: α, β, and γ. It circulates in plasma at concentrations of 200 to 400 mg percent, and it is also localized in the α granules of platelets. The biologic half-life of fibrinogen is 72 h, which has to be taken into account when replacement therapy is considered. Thrombin splits fibrinopeptides A and B from α and β chains of fibrinogen, respectively. These fibrin monomers polymerize to form fibrin. Fibrinogen molecules also play a crucial role during platelet aggregation, since they serve a ligand role after attachment to the platelet membrane receptor GPIIb/IIIa. Fibrinogen is also proteolyzed by plasmin, resulting in fibrinogen split products (FSPs) of variable molecular weight, known as fragments X, Y, D, and E.

Factors II, VII, IX, and X are vitamin K-dependent factors. During synthesis, an inert precursor protein is produced by the liver. Within this precursor, vitamin K then induces the γ carboxylation of 10 to 12 glutamic acid residues. Once carboxylation takes place, these zymogens are ready to be activated by the presence of other coagulation factors converted

Table 15-3
PLATELET COMPONENTS

Location	Components	Main Function
Membrane receptors	GPI/GPIX	Binding sites for vWF, thrombin
	GPIIb/III	Receptor for fibrinogen, fibronectin, and thrombospondin binding
Platelet membrane phospholipids	Phosphatidylcholine, phosphatidylinositol, phosphatidylethanolamine (PC, PI, and PE)	Template site for the binding of activated coagulation factors
Membrane and cytoplasm	Fatty acid pathway, thromboxane A_2	Platelet aggregation
Granules		
Dense bodies	Adenine nucleotides	Platelet aggregation
	Serotonin	Vasoconstriction
α granules	Factors I and V	Coagulant activity
	vWF	Coagulant function
	PDGF	Fibroblast proliferation
	PF-4 and thrombospondin	Heparin inactivation
Lysozomes	Hydrolases and proteases	Enzymatic activation or degradation

into enzymes by previous proteolysis (cascade effect). The biologic half-lives of vitamin K-dependent factors are variable. The approximate half-life of factor II is 60 h, factor X 36 h, factor IX 18 h, and factor VII, 9 h. Two other vitamin K-dependent factors, protein C and protein S, will be considered separately.

Factor VIII coagulant (VIII:C) is also known as antihemophiliac factor. It is produced by the liver in cells other than the hepatocyte. It circulates complexed to a large-molecular-weight carrier protein recognized as von Willebrand Factor. Factor VIII:C is activated by thrombin and destroyed by plasmin or activated protein C. Factor VIII:C deficiency has been reported to occur in hemophilia A, von Willebrand's disease, and carriers of the defective gene, and rarely, it is due to factor VIII:C antibodies. Factor VIII:C has been cloned and is now available as a synthetic product.

Factor V has some structural similarities to factor VIII, but unlike factor VIII it is produced by the hepatocyte. It is not a vitamin K-dependent factor. Its biologic half-life is 10 to 12 h. Factor V is a cofactor in the activation of prothrombin.

Factor XI circulates in the plasma as a complex of high-molecular-weight kininogen. Its biologic half-life varies between 48 and 84 h. It is now believed that factor XI activa-

tion occurs mostly by the action of thrombin and not by the action of factor XIIa stimulation.

It is a known fact that the degree of factor XI deficiency does not necessarily correlate well with the tendency to bleed. This has been extensively studied and recently proposed to be due to two factors: (1) mutations in factor XI, leading to a dysfunctional molecule or resulting in a molecule that is secreted poorly, and (2) procedure-specific risk. Hemorrhagic risk in part depends upon the type of procedure contemplated (i.e., increased risk with surgeries such as tooth extractions, tonsillectomy, and nasal surgery). These tissues in particular have been found to have relatively high local fibrinolytic activity.

Finally, deficiencies of the contact factors (factor XII, high-molecular-weight kininogen, and prekallikrein) result in a prolonged partial thromboplastin test (PTT) result but without an associated bleeding diathesis.

Von Willebrand Factor (vWF) is a large-molecular-weight glycoprotein produced by endothelial cells and is stored in the Weibel-Palade bodies. It is also stored in the α granules of platelets. The basic structure is a subunit of molecular weight 260,000, but this subunit polymerizes to multimers of higher molecular weight. Von Willebrand factor performs a variety of biologic functions. It serves as a carrier protein for factor VIII:C while also playing a role in maintaining factor VIII:C stability. In addition, the role of vWF in platelet-endothelium interactions has already been described. This glycoprotein can be quantitated in terms of its biologic function or antigenic expression. Von Willebrand's disease is either due to a low level of functionally active high-molecular-weight multimers or secondary to a true deficiency of the vWF. Since treatment modalities vary, a correct classification of the type of disease should be attempted in all cases.

FIBRINOLYTIC SYSTEM

Equally important to clot formation is clot dissolution. The fibrinolytic mechanism starts as soon as a fibrin clot is formed. This is a much slower process and physiologically gives enough time for the vascular injury to be reendothelialized. This system is critical for the dissolution of pathologic thrombi as well.

Plasminogen is an inactive protein produced by the liver, and its plasma concentration is around 20 mg percent. It is a single-chain glycoprotein of molecular weight 92,000. It has five kringles (triple-loop structures) and a serine protease domain. Native plasminogen is glu-plasminogen that undergoes plasmic digestion to form lys-plasminogen. The lysine binding sites of lys-plasminogen are the receptors for fibrin, the latter being the template as well as the substrate for plasmin-mediated clot dissolution. The lys-plasminogen is converted to plasmin by the cleavage of a single peptide bond.

Plasmin, still bound to the fibrin surface, proteolytically lyses the clot. In addition, it can also degrade factors V, VIII, and fibrinogen. The cleavage of fibrinogen and fibrin produces fragments of variable molecular weight collectively known as the fibrin-fibrinogen split or degradation

Table 15–4
COAGULATION INHIBITORS AND THEIR DEFICIENCIES

Component	Biologic Actions	Associated Deficiency
Antithrombin III	Inhibition of serine proteases IIa, IXa, Xa, and XIa	Thrombosis
Heparin cofactor II	Inhibition of IIa	Thrombosis
α_2 macroglobulin	Inhibition of plasmin	Unknown
Activated protein C	Inhibition of Va and VIIIa, increased fibrinolysis	Thrombosis
Protein S	Cofactor for activated protein C	Thrombosis

products (FSP or FDP). Four clinically relevant FSPs are recognized, denoted as fragments X, Y, D, and E; by a variety of mechanisms, all of these fragments have been implicated in the production of coagulopathic states. The fibrinolysis of clots transaminated through the action of XIIIa cannot progress to the formation of the terminal fragments D and E but instead gives the intermediate degradation product D2E, referred to as the D-dimer. This peptide is one of the best markers in the diagnosis of disseminated intravascular coagulation (DIC).

There are two well-recognized endogenous activators of fibrinolysis: tissue plasminogen activator (tPA) and single-chain urokinase (scUK). Both moieties participate in the conversion of plasminogen to plasmin, with resultant thrombolysis. Tissue plasminogen activator has a molecular weight of 70,000. It binds to endothelial cells and fibrin (with lys-plasminogen). The proteolytic effect of tPA increases in the presence of fibrin. This high-affinity effect allows efficient activation by fresh clots. Tissue plasminogen activator is released into circulation from endothelial cells in response to several stimuli, including exercise, venous occlusion, stress, or thrombin. The half-life of tPA is 6 min. Single-chain urokinase is a protein of molecular weight 54,000. Urokinase is cleared by liver metabolism and has a half-life of around 4 min after intravenous infusion. Several other exogenous fibrinolytic activators are recognized and commercially available. Best known among these is streptokinase, either alone or combined with other products (i.e., APSAC or anisoylated plasminogen-streptokinase activator complex).

Physiologically, the inhibition of the fibrinolytic system occurs at the level of plasmin or that of plasminogen activator. Alpha-2 antiplasmin freely circulates in the plasma and has a biologic half-life of approximately 2 days. It forms a 1:1 molar complex with plasmin by binding to its lysine binding sites; as may be recalled, these binding sites also serve as the receptors for fibrin binding. In other words, fibrin-bound plasmin is saved from inactivation owing to this common receptor. The overall effect is to ensure that plasmin activity is limited to the area of the clot and also to prevent free plasmin from circulating.

A severe deficiency of α_2 antiplasmin is associated with a bleeding diathesis. Other circulating plasmin inhibitors that have been identified include α_2 macroglobulin and α_1 antitrypsin. Other naturally occurring inhibitors functioning at the plasminogen activator level are the plasminogen activator inhibitors 1, 2, and 3 (PAI-1, PAI-2, and PAI-3) produced by endothelial cells. PAI-1 can be inactivated by the activated protein C (APC), this being the proposed mechanism of the fibrinolytic effect of APC. Several commercial fibrinolytic inhibitors are currently available, including ϵ amino caproic acid (Amicar), tranexamic acid, and aprotinin.

COAGULATION INHIBITORS

Several coagulation inhibitors are present in the plasma (Table 15–4). The most important is antithrombin III (ATIII), which, with heparin, inhibits the serine proteases, such as factors IIa, IXa, Xa, and XIa. The predominant effect

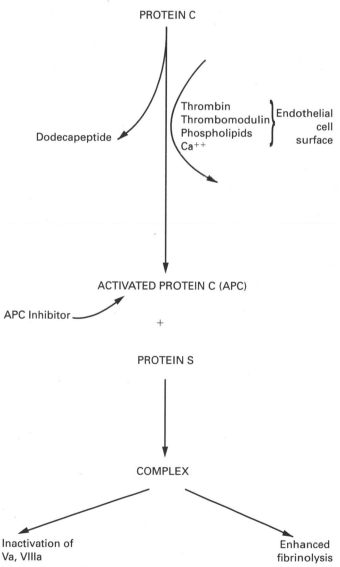

Figure 15–2   The role of activated protein C and proteins in coagulation and fibrinolysis.

of ATIII is to inactivate IIa and Xa. The rate of inactivation is slow if ATIII is alone but very rapid when it is complexed to heparin.

Antithrombin III is a single-chain molecule of molecular weight 50,000. It is not a vitamin K-dependent factor. Thirty percent of the 424 amino acid sequence for ATIII has a structural homology to α_2 antitrypsin. It is a part of the so-called serine protease inhibitor superfamily, since all of these inhibitors possess quite similar amino acid distributions and complementary DNA structure. Heparin binds to ATIII, forming a 1:1 molar complex, and exposes a serine receptor site that can bind to the activated factors, resulting in their inactivation. Antithrombin III has a plasma half-life of 72 h. Patients with ATIII deficiency suffer a tendency to thrombose. Modalities of treatment for these patients include anticoagulation and factor replacement (plasma or ATIII concentrate). However, ATIII deficiency has also been reported in patients with liver disease (decreased production), active thrombosis (increased inactivation), DIC (increased inactivation), and nephrotic syndrome (urinary loss).

Protein C and protein S (Fig. 15–2) act as important inhibitors of the procoagulant system. In contrast to the other vitamin K-dependent factors, a deficiency of either protein C or S is associated with thrombosis. It is a well-known fact that activated protein C is a powerful anticoagulant. The activation of protein C is initiated by the effect of thrombin on an endothelial cell membrane receptor, thrombomodulin. This activation requires calcium and a phospholipid surface. During the activation, a dodecapeptide is released. Currently, the measurement of circulating levels of this peptide is being investigated for use in clinical practice. Activated protein C is either neutralized by APC inhibitor or complexes with protein S. This complex has anticoagulant properties, since it inactivates factors Va and VIIIa and also inactivates plasminogen activator inhibitor 1 (PAI-1), thus inducing fibrinolysis.

Both protein C and protein S are produced by the liver and are vitamin K-dependent. Coumadin blocks their synthesis in a manner similar to the other vitamin K-dependent factors. The half-life of protein C is about 8 h, and that of protein S is about 24 h. Protein S is either free or bound to C_4B binding protein, a component of the complement system. It seems that under conditions of stress, there is a shift from bound to unbound protein S; this appears to affect the measurement of circulating protein S levels under stress or during active thrombosis. Congenital deficiencies of either protein C or S have been associated with a tendency to thrombosis. However, a recently described disorder involves the inability of APC to proteolyze factor V due to a mutation in factor V. This has been termed APC resistance.

REFERENCES

Asakai R, Chung DW, Davie EW, Seligsohn V: Factor XI deficiency in Ashkenazi Jews in Israel. *N Engl J Med* 325: 153–158, 1991.

Asakai R, Chung DW, Ratnoff OD, Davie EW: Factor XI deficiency in Ashkenazi Jews is a bleeding disorder that can result from three types of point mutations. *Proc Natl Acad Sci USA* 86:7667–7671, 1989.

Broze AG Jr: The role of tissue factor pathway inhibitor in a revised coagulation cascade. *Semin Hematol* 29:159–169, 1992.

Chediak J, Kraines J, Hahn A, Telfer MC: Survival of infused antithrombin in a patient with hepatic failure. *Clin Res* 24:539A, 1976.

Dahlback B: Physiological anticoagulation: Resistance to activated protein C and venous thromboembolism. *J Clin Invest* 943:923–927, 1994.

Furie B, Furie BC: Molecular and cellular biology of blood coagulation. *N Engl J Med* 326:800–806, 1992.

Gandhi CR, Berkowitz DE, Watkins DW: Endothelins: Biochemistry and pathophysiologic actions. *Anesthesiology* 80: 892–903, 1994.

Hessing M: Interaction between complement component C4B-binding protein and protein S as a link between coagulation and the complement system. *Biochem J* 277:581–592, 1991.

Mark G, Davies PH, Per-Otto Hagen: The vascular endothelium: A new horizon. *Ann Surg* 218:593–609, 1993.

Meyer D, Pietu G, Fressinand E, Girma JP: Von Willebrand factor: Structure and function. *Mayo Clin Proc* 66:516–523, 1991.

Nieuwenhuizen W, Voskuilen M, Vermond A, et al: The influence of fibrin (ogen) fragments on the kinetic parameters of the tPA mediated activation of different forms of plasminogen. *Eur J Biochem* 174:163–169, 1988.

Osterud B, Rapaport SI: Activation of factor IX by the reaction product of tissue factor and factor VII: Additional pathway for initiating blood coagulation. *Proc Natl Acad Sci USA* 74:5260–5264, 1977.

Svensson PJ, Dahlback B: Resistance to activated protein C as a basis for venous thrombosis. *N Engl J Med* 330:517–522, 1994.

Ware JA, Heistad DA: Platelet endothelium interactions. *N Engl J Med* 328:628–635, 1993.

CHAPTER
16

Physiology of Pregnancy

David Young and Nancy Burk

The physiologic changes that occur as pregnancy advances are dramatic. As the metabolic demands of the fetus increase and as the conceptus grows, the anatomic and physiologic state of the mother undergo profound evolution.

☐ CARDIOVASCULAR CHANGES IN PREGNANCY

There is an increased cardiac output during pregnancy. At the time of the first missed menses, cardiac output has already risen by 1L, or 22% above the preconception level. Previously, it was felt that the increase in heart rate was the predominant reason for the increased cardiac output in the first trimester. However, newer data point to an increase in the stroke volume as the predominant etiology for this change.

As pregnancy progresses through the second trimester, the cardiac output increases by approximately 35 to 50% above preconception values. This change remains stable until the onset of labor. The modification is about equally due to increases in heart rate and in stroke volume. The heart rate usually reaches between 80 to 90 beats per minute (BPM), and heart rates that exceed 100 should be considered abnormal. Figure 16–1 and Table 16–1 summarize these dramatic changes.

During labor, further dramatic adaptations in the cardiovascular system are seen. Early in labor, the cardiac output between uterine contractions increases by 12%. Cardiac output continues to rise another 25% late in the first stage of labor and up to 40% above term pregnancy values at full cervical dilatation (end of stage I). This is mainly due to an increase in stroke volume postulated to be a result of elevated sympathetic tone (from painful contractions) and myocardial contractility. The maternal sympathetic tone increases while at the same time uterine contractions augment the central intervascular blood volume by 300 to 500 mL with blood that has been shifted from the intervillous spaces during contractions.

Initially after delivery, aortocaval compression is alleviated, and the increase in cardiac output transiently may reach a full 150% higher than pregnancy levels. These changes are then quickly reversed after delivery by a decrease in maternal sympathetic tone and subsequent decreases in both heart rate and stroke volume. Stroke volume is reduced because of an obligatory 500 to 1000 mL blood loss that occurs at time of delivery. Full resolution of all the maternal cardiovascular changes does not occur until 24 to 30 weeks postpartum.

Despite the increase in cardiac output discussed, studies have shown a nearly complete obstruction of the inferior vena cava (IVC) and the aorta when the patient is supine at term. The aortocaval compression is produced by the mechanical obstruction of the IVC and aorta by the gravid uterus. In late pregnancy, this compression may result in a 25% decline in both cardiac output and stroke volume. This decline in cardiac output is secondary to a decrease in the venous return of blood to the right atrium. Therefore, to prevent supine hypotension, displacement of the gravid uterus is needed. Clinically, this is usually accomplished via shifting the uterus leftward by either a wedge placed under the patient's right hip, or tilting of the operating room table. Serious consequences may result to both the mother and fetus if displacement is not accomplished.

Anatomically, by 12 weeks gestation, the total ventricular wall thickens by 28% in comparison to prepregnancy values, and the left ventricular mass increases by 52%. As blood volume expands during pregnancy, the end-diastolic volume increases, but the end-systolic volume remains unchanged (because of an increase in ejection fraction). The increased left

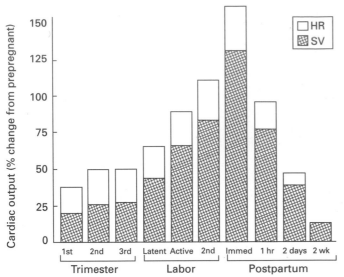

Figure 16–1 Graph of the cardiac output changes during pregnancy. (With permission from Chestnut, p 21, 1994.)

and to the left. Concomitant electrocardiogram changes include sinus tachycardia, leftward axis, and a shortening of the PR interval. Low-voltage T waves and minor ST-segment depression in both the precordial and the limb leads are not uncommon.

Auscultatory changes in pregnancy may actually mimic cardiac disease. At 12 weeks gestation, the aortic, pulmonary, and mitral valve surface areas are all increased. This change continues until the third trimester, when valvular surface areas are dilated to approximately 20% higher than prepregnancy values. Nearly all parturients develop systolic flow murmurs, and a small proportion (20%) will have diastolic murmurs without known cardiac pathology. In addition, a loud S_3 is also heard in many pregnant women.

☐ BLOOD VOLUME

The maternal blood volume is increased by 50% above prepregnancy values; one-third of the increase occurs during the first trimester ($\sim$15%). This increase in blood volume is needed to attenuate several changes that occur both during the development of the conceptus and at the time of delivery. The red blood cell volume increases by 30 to 35%, while plasma volume increases 50 to 55%. The resulting dilution of the red blood cell mass causes the physiologic anemia of pregnancy. This anemia may occur as early as 16 weeks gestation and reaches its relative red blood cell mass nadir at 32 weeks, when the hematocrit equals roughly 35%. This hemodilution will enhance oxygen delivery to the fetus by improving in vivo flow. This occurs because of the improved rheologic properties and reduced viscosity of blood. In addition, this reduced blood viscosity will preserve the patency of the uteroplacental circulation. Finally, the increase in blood volume is needed to compensate for the obligatory 500 to 1000 mL blood loss that occurs at the time of delivery.

J. Pritchard summarizes this point: "The hypervolemia induced by pregnancy seems to meet the metabolic demands of the enlarged uterus with its greatly enlarged vascular system, to protect the mother and, in turn, the fetus against the deleterious effects of impaired venous return and reduced cardiac output when in the supine and erect positions." The hypervolemia of pregnancy is also of considerable importance in safeguarding the mother against the adverse effects of hemorrhage during parturition and puerperium. These points are summarized in the Tables 16–2 and 16–3.

The plasma volume increases in response to increased serum levels of the hormones estrogen and progesterone. Estrogen increases renin activity, which stimulates renal reabsorption of water and sodium. Progesterone also increases aldosterone production, and therefore sodium retention occurs.

ventricular end-diastolic volume can be accommodated without concurrent increase in end-diastolic pressure because of the ventricular dilation and hypertrophy. The increased ejection fraction occurs because of decreased systemic vascular resistance (SVR), or afterload (at term, the SVR decreases approximately 30%), and not because of increased myocardial contractility.

The fall in SVR is accompanied by a fall in blood pressure. Although affected by position (lowest in the lateral decubitus position and highest when upright), blood pressure decreases serially during pregnancy, reaching a nadir at 20 to 26 weeks. The fall is greater in diastolic than in systolic blood pressure. After 26 weeks of gestation, there is a small increase in blood pressure until term.

Radiographic evaluation of the chest during pregnancy reveals that the cardiac silhouette is shifted upward, anteriorly,

Table 16–1
CENTRAL HEMODYNAMICS
AT TERM GESTATION

Parameter	Change[a]
Cardiac output	+50%
Stroke volume	+25%
Heart rate	+25%
Left ventricular end-diastolic volume	Increased
Left ventricular end-systolic volume	No change
Ejection fraction	Increased
Left ventricular stroke work index	No change
Pulmonary capillary wedge pressure	No change
Pulmonary artery diastolic pressue	No change
Central venous pressure	No change
Systemic vascular resistance	−20%

[a]Relative to nonpregnant women.
SOURCE: Adapted with permission from Conklin KA: Maternal physiological adaptations during gestation, labor, and the puerperium. *Semin Anesth* 10:221–234, 1991.

☐ PULMONARY ADAPTATION

There is a marked increase in the basal metabolic rate during pregnancy, which requires changes in pulmonary mechanics in order to prevent hypoxemia and respiratory acidosis. By

Table 16–2
BLOOD AND RED BLOOD CELL VOLUMES IN NORMAL WOMEN LATE IN PREGNANCY AND AGAIN WHEN NOT PREGNANT

Value	SINGLE FETUS (50)			
	Late Pregnant	Non-pregnant	Increase mL	Increase %
Blood volume	4820	3250	1570	48
RBC volume	1790	1355	430	32
Hematocrit	37.0	41.7		
TWINS (30)				
Blood volume	5820	3865	1960	51
RBC volume	2065	1580	485	31
Hematocrit	35.5	41.0		

SOURCE: With permission from Pritchard, p 394, 1965.

the end of the first 7 weeks of gestation, maternal oxygen consumption increases by 10%. This will rise to 40% above prepregnancy levels by term.

To accommodate the increased oxygen demand, there is an accompanying increase in the minute ventilation by 20 to 50% by the end of the first trimester. This is presumably secondary to the increased levels of progesterone. Ventilation of the parturient exceeds the needed amount to attenuate the increase in oxygen consumption, resulting in hyperventilation and hypocapnia. As the Pa_{CO_2} decreases and approaches 30 mmHg, there is a compensatory decrease in the serum bicarbonate level (18 to 21 mEq/L), with a resultant pH increase to approximately 7.44.

Anatomic changes occur within the thoracic cavity to accommodate the enlarging uterus. The diaphragm is elevated by 4 cm without any marked changes in function. The excursion of the diaphragm is greater in pregnancy because of decreased thoracic cage muscle tone. However, because of diaphragmatic elevation (from the gravid uterus), the functional residual capacity (FRC) is reduced. In addition, there is a 5 to 7 cm increase in the chest circumference, with a change

Table 16–3
MATERNAL BLOOD LOSS ASSOCIATED WITH DELIVERY

Method	RBC Loss	Hematocrit	Blood Loss
Vaginal delivery			
Single fetus (75)	190	37.5	505
Twins (20)	320	35.5	905
Repeat cesarean section (40)	340	36.5	930
Repeat cesarean section, hysterectomy (35)	425	36.5	1435

SOURCE: With permission from Pritchard, p 395, 1965.

in both the anteroposterior and transverse diameter of about 2 cm.

As noted in Fig. 16–2, the tidal volume increases during pregnancy from 450 to 650 mL. This increase will accommodate the expanded metabolic needs of the parturient. In order for the tidal volume to expand, there is an accompanying decrease in the expiratory reserve volume (ERV) by up to 40%. This results in the decreased FRC, as illustrated by the formula FRC = ERV + Residual Volume.

The upper airway mucosa becomes engorged, with resultant nasal congestion and, occasionally, voice changes. Although airway resistance would be expected to increase in the face of a decreased Pa_{CO_2}, mild hypoxemia, and decreased FRC, airway resistance is actually decreased. This is most likely an effect of progesterone and relaxin on the bronchial smooth muscle.

The total chest wall compliance decreases late in pregnancy because of the encroachment of the fetus; however, lung compliance remains unchanged. There is no change in the closing capacity (CC = Closing Volume + RV), but, because of the reduction of the FRC to a level below the closing capacity, the pregnant mother is at risk for mild hypoxemia with an A-a gradient increase of 5 to 10 mmHg. When the closing capacity exceeds the FRC, then shunting will occur during normal tidal volumes and cause hypoxemia. In one study, airway closure occurred during normal tidal volumes in greater than 50% of term patients in the supine position. Table 16–4 summarizes these pulmonary adaptations during pregnancy.

☐ RENAL ADAPTATION

As the cardiac output increases during gestation, there is a concomitant increase in the effective renal plasma flow. Accompanying changes in renal anatomy occur, including dilation of the renal pelvis, calyces, and ureters. In early pregnancy, this is probably a hormonal response (primarily to progesterone); however, as pregnancy progresses it is a result of compression of the ureter by the enlarging uterus. The renal plasma flow reaches an increase of 60 to 80% over the nonpregnant state during the second trimester but declines to about 50% by the end of pregnancy.

The glomerular filtration rate (GFR) rises 40 to 50% above prepregnancy levels and maintains this increase until 36 weeks of gestation. The creatinine clearance increases to over 100 mL/min. Normal laboratory values for the term pregnant patient include a blood urea nitrogen (BUN) level of 8.5 mg/dL and a creatinine level of 0.46 mg/dL. Despite this increase in filtration, there is an accumulation of about 7 L of excess water and 500 to 900 mEq/L of sodium. This excess of water and sodium causes a decrease in the total body osmolality of about 10 mOsm below the nongravid state. Tubular flow may exceed tubular reabsorption of glucose, proteins, and some amino acids, resulting in greater urinary excretion of these compounds. In the second and third trimesters, protein excretion of 150 to 180 mg/24 h is considered normal. Finally, the compensation of the previ-

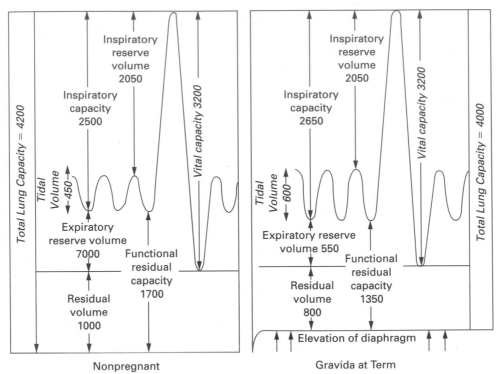

Figure 16-2 Pulmonary volumes during pregnancy. (With permission from Shnider, p 5, 1993.)

ously discussed respiratory alkalosis occurs. The kidneys increase the excretion of bicarbonate so that the normal value decreases from approximately 24 to 20 mEq/L.

☐ MUSCULOSKELETAL CHANGES

Numerous stresses and changes occur as a result of pregnancy and its hormonal influences. The sacroiliac joints loosen and the pelvic symphysis widens. In addition, parturients frequently complain of inguinal pain secondary to stretching of the round ligament. Also, secondary to both increased weight and an increase in the lumbar lordosis, patients complain of back, ankle, and knee pain.

Table 16-4
PULMONARY CHANGES DURING PREGNANCY

Value	Change
Dead space	No change
Minute ventilation	Increased 20-50%
Tidal volume	Increased 40%
Alveolar ventilation	Increased 70%
Maximum breathing capacity	No change
FVC	No change
FEV$_1$	No change
FEV$_1$/FVC	No change
Lung compliance	No change
Chest wall compliance	Decreased
Total pulmonary compliance	No change
Airway resistance	Decreased 50%
Diffusion capacity	No change

☐ GASTROINTESTINAL AND HEPATIC CHANGES

During pregnancy there is a decrease in the volume of gastric acid produced. However, despite the decrease in gastric acid, in several studies, pH has been found below 2.5 in 80% of parturients. There are conflicting data about gastric emptying, but it is felt that it is unchanged in pregnancy. Esophageal barrier pressure is reduced during pregnancy (dramatically during active labor), increasing the risk of heartburn and aspiration of gastric contents. In labor, gastric motility slows and gastric volume increases; however, the stomach may continue to demonstrate a reduction in secretion of gastric acid.

The liver demonstrates marked changes in protein production. The total serum protein and albumin levels decrease, while globulin levels increase, resulting in a reverse albumin-to-globulin ratio. The liver enzyme levels remain at the upper limits of normal except for a marked increase in the alkaline phosphatase level produced primarily by the placenta.

Estrogen is felt to be primarily responsible for the increased protein production. There is an increase in the level of thyroid-binding globulin, which causes a rise in total T3 and T4 levels. However, free T3, T4, and thyroid-stimulating hormone (TSH) levels remain normal. Of particular interest to the anesthesiologist is the decrease in plasma cholinesterase levels by 25% in the first trimester, with persistently low levels until after delivery.

Pregnancy is known to produce a state of hypercoagulability, with a decrease of the prothrombin time (PT) and partial thromboplastin time (PTT) by 20% and bleeding time by 10%. Platelet count increases modestly to about 450,000 cells per mm^3, and fibrinogen levels are increased to 500 to

600 mg/dL by the last trimester. This results in an increased sedimentation rate, with estrogen being the most likely cause. All the clotting factors are increased except for factors II and V, which remain unchanged, and factors XI and XIII, which are decreased.

☐ PHYSIOLOGY OF THE PLACENTA

The placenta is the sole source of nutrition and gas exchange for the developing fetus. Uterine blood flow (UBF) increases from less than 2% of cardiac output to greater than 10% of cardiac output at term. This change increases UBF from its baseline of 100 mL/min to 700 mL/min, of which 90% passes through the placental intervillous space. Since uterine spiral arteries are near maximal vasodilation, blood flow depends on maternal perfusion pressure entirely. The formula for determining uterine blood flow is as follows:

$$UBF = \frac{\text{uterine arterial pressure} - \text{uterine venous pressure}}{\text{uterine vascular resistance}}$$

Therefore, a decrease in systemic blood pressure, which may occur with the supine hypotensive syndrome or after regional blockade (e.g., spinal or epidural anesthesia), is a major source for decreased UBF. Similarly, an elevation in uterine venous pressure, which may occur with uterine contractions, caval compression, second-stage pushing, or uterine hyperstimulation, may decrease UBF.

Placental transfer of nutrients, oxygen, and drugs is dependent upon the same principles of transport seen in any membrane barrier. Oxygen transfer across the placenta to the fetus is driven by the difference of partial pressures of oxygen between maternal and fetal blood. Dissolved oxygen and that bound to maternal hemoglobin is released and transferred across the placental membrane. The placenta needs to supply at least 8 mL of oxygen per minute per kilogram of fetal weight for adequate growth and development.

Because of the morphologic differences in fetal hemoglobin, the oxyhemoglobin dissociation curve is shifted to the left, resulting in a lower P_{50} for fetal hemoglobin. P_{50} is the partial pressure of oxygen at which hemoglobin oxygen saturation is 50%. P_{50} is a useful measure of hemoglobin affinity for oxygen, as a low P_{50} indicates high affinity and high P_{50}

Table 16–5
NORMAL UMBILICAL CORD BLOOD GAS VALUES

Value	Artery	Vein
pH	$7.24 \pm .07$	$7.32 \pm .06$
P_{O_2} (mmHg)	17.9 ± 6.9	28.7 ± 7.3
P_{CO_2} (mmHg)	56.3 ± 8.6	43.8 ± 6.7
Bicarbonate (mEq/L)	24.1 ± 2.2	-2.6 ± 2.1
Base excess (mEq/L)	-3.6 ± 2.7	-2.9 ± 2.4

NOTE: Data are expressed as mean ± 1 SD.
SOURCE: With permission from Creasy and Resnick, p 354, 1994.
Thorp et al: *Am J Obstet Gynecol* 161:600, 1989.

implies low hemoglobin affinity for oxygen binding. The low P_{50} of fetal hemoglobin enhances uptake of oxygen by fetal hemoglobin from maternal hemoglobin, which has a lower affinity for oxygen. In addition, there are local placental pH differences caused by CO_2 transfer across this physiologic membrane. This makes placental maternal blood more acidic and fetal placental blood more basic. This causes a rightward shift in the maternal curve and a leftward shift of the fetal curve, which enhances transfer of oxygen to the fetus. This is known as the double Bohr effect.

Clinically, umbilical cord blood gas values are used as the most readily sensitive indicator of birth asphyxia and acidosis. Normal umbilical cord blood gas values are noted in Table 16–5.

One transport mechanism used by the placenta is diffusion, or passive transport. Oxygen, CO_2, ions, and fatty acids are transported in this way. This mechanism involves the transfer of materials down concentration gradients without expenditure of energy. Glucose, however, is transferred via facilitated diffusion, which is a carrier-mediated, non-energy-requiring transport of relatively lipid-insoluble substances. Active transport involves energy utilization and is responsible for movement of larger anions, such as calcium, iron, and amino acids. Finally, water transport occurs by a means known as bulk flow, which is transport down hydrostatic or osmotic gradients. Factors that favor transfer of drugs across the placental membrane include high concentrations of non-ionized, non-protein-bound, and lipid-soluble substances.

BIBLIOGRAPHY

Branch DW: Physiologic adaptations of pregnancy. *Am J Reprod Immunol* 28:120–122, 1992.

Capeless E, Clapp J: Cardiovascular changes in early phase of pregnancy. *Am J Obstet Gynecol* Dec:1449–1453, 1989.

Chestnut D: *Obstetrics Anesthesia*. St. Louis, Mosby, 1994.

Creasy RK, Resnick R: *Maternal-Fetal Medicine: Principles and Practice*, 3d ed. Philadelphia, Saunders, 1994.

Elkus R, Popovich J: Respiratory physiology in pregnancy. *Clin Chest Med* 13:555–565, 1992.

Hunter S, Robson S: Adaptations of the maternal heart in pregnancy. *Br Heart J* 68:540–543, 1992.

Koller O: The clinical significance of hemodilution during pregnancy. *Obstet Gynecol Surv* 37:649–652, 1982.

Pritchard J: Changes in the blood volume during pregnancy and delivery. *Anesthesiology* Jul–Aug:393–399, 1965.

Shnider S, Levinson G: *Anesthesia for Obstetrics*, 3d ed. Baltimore, Williams & Wilkins, 1993.

17

Neonatal Physiology

Timothy B. McDonald
and Richard A. Berkowitz

The study of newborn and infant physiology reveals the scientific basis for the well-established axiom that children are not just little adults. The development of the fetus into the adult human is not complete until all organ systems have matured into their adult state. The rate of maturity of these organ systems varies from system to system. Physicians have long recognized that endocrine function does not become "adultlike" until the completion of puberty (14 to 19 years of age), whereas adult-equivalent renal function is established by the age of 2 years. The proper administration of anesthesia requires an in-depth understanding of this maturation process.

The anesthesiologist must be aware that many newborns, despite their immature physiologic status, require immediate surgery. Surgery on newborns most often involves the correction of congenital defects of major organ systems. The most serious of these defects include structural heart anomalies, diaphragmatic hernia, congenital bowel malformation, and central nervous system maldevelopment. While the incidence of any single specific defect may be low (congenital diaphragmatic hernia occurring in 1:100,000 live births), the likelihood of the occurrence of at least one of these defects in a newborn is 1 to 2%. This relatively high incidence of congenital defects dictates an awareness and appreciation for the subtleties of fetal and newborn physiology.

Beyond the newborn period, children may present with less serious but more common surgical conditions, such as inguinal hernia or pyloric stenosis. In some groups of prematurely born infants (born less than 37 weeks gestation), the incidence of inguinal hernia may be as high as 20%.

Drug effects and drug metabolism necessarily depend upon the state of maturity of the various organ systems. The appropriate use of pharmacological agents, therefore, depends upon an awareness of newborn and infant physiology and the interaction between pharmacological agents and those immature organ systems. The following discussion explores that interaction.

☐ CARDIOVASCULAR PHYSIOLOGY

The discussion of pediatric cardiovascular physiology begins with the intrauterine development of the fetal heart and fetal circulation. The structural development of the fetal heart and major blood vessels is generally complete at 2 months' gestation. This early development of the circulatory system is essential to the development of other fetal organ systems. The growth and maturation of these other systems require a well-functioning circulatory system to provide adequate oxygen delivery and nutrient transport.

Fetal circulation consists of parallel circuits that, unlike circulation after birth, mix the streams of oxygenated and unoxygenated blood. The right and left ventricle provide the force for perfusing these two circuits. Fetal blood is oxygenated in the placenta and passes through the umbilical vein, the ductus venosus, and the inferior vena cava and into the right atrium. Oxygenated blood in the right atrium then passes into the aorta either via the foramen ovale and left ventricle or via the right ventricle, pulmonary artery, and ductus arteriosus pathways. Oxygenated blood in the aorta may then follow one of several routes to capillary beds in the fetus or the placenta and then pass back to the heart and through either ventricle. Before birth, the right ventricle pumps in excess of 60% of the total combined blood volume pumped by both the right and left ventricles (Fig. 17-1).

Because the resistance to blood flow through the lungs is relatively great, only minimal blood flow through the lungs occurs in utero. Almost all of the right ventricular output into the pulmonary artery passes through the ductus arteriosus to the descending aorta. Only 5% of the blood entering the pulmonary artery enters the lung, whereas the other 95% passes through the ductus arteriosus into the descending aorta, again, a reflection that gas exchange for the fetus takes place in the placenta.

Immediately before birth, the pulmonary arterioles are relatively muscular and constricted. With the first breath, total pulmonary vascular resistance falls rapidly because expansion of the lungs causes anatomic unkinking of pulmonary blood vessels and because inspired oxygen vasodilates pulmonary blood vessels. Conversely, at birth, total systemic vascular resistance increases as the low-resistance placenta is removed from the systemic circuit (Fig. 17–2).

As a result of the decrease in the right-sided pulmonary vascular resistance and the increase in the left-sided systemic vascular resistance, blood flow through the ductus arteriosus reverses direction and becomes left-to-right. By 30 days of age, the pulmonary vascular resistance has usually fallen to adult levels. In the normal infant, the ductus arteriosus has anatomically and physiologically closed by the tenth day of life because of the effects of increased blood oxygen levels and decreased prostaglandin levels (Table 17–1).

Caregivers of newborns and small infants must be mindful of the transition from fetal to infant circulation. After birth, the reversal of blood flow from right-to-left to left-to-right through the foramen ovale and the ductus arteriosus prevents deoxygenated blood from entering the oxygenated systemic circulation. In the newborn, pharmacological therapy is designed to facilitate and maintain the transition to extrauterine life. In order to prevent right-to-left shunting through the ductus arteriosus, therapeutic agents should be used with an eye toward maintaining the proper ratio of pulmonary vascular resistance to systemic vascular resistance. Pulmonary vascular resistance should be kept low relative to systemic vascular resistance. Inappropriately high pulmonary vascular resistance causes a condition known as persistent pulmonary hypertension of the newborn (PPHN), a potentially lethal condition that is not uncommon in children with congenital diaphragmatic hernia and severe meconium aspiration. In these conditions, high pulmonary vascular resistance prevents adequate pulmonary blood flow (Table 17–2).

Adequate oxygenation is necessary to keeping pulmonary vascular resistance low in addition to assisting in the closure

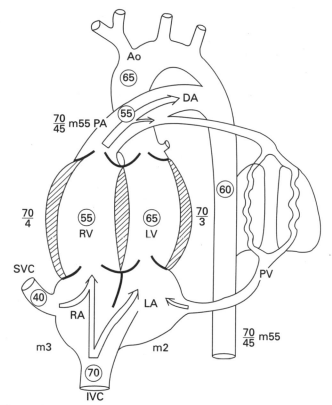

Figure 17–1 Circulatory patterns, intracardiac pressures, and oxygen saturations in the fetal lamb. (With permission from Rudolph AM: *Congenital Diseases of the Heart.* Chicago, Year Book Medical Publishers, 1974.)

of the ductus arteriosus. Both metabolic and respiratory acidosis and increased catecholamine levels caused by pain, hypothermia, or other stress may adversely affect pulmonary vascular resistance. Although all of the factors listed in Table 17–2 contribute to an increase in pulmonary vascular resistance, the combination of hypoxemia and acidosis contributes significantly more than any other single factor (Fig. 17–3). In most instances, elevated pulmonary vascular resistance is amenable to conservative therapy with adequate ventilation, sodium bicarbonate, narcotic analgesia, and sedation. In the most severe cases of PPHN, extracorporeal membrane oxygenation and/or nitric oxide may be necessary.

Regarding the ductus arteriosus, prostaglandin inhibition with indomethicin may be necessary to help close the ductus

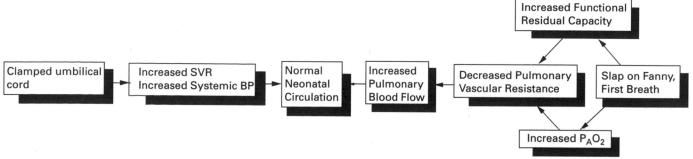

Figure 17–2 Cardiovascular and respiratory events at birth resulting in normal neonatal circulation.

Table 17–1
IN UTERO PHYSIOLOGIC SHUNTS AND SUBSEQUENT FATES

Structure (Vestigial)	Functional Closure	Anatomic Closure	Stimuli	Reversible
Ductus arteriosus (ligamentum arteriosum)	10–15 h	2–3 weeks (term)	O₂, epinephrine, norepinephrine, acetylcholine, bradykinin	Yes
Foramen ovale (fossa ovalis)	12–24 h	3–12 months	Increase systemic vascular resistance, decrease pulmonary vascular resistance	Yes
Ductus venosus (ligamentum venosum)	3–7 days	2–3 months		

arteriosus in premature newborn infants. For circumstances in which it is necessary to keep the ductus arteriosus open, as is the case with transposition of the great arteries or other "ductal-dependent" congenital heart defects, prostaglandin infusions have proved lifesaving.

Once the infant has survived the transition to extrauterine life, the primary cardiovascular goal becomes the maintenance of appropriate cardiac output. In maintaining cardiac output, it is crucial to remember the equation:

$$\text{Cardiac output (CO)} = \text{heart rate (HR)} \times \text{stroke volume (SV)} \quad (1)$$

The sympathetic nervous system, which provides chronotropic and inotropic support for the mature heart, is much less mature and therefore more limited in the newborn than in the adult. Because infants possess relatively high parasympathetic (vagal) tone and a predilection for bradycardia when stressed with hypoxia, laryngoscopy, and intubation, or surgical stress, pharmacological interventions must first be geared toward preserving and maintaining heart rate. The routine use of anticholinergic agents to prevent infant bradycardia during periods of possible vagal stimulation is recommended. Atropine is the most commonly used anticholinergic agent in infants. Unlike older adults and adults with coronary artery disease, infants easily tolerate heart rates in excess of 200.

It is traditionally taught that an infant's cardiac output is heart rate dependent; however, it is incorrect to assume that an infant's stroke volume cannot be augmented. Although the neonatal myocardium may have limited contractile mass, proper manipulation of preload, afterload,

Table 17–2
FACTORS INCREASING PULMONARY VASCULAR RESISTANCE

Hypoxemia
Acidosis
    Metabolic
      Respiratory
Pain
Cold Stress

and contractility can significantly improve a child's stroke volume and therefore cardiac output. However, as the child grows older, cardiac output becomes less dependent on heart rate. In addition, as the child grows older, the resting heart rate gradually decreases while the stroke volume increases up until the child reaches puberty (Tables 17–3 and 17–4).

With regard to the child's circulation, the actual amount of circulating blood volume (CBV) in relation to body mass in the newborn is quite large compared to the adult and gradually decreases over time. The very premature infant may have a CBV as high as 120 mL/kg. The healthy full-term newborn will have a CBV approximately equal to 100 mL/kg, whereas the 5-year-old's CBV is about 80 mL/kg. This value begins to approximate the adult CBV of 70 mL/kg. The anesthesiologist should consider these values during the calculation of an infant's fluid and electrolyte requirements as well as allowable blood loss during major surgical procedures (Fig. 17–4).

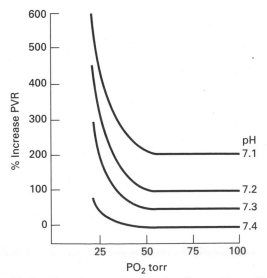

Figure 17–3 The adverse effects of low P_{O_2} and low pH on the pulmonary vascular resistance in the newborn calf. (With permission from Rudolph AM: *Congenital Diseases of the Heart.* Chicago, Year Book Medical Publishers, 1974.)

Table 17–3
HEART RATE ACCORDING TO AGE

Age	Heart Rate beats/min
Preterm	150 ± 20
Term	133 ± 18
6 months	120 ± 20
12 months	120 ± 20
2 years	105 ± 25
5 years	90 ± 10
12 years	70 ± 17
23 years	77 ± 5

(With permission from Gregory GA: Monitoring During Anesthesia, in Gregory GA (ed): *Pediatric Anesthesia.* New York, Churchill Livingstone, Figure 10.1, p. 262, 1994.)

☐ RESPIRATORY PHYSIOLOGY

As with the cardiovascular system, fetal lung development begins within the first weeks of conception and continues for some years beyond birth. From the pulmonary point of view, the transition from intra- to extrauterine life occurs quite rapidly. The adaptation to extrauterine life is associated with significant changes in lung mechanics and the control of respiration. Appropriate intraoperative care of the newborn requires an in-depth understanding of the changes in lung mechanics and the control of respiration as well as the differences in pulmonary anatomy between neonates and older children.

By 10 to 20 min of life, the newborn will have achieved nearly normal functional residual capacity and stable blood gas levels. As stated earlier, pulmonary vascular resistance drops substantially during the next 30 days of life. In part, this rapid transition to extrauterine life, with the drop in pulmonary vascular resistance, is due to the rapid expansion of the pulmonary parenchyma, with the associated unkinking of pulmonary blood vessels. This unkinking occurs when alve-

$$\text{Allowable Blood Loss (ABL)} = \text{weight (kg)} \times \text{EBV (cc/kg)} \times \frac{(H_i - H_f)}{H_i}$$

EBV = estimated blood volume
H_i = initial hematocrit
H_f = final hematocrit

Figure 17–4 Allowable blood loss equation.

oli change from fluid-filled to air-filled. In addition, increased blood oxygen levels vasodilate the pulmonary vasculature. All of these changes allow for improved blood flow to the infant's alveoli. In addition to improved pulmonary blood flow, the infant also has anatomic and physiologic features that provide for optimal gas flow into the alveoli (Table 17–5).

The newborn's respiratory rate is substantially higher than the adult's (40 versus 12 breaths per minute), and the ratio of minute ventilation to weight is also higher in order to meet the oxygen demands of the newborn. The infant's oxygen consumption can be as high as 6 to 12 mL/kg of body weight per minute. This high oxygen requirement increases in babies with cardiorespiratory disease or babies exposed to cold. This oxygen requirement contrasts significantly with the adult's oxygen consumption of 3 to 4 mL/kg of body weight per minute. Obviously, maintaining adequate minute ventilation and inspired oxygen concentration is of paramount importance in newborns and small infants.

Extreme caution and vigilance must be maintained when infants are administered medications that depress respiratory drive. The apneic or hypoventilating newborn experiences rapid arterial desaturation because of the child's high oxygen consumption coupled with the relatively high minute ventilation requirement. A newborn breathing room air who becomes apneic may begin to desaturate in less than 20 s, whereas an adult may maintain adequate oxygen saturation for 80 s or longer. Therefore, drugs that depress respiration,

Table 17–4
ARTERIAL BLOOD PRESSURE ACCORDING TO AGE

Age	ARTERIAL BLOOD PRESSURE	
	Systolic mmHg	Diastolic mmHg
Preterm	50 ± 3	30 ± 2
Term	67 ± 3	42 ± 4
6 months	89 ± 29	60 ± 10
12 months	96 ± 30	66 ± 25
2 years	99 ± 25	64 ± 25
5 years	94 ± 14	55 ± 9
12 years	109 ± 16	58 ± 9
23 years	122 ± 30	75 ± 20

(With permission from Gregory GA: Monitoring During Anesthesia, in Gregory GA (ed): *Pediatric Anesthesia.* New York, Churchill Livingstone, Figure 10.3, p. 263, 1994.)

Table 17–5
MEAN PULMONARY FUNCTION VALUES

Value	Neonate (3 kg)	Adult (70 kg)
Oxygen consumption (mL/kg/min)	6.4	3.5
Alveolar ventilation (mL/kg/min)	130	60
Carbon dioxide production (mL/kg/min)	6	3
Tidal volume (mL/kg)	6	6
Breathing frequency (min)	35	15
Vital capacity (mL/kg)	35	70
Functional residual capacity (mL/kg)	30	35
Tracheal length (cm)	5.5	12
Pa_{O_2} (FI_{O_2} 0.21, mmHg)	65–85	85–95
Pa_{CO_2} (mmHg)	30–36	36–44
pH	7.34–7.40	7.36–7.44

(With permission from Stoelting RK, Dierdorf SF (eds.): Diseases Common to the Pediatric Patient, in *Anesthesia and Co-Existing Disease.* New York, Churchill Livingstone, Figure 32.2, p. 580, 1993.)

such as narcotics, barbiturates, benzodiazepines, vapor anesthetics, or muscle relaxants, must be used in controlled and well-monitored settings.

Furthermore, in the event apnea-producing drugs are used, it is prudent to administer supplemental oxygen prior to drug administration. Obviously, when the newborn breathing 100% oxygen is compared with the infant breathing room air (21% oxygen), there is a signifigant difference in the amount of time before desaturation will occur following the onset of apnea. This additional "safety" period allows therapeutic maneuvers, such as endotracheal intubation, to take place without the infant's experiencing significant arterial desaturation and the associated complications.

After the newborn's rapid transition to extrauterine life has occurred, gradual maturation of the pulmonary system occurs over the next several months. By 1.5 years of age, the child's pulmonary system approaches miniature adult pulmonary physiology. Blood gases have reached adult values by this age. However, children continue to develop new alveoli for several years. By age 3, children will have approximately 80% of the number of alveoli they will have as adults. This is a vital consideration for formerly premature infants who required mechanical ventilation as newborns and developed bronchopulmonary dysplasia. These children can expect significant improvement in their pulmonary function as they develop more alveoli from 6 months to 5 years of age. It is estimated that the newborn is born with 30×10^6 saccules and that this number increases to the adult value of 300×10^6 saccules by 5 years of age.

With regard to the upper airway, there are many anatomic differences between the neonate and the older child or adult (Fig. 17–5). First, the neonate is an obligate nose breather. With relatively small nasal passages, any obstruction caused by secretions may make spontaneous ventilation difficult. In addition, the neonate has a large occiput, which causes the neck to naturally rest in a slightly flexed position when the

child is supine. The neonatal glottis is located at the level of the second or third cervical vertebra, while in the adult it is found at the fourth to fifth cervical level. With the neonatal glottis, the vocal cords angle slightly anteriorly.

With regard to intubation of the trachea, clinicians must recognize that the narrowest portion of the adult airway is at the vocal cords. However, in the neonate, the narrowest part of the airway beyond the nares is the subglottic area. Therefore, in a small child, an endotracheal tube that easily passes through the cords may fit too tightly in the subglottic region. To avoid subglottic edema, clinicians should intubate all children less than 6 years of age with uncuffed endotracheal tubes that manifest a leak around the endotracheal tube at less than 30 cmH₂O pressure.

RENAL PHYSIOLOGY AND BODY WATER COMPOSITION

With regard to the transition from intra- to extrauterine life, there are many similarities between the lungs and the kidneys. Like the lungs, the kidneys are functionally supported by the placenta. Also similar to the pulmonary system, limited renal blood flow causes a decreased glomerular filtration rate (GFR), with an associated high renal vascular resistance. At birth, the elevation of systemic blood pressure and increased blood oxygenation decrease renal vascular resistance and increase renal blood flow. These changes facilitate the waste-removing functions of the newborn's kidneys, previously provided by the placenta.

It is well-recognized that the newborn's kidneys have limited ability to concentrate urine. This limited concentrating ability is secondary to the newborn's limited GFR. However, with the increase in systemic blood pressure, decrease in renal vascular resistance, and associated increased GFR, the newborn rapidly gains the ability to concentrate urine. One-month-old infant kidneys possess 70% of the adult kidney concentrating ability. By 2 to 3 years of age, the child's kidneys have matured to adult levels (Table 17–6).

The immature newborn kidney not only concentrates urine less well but also possesses a decreased ability to reabsorb glucose and bicarbonate. In addition, the neonatal kidney is

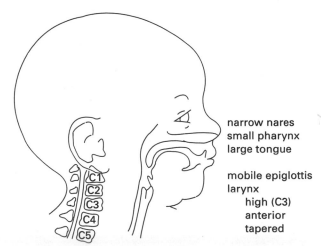

Figure 17–5 Schematic representation of neonatal anatomic characteristics as they relate to airway management. (With permission from Stoelting RK, Dierdorf SF (eds): Diseases Common to the Pediatric Patient, in *Anesthesia and Co-Existing Disease*. New York, Churchill-Livingstone, p 580, 1993.)

narrow nares
small pharynx
large tongue

mobile epiglottis
larynx
  high (C3)
  anterior
  tapered

Table 17–6
PEDIATRIC RENAL FUNCTION VALUES

Age	GFR, mL/kg/min
Neonate (preterm)	16
Neonate (term)	20
3–5 weeks	60
1 year	80
Adult	120

(With permission from Stoelting RK, Dierdorf SF (eds.): Diseases Common to the Pediatric Patient, in *Anesthesia and Co-Existing Disease*. New York, Churchill Livingstone, Figure 32.5, p. 582, 1993.)

unable to conserve sodium. Therefore, newborns are more predisposed to dehydration, renal tubular acidosis, and hyponatremia. Newborns are also more predisposed to the adverse effects of hyperglycemia. These factors make it imperative that the small infant scheduled for elective surgery not be subjected to prolonged periods (>4 h) of nothing by mouth (NPO) status and that intraoperative blood sugar levels be routinely monitored.

As a percentage of body weight, total body water and extracellular water decrease in parallel with fetal maturation. The full-term infant possesses total body water of approximately 80% and extracellular water of about 45%. Both total body water and extracellular water decrease to adult levels by 2 years of age. In the 2-year-old, total body water has decreased to 60%, and extracellular fluid has decreased to about 20% of total body weight. Conversely, intracellular fluid increases from 33% to 44% of body weight by 3 months of age. Figure 17–6 demonstrates these changes.

Obviously, the newborn, with this excessive amount of extracellular fluid, undergoes a significant amount of water unloading during the first weeks of life. The premature infant has even greater amounts of total body and extracellular water. Water unloading in premature babies must be completed by marked natriuresis and diuresis.

For the clinician, these changes in total body water have important implications. The administration of large volumes of intravenous fluids may interfere with the premature infant's physiologic transition to a lower total body and extracellular fluid status. Fluid overload in such infants may complicate or create problems of respiratory distress syndrome, left ventricular failure, or patent ductus arteriosus.

Furthermore, the maturation of the infant's renal system and body water composition has important implications in the kinetic and dynamic effects of various pharmacological agents. These effects are discussed below.

☐ NERVOUS SYSTEM

Aside from the obvious cognitive differences between infants and adults, it is important to consider other central nervous system differences between these age groups.

The difference between infant and adult cerebral blood flow is one important consideration. The small child's brain makes up a much greater percentage of the total body weight than does the adult brain. In fact, the 2-year-old's brain weighs about 80% of what the adult brain will weigh. In addition, cerebral blood flow in the child is 2.5 times greater per 100 g of brain tissue than the cerebral blood flow of the adult. These two factors combine to provide the 2-year-old with up to 1000 mL/min of cerebral blood flow. This means that up to 50% of the child's cardiac output is directed to the young child's head. Successful anesthetic management demands knowledge and anticipation of the potential effects of decreased cardiac output on the child's brain (Table 17–7).

Cerebral autoregulation is the process whereby cerebral vasodilation or vasoconstriction occurs and alters cerebral blood flow in order to meet the infant's present demands for cerebral oxygenation. In the newborn, cerebral autoregulation may be impaired or lost completely under conditions of severe stress. Obviously, the loss of cerebral blood flow may lead to significant intracranial catastrophes.

Regarding the loss of cerebral autoregulation in premature infants, another important feature to consider is the fragility of the vascular structures that comprise the germinal matrix in the cerebral ventricles within the infant's brain. This fragile germinal matrix is sensitive to fluctuations in cerebral blood flow. Pharmacological interventions or surgical events that cause wide circulatory changes may cause rupture of vessels within the germinal matrix. Germinal matrix rupture is more common in infants who weigh less the 1500 g because of their immature germinal matrix. Severe intraventricular hemorrhages may be catastrophic for the baby. This potential complication must be considered whenever pharmacological choices are made that alter cerebral blood flow.

As mentioned under "Cardiovascular Physiology," the infant's nervous system possesses relatively high vagal tone because of the immaturity of the sympathetic nervous system. Stressful circumstances may cause the infant to experience severe bradycardia and, therefore, severely decreased cardiac output to all vital organs, including the brain. Thus, it is important to prevent episodes of severe bradycardia with the liberal use of anticholinergic medications, specifically, atropine.

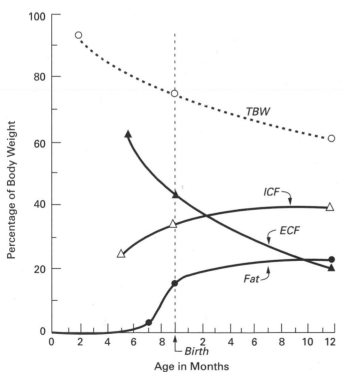

Figure 17–6 Total body water (TBW), intracellular fluid (ICF), extracellular fluid (ECF), and fat as proportions of patient weight. Age-related changes are noted. (With permission from Liu LMP: *Pediatric Blood and Fluid Therapy,* in Hersey SG (ed): *Refresher Courses in Anesthesiology,* vol 12. Philadelphia, Lippincott, pp 109–120, 1984.)

Table 17–7
CHILD VERSUS ADULT CEREBRAL BLOOD FLOW (CBF)

Age	Brain Weight, g	CBF, mL/100 g/min	Total CBF, mL/min	Total Cardiac Output, mL/min	Central Nervous System Cardiac Output, % to Brain
Newborn	400	60	240	500	50
Child (2 years)	1000	100	1000	2000	50
Adult	1400	40	550	5000	10

(With permission from McDonald TB, Berkowitz RA: Massive Transfusion in Children, in Jefferies LC, Brecher ME (eds.): *Massive Transfusion*. Bethesda, American Association of Blood Banks, Table 5.1, p. 102, 1994.)

☐ HEMATOLOGIC PHYSIOLOGY

Any discussion of pediatric hematology must include an analysis of the oxygen delivery equation. The oxygen delivery equation allows one to use an infant's oxygen saturation, arterial oxygen level (Pa_{O_2}), hemoglobin (Hb) level, and cardiac output to calculate the total amount of oxygen delivered to an infant's tissues, at any given time. The oxygen delivery equation is

$$\text{Oxygen delivery} = \text{cardiac output} \times \text{oxygen content}$$

$$\text{Cardiac output} = \text{heart rate (HR)} \times \text{stroke volume (SV)}$$

$$\text{Oxygen content} = [\text{Hb} \times 1.34 \times \% \text{ oxygen saturation (O}_2\text{ sat)} + (.003 \times Pa_{O_2})]$$

Therefore,

$$\text{Oxygen delivery} = [\text{HR} \times \text{SV}] \times [(\text{Hb} \times 1.34 \times \% \text{ O}_2 \text{ sat}) + (.003 \times Pa_{O_2})]. \quad (2)$$

From this equation, it is easy to see why Hb level and oxygen saturation play such an important role in oxygen delivery. Because fetal blood is oxygenated in the placenta, the fetus's intrauterine arterial oxygen saturation is low relative to extrauterine arterial oxygen saturation (fetal arterial oxygen saturation approximates 70 to 75%). The maintenance of adequate oxygen delivery therefore requires a relatively high intrauterine Hb level. However, after the first few moments of life and after the first extrauterine breaths, the newborn's arterial oxygen saturation increases to greater than 95%. Referring to Eq. 2, this increase of approximately 30% in arterial oxygen saturation necessarily increases the newborn's oxygen delivery approximately 30%.

The substantial increase in oxygen delivery that occurs with the first breath of life is associated with an abrupt decrease in erythropoietin production. Subsequently, erythropoiesis almost ceases shortly after birth. The cessation of erythropoiesis is one of the most important factors for the development of physiologic anemia of infancy. It is interesting to note that, after birth, the 30% increase in the infant's arterial oxygen saturation is followed by an associated 30% *decrease* in the infant's Hb level over the next 2 to 3 months. Again, referring to Eq. 2, it is also interesting to note that there is no net effect on oxygen delivery if the oxygen saturation increases 30% while the Hb level decreases 30%! It is

not surprising, then, that infants tolerate the physiologic Hb nadir quite well (Table 17–8).

Approximately 80% of the newborn's Hb is HbF. After 2 to 3 months of age, erythropoiesis begins anew, and the normal bone marrow converts to creating red blood cells containing HbA instead of HbF. By 6 months of age, the percentage of HbF has decreased to the adult level, approximately 2%.

The conversion from HbF to HbA production follows a logical physiologic pattern. HbF possesses a higher affinity for oxygen than does HbA. The P_{50} for HbF is 19, compared to 26 for HbA. The P_{50} is defined as the arterial partial pressure of oxygen at which hemoglobin is fifty percent saturated. P_{50} is used as a measure of affinity of hemoglobin for oxygen. The higher HbF oxygen affinity is necessary for the fetal red blood cells to extract oxygen from the maternal HbA-containing red blood cells in the placenta. The lower systemic pH in the distal fetal tissues allows these HbF-containing fetal red blood cells to unload oxygen once it is delivered to the slightly acidic tissues (Fig. 17–7).

Once the infant becomes independent from the placenta, the need for HbF ceases. Therefore, with the cessation of erythropoiesis, it is logical that the production of HbF would cease and be followed by the production of Hb with less oxygen affinity. It is interesting to note that the subsequent production of HbA (with its decreased affinity for oxygen) coincides with the infant's maintaining adequate oxygen

Table 17–8
NORMAL HEMOGRAM VALUES

Age	Hemoglobin, g/dL	Hematocrit, %	Leukocytes, cells/mm³
1 day	19.0	61	18,000
2 weeks	17.3	54	12,000
1 month	14.2	43	———
2 months	10.7	31	———
6 months	12.3	36	10,000
1 year	11.6	35	———
6 years	12.7	38	———
10–12 years	13.0	39	8,000

(With permission from Stoelting RK, Dierdorf SF (eds.): Diseases Common to the Pediatric Patient, in *Anesthesia and Co-Existing Disease*. New York, Churchill Livingstone, Figure 32.6, p. 583, 1993.)

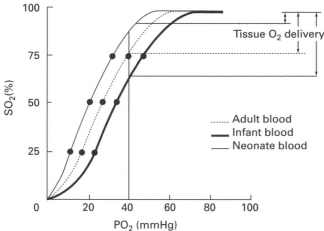

Figure 17-7 Differences in hemoglobin oxygen affinities in neonatal, infant, and adult blood. Neonatal oxygen delivery to tissues is decreased for a given P_{O_2} relative to older children or adults whose hemoglobin has a higher P_{50}, implying lower O_2 affinity. (Reproduced with permission from Motoyama EK, Cook CD: Respiratory Physiology, in Smith RM (ed): *Anesthesia for Infants and Children.* St. Louis, Mosby, pp 38–86, 1980.)

unloading ability despite an increase in tissue pH that follows birth.

As previously stated, normal newborns easily tolerate the transition from HbF to HbA and the associated physiologic anemia of infancy. However, in premature infants, the rapidity with which the Hb level falls is greater. In addition, the nadir to which the Hb level falls is much lower in premature infants. In these babies, it is not unusual for Hb levels to fall as low as 7 mg/dL within 6 weeks of age.

Pediatric anesthesiologists and pediatric surgeons have long recognized that formerly premature infants in general, and particularly those with Hb levels less than 8 to 10 mg/dL, are predisposed to postoperative apnea and other hypoxic events. It is therefore recommended that elective surgery in formerly premature infants be delayed until the Hb level is at least 10 mg/dL. If surgery cannot be delayed on an anemic, formerly premature infant, one must be vigilant for postoperative apnea and even consider, in certain circumstances, appropriate medical therapy. Therapeutic possibilities include postoperative intubation, red blood cell transfusion to bring the Hb level to 10 or greater, and the administration of methylxanthines, such as theophylline or caffeine, upon the induction of anesthesia. These drugs may help prevent apnea in formerly premature infants.

☐ THERMOREGULATION

Maintaining a core body temperature is another significant physiologic challenge involved in the transition from fetus to newborn. Although neonates possess some ability to thermoregulate, the lowest environmental temperature at which an unclothed, unanesthetized baby can maintain a normal core body temperature is approximately 23°C. In contrast, the unclothed, unanesthetized adult can maintain a core body

temperature at an ambient temperature of 1°C. In newborns, failure to maintain core temperature is associated with peripheral and pulmonary vasoconstriction, metabolic acidosis, hypoxemia, hypoventilation, apnea, and, in extreme cases, death.

In analyzing heat loss, it is important to consider the equation for the rate of heat loss:

$$\text{Heat loss} = [T(s) - T(e)]h \times SA \qquad (3)$$

where $T(s)$ and $T(e)$ are skin and environmental temperatures, respectively, h is the thermal transfer coefficient, and SA is the body surface area. The thermal transfer coefficient is controlled by tissue thickness, body size, and blood flow. Infants have large surface-to-volume ratios and a relative lack of subcutaneous tissue. Therefore, neonates are much more susceptible to heat loss than are adults.

The four types of heat loss are conductive, radiant, convective, and evaporative. Conductive heat loss involves the transfer of heat from the baby to the surrounding objects it is in contact with. This may include the operating table or room air and does not depend on airflow. Radiant loss, in contrast, does not require contact, can occur in a vacuum, and depends on the surface to volume ratio of the patient. Convective loss is the loss of heat to the air that depends on airflow; evaporative loss occurs through the skin and respiratory system and correlates with the latent heat of vaporization of water. The two major mechanisms for heat loss in neonates are radiation and evaporation. Clinicians can reduce heat loss in infants by providing warm, dry bedding, radiant warmers, an increased ambient temperature, and heated, humidified ventilation.

In response to cold stress, infants attempt to increase their metabolic rate, and hence oxygen consumption, in order to maintain body temperature. It has been shown that maintenance of a neutral thermal environment is essential to minimizing oxygen consumption in the neonate. Furthermore, a direct correlation exists between the environmental temperature-skin temperature gradient and oxygen consumption. Oxygen consumption is minimal if this gradient is maintained at 2 to 4°C (Fig. 17-8).

Metabolic rate can be increased by voluntary and involuntary muscle activity (shivering) in addition to nonshivering thermogenesis. Unlike adults, infants have little capacity for shivering. Instead, small babies rely on nonshivering thermogenesis to maintain body temperature. Cold stress stimulates a rise in serum concentrations of catecholamines, glucocorticoids, and thyroxine, resulting in fatty acid and glucose metabolism and generating the heat provided by nonshivering thermogenesis. Norepinephrine, the principal mediator, stimulates fatty acid metabolism of brown fat, the primary site of nonshivering thermogenesis in neonates. In babies, areas of brown fat can be found between the child's scapulae, in the axillae, around major blood vessels of the neck, and around the kidneys, adrenals, and vertebrae. After the child reaches 1 year of age the importance of nonshivering thermogenesis significantly diminishes, while shivering begins to play the most significant role in the maintenance of body temperature.

Regardless of the means by which infants attempt to main-

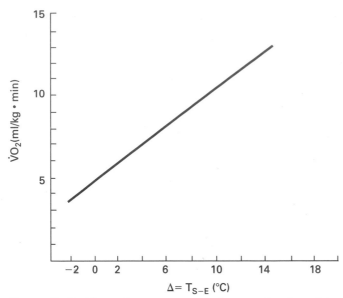

Figure 17-8 Neonatal oxygen consumption as a function of the gradient between the neonatal skin temperature and the enviromental temperature. (Reproduced with permission from Adamson K Jr, Gandy G, James L: The influence of thermal factors upon oxygen consumption of the newborn human infant. *J Pediatr* 66:495–508, 1965.)

tain their core temperature under conditions of physiologic stress and surgery, the infant is unable to maintain temperature without assistance. It is essential for the infant's overall physiologic homeostasis that all possible attempts are made to keep the infant warm.

☐ PHARMACOKINETICS AND PHARMACODYNAMICS

During the first several months of life, there are rapid physical growth and rapid change and maturation in the factors involved in the uptake, distribution, redistribution, metabolism, and excretion of drugs. Thus, there are significant differences between infants and adults in their requirements for and responses to various pharmacological agents.

With regard to the uptake and distribution of vapor anesthetics, such as halothane, infants and small children experience a much more rapid uptake than do adults. In part, this difference in uptake can be explained by looking at some of the fundamental physiologic differences between infants and adults previously discussed in this chapter.

Vapor anesthetic uptake and distribution are influenced by the solubility of the vapor anesthetic, alveolar ventilation, and distribution of cardiac output. Evidence suggests that increased water content, increased alveolar ventilation, and increased brain blood flow all increase the uptake of vapor anesthetics. It is therefore not surprising that the uptake of vapor anesthetics is more rapid in small infants because, as previously demonstrated, such babies have increased total body water content, increased alveolar ventilation, and relatively increased brain blood flow. In addition, research indi-

cates that the solubility of vapor anesthetics is lower in neonates, which causes a faster rise in the F_A/F_I ratio. $F_A =$ the alveolar concentration of volatile anesthetic, and $F_I =$ the inspired concentration of volatile anesthetic. The faster the F_A (alveolar concentration of volatile agent) approaches F_I or the faster F_A/F_I approaches 1 the faster the onset of induction of anesthesia with a particular volatile agent. More insoluble anesthetic agents characteristically approach an F_A/F_I of 1 faster than soluble agents.

In addition to these factors, brain uptake of the lipid-soluble drugs may be influenced by the blood-brain barrier, a lipid membrane interface between the endothelial cells of the brain vasculature and the extracellular fluid of the brain. In small infants, the blood-brain barrier is considered immature, and it is therefore not surprising that the brain concentration of many drugs is higher in the infant than in the adult.

This increased brain permeability in infants may partially explain why infants are more sensitive to narcotics, such as morphine and meperidine. Animal research demonstrates that morphine concentrations are four times higher in animals with "immature" blood-brain barriers despite equal blood concentrations. Consequently, extra care must be used in the dosing and timing of narcotics in infants.

An analysis of drug distribution involves the processes whereby drugs reach various concentrations in various tissues. The drug distribution process is controlled by the degree of protein binding, tissue volumes, and blood flow to these various tissues. As previously stated, the neonate has relatively larger total body water, extracellular fluid, and blood volume than the adult. In addition, the neonate has lower levels of albumin and other serum glycoproteins that bind many drugs. All of these factors contribute to the larger volume of distribution of parenterally administered drugs.

Since drug concentration is equal to dose of drug divided by volume of distribution, the neonate's larger volume of distribution may partially explain why neonates require a larger dose (on a per-kilogram basis) of many anesthetic drugs in order to produce the desired effect:

Drug concentration = drug dose/volume of distribution   (4)

Examples of such drugs include the sedative-hypnotics and muscle relaxants. The amount of ketamine per kilogram of body weight required to prevent gross movements is four times greater in the 6-month-old than in the 6-year-old. In part, this is because the volume of distribution is much higher in the 6-month-old than in the 6-year-old. Similarly, induction doses of thiopentone and succinylcholine are significantly higher on a milligram-per-kilogram basis in neonates and infants than in adults.

The major process that leads to the termination or alteration of pharmacological activity is drug metabolism. The liver is the principal organ of drug metabolism, although the lungs and kidneys have considerable metabolic activity. Metabolism in the liver depends upon liver size and the maturation of microsomal enzymes. Enzyme systems that are responsible for the metabolism of drugs are immature or absent in the neonate.

Neonates are significantly impaired in the ability to oxidize drugs but are not as impaired in the reduction or hydrolysis biotransformation processes. In addition, the infant is severely limited in the ability to conjugate drugs with sulfate, acetate, glucuronic acids, or amino acids. Research suggests that this hepatic immaturity or decreased enzyme activity results from a lack of stimulation rather than an inability of the enzyme system to be stimulated.

Premature infants and full-term infants with the same "postbirth" age possess the same enzymatic activity and ability to handle various drug substrates. This suggests that the age since birth, not the gestational age, is most important for the maturation of these enzyme systems.

All of these pharmacological considerations create a paradoxical situation for the clinician. On one hand, because of the neonate's larger volume of distribution, the neonate requires a larger initial dose of drug. On the other hand, the baby's immature enzyme system often results in an undesirable prolonged duration of action following these initially large doses.

CHAPTER 18

Physiology of Advanced Age

Janet R. Newman

The medical definition of *elderly* is continually revised, but people over 65 years of age are arbitrarily designated geriatric patients by multiple sources. The most rapidly increasing component of our society are the elderly, who comprise over 10% of the American populace. In 1900, only 4% of the population was older than 65; by 2030, 17% of the population will be older than 65. Daily, 5000 Americans celebrate their sixty-fifth birthday, and these people can anticipate living another 15 to 20 years.

Because life expectancy has increased, more geriatric patients present for surgery. It is estimated that 50% of those who reach 65 will require surgery. Currently, approximately 25% of surgical procedures involve elderly patients. Cataract extraction, transurethral resection of the prostate (TURP), herniorrhaphy, cholecystectomy and reduction of a hip fracture are the most common operations associated with the elderly.

Age alone is not a contraindication to surgery. However, morbidity and mortality rates are increased in geriatric patients if they have coexisting diseases that alter their American Society of Anesthesiologists (ASA) classification and if they are undergoing an emergency operation. In order to minimize the risk of anesthesia and surgery in the elderly patient, it is necessary to understand the physiologic changes associated with aging and how these changes will affect anesthetic management.

Aging is variable among individuals, and chronologic and biologic ages often are not equivalent. The process of aging includes atrophy, loss of tissue elasticity, and reduced functional reserve of most organ systems. The physiologic function of most organ systems begins to decline in the late twenties or early thirties and continues at a linear rate until age 85, when the rate of decline accelerates. Generally, most organ systems lose 5 to 10% of their function per decade after

age 30. These changes in organ structure and function are usually appreciated when elderly patients are stressed beyond the limits of their usual lifestyle (e.g., by surgery, perioperative anemia, or infection). Stress is less well-tolerated because of the decreased ability of compensatory mechanisms to maintain physiologic equilibrium. Therefore, perioperative care of the elderly patient must be tailored to the age-related physiologic changes of major organ systems and the age-related responses to drugs. The following discussion reviews these physiologic, pharmacokinetic, and pharmacodynamic changes.

☐ CARDIOVASCULAR SYSTEM

Cardiovascular changes in the elderly population reflect a combination of the aging process per se, age-related disease, and lifestyle. The effects of these variables are interactive, making it difficult to assess the influence of "aging" alone on the cardiovascular system. Greater than half the morbidity rate in the elderly population is due to cardiovascular disease. Therefore, an understanding of the physiologic changes occurring in cardiovascular structure and function is important to any practitioner dealing with this population.

Anatomic changes occur within this organ system. There is atrophy of the myocardium, and myofibers are replaced by connective tissue. Increasing endocardial thickening and stiffness result from fibrosis of the endocardial lining. Valvular calcification leads to changes in leaflet configuration, resulting in valvular incompetence and perivalvular turbulence.

The cardiac conduction system also undergoes age-related changes, including degeneration of the sinoatrial node and conducting tissue, and attrition of the pacemaker cells. Supraventricular and ventricular dysrhythmias and block occur more frequently in elderly persons; sick sinus syndrome and trifasicular block are predominantly geriatric diseases. Common electrocardiographic (ECG) findings among the elderly population include first-degree heart block, left anterior hemiblock, and right bundle branch block. Other ECG changes involve decreased T-wave amplitude; T-wave inversions, especially in leads I, AVL, V_5, and V_6; and left axis deviation.

There is a generalized loss of elasticity throughout the vasculature. This vascular stiffness occurs as a result of changes in the vascular media. There is progressive dilation and elongation of the aorta and increased wall stiffness. With this decrease in vascular compliance, the arterial pulse pressure increases, a result of a greater increase in systolic pressure relative to the change in diastolic pressure.

Progressive left ventricular hypertrophy occurs with aging, probably in response to the chronic increase in afterload due to the elevated peripheral vascular resistance. Left ventricular wall thickness increases approximately 30% between the fourth and ninth decades. Autopsy data from patients in this age range shows that the heart mass increases an average of 1 g/year in men and 1.5 g/year in women. This hypertrophy appears to be a compensatory mechanism to maintain normal cardiac volume, wall stress, and systolic function in the face of increased arterial pressure.

Decreased left ventricular compliance leads to left atrial enlargement. With aging, the contribution of atrial contraction to ventricular filling almost doubles, providing 10% of ventricular filling in a young adult versus 18% of ventricular filling in an elderly person. Therefore, a normal sinus rhythm becomes increasingly important in ensuring optimal ventricular filling in the older patient.

The coronary arteries also become less distensible and have decreased caliber, thereby reducing maximum coronary blood flow. Coronary artery disease becomes more severe throughout an adult life span but may not manifest until a critical stenosis is reached. At autopsy, there is a higher incidence of coronary stenosis (50 to 60%) among the elderly over age 75, compared to the incidence of coronary artery disease (30%) that is diagnosed via clinical symptoms (e.g., angina, myocardial infarction, or resting ECG) in a similar population. Therefore, coronary artery disease is latent or occult in a significant portion of the geriatric population. Regardless of symptoms, people over 70 years of age have a 50% or greater chance of developing coronary artery disease.

Many studies propose that cardiac output decreases or remains unchanged in the elderly population. It is stated that cardiac output decreases about 1% per year after age 30, possibly due to decreased oxygen requirements of organ systems. These conclusions are based on studies that included hospitalized patients with sedentary lifestyle and acute or chronic diseases. The Baltimore Longitudinal Study on Aging demonstrated no significant age-related decrease in cardiac output at rest or with exercise. This study involved rigorously screened, healthy subjects, 30 to 80 years old. Due to a decline in physical activity, or to age-related disease, the older patient may suffer decreased cardiac output. However, the healthy elderly patient who has remained active does not necessarily have a decline in cardiac output secondary to aging alone.

The effects of aging on the cardiovascular system may be anticipated when the system is stressed (i.e., during exercise). In the Baltimore Longitudinal Study on Aging (where the subjects are screened to exclude coronary artery disease or other cardiac disease), there was no decrease in cardiac output during exercise in the elderly population studied as compared to younger subjects. However, the increase in cardiac output in response to stress in the elderly is achieved by a different mechanism than in younger subjects.

The maximum heart rate attained by an elderly person is less than that of a younger person and is estimated by the following formula: maximum heart rate $= 220 - $ age. To compensate for this lower maximum heart rate, stroke volume increases more in the elderly during exercise than in younger individuals. The Frank-Starling mechanism augments cardiac output in the elderly as workload increases. Venous return increases, thereby enhancing cardiac filling. End-diastolic volume increases more than end-systolic volume, and therefore a larger stroke volume is ejected.

However, this mechanism has a price in greater wall tension, which increases myocardial oxygen consumption. In addition, the increase in end-diastolic volume causes an increase in left ventricular filling pressure. Because of progressive age-related myocardial hypertrophy, elderly patients have a steeper pressure-volume curve. Therefore, when elderly persons increase cardiac output by increasing left ventricular filling volumes, left ventricular filling pressures increase, predisposing to congestive heart failure if large filling volumes are necessary.

Several components of the cardiovascular response to maximal aerobic exercise decrease with aging. There are age-related declines in maximal work capacity, maximal oxygen consumption, and maximum heart rate. The degree of decrease depends on the subjects studied.

Studies in animal and human subjects suggest that the age-related cardiovascular response to stress may be due to a reduction in β-adrenergic effects on cardiovascular function. During stress, elderly subjects generate a reduced maximal heart rate and ejection fraction compared to younger subjects. However, measured catecholamine levels in these elderly subjects are greater than those levels measured in the younger subjects. There are diminished chronotropic and inotropic effects of β-agonist drugs in the elderly. Vascular relaxation and constriction mediated by adrenoreceptors are also reduced in the elderly. Thus, elderly patients respond to stimulation as if they have an intrinsic β blockade. Proposed mechanisms for this decreased responsiveness include a decrease in receptor number, a decrease in receptor affinity for agonist molecules, or a change in the adenylate-cyclase system. Therefore, the cardiovascular changes associated with aging may reflect a decreased responsiveness to stimulation by the autonomic nervous system. In summary, recent studies in healthy geriatric patients demonstrate that cardiac output at rest and in response to stress does not change significantly between 30 and 80 years old. Cardiac output is maintained by the Frank-Starling mechanism in the elderly and by an increase in heart rate in the younger population.

RESPIRATORY SYSTEM

The effects of aging on the respiratory system involve alterations in the mechanical properties of the lung, alveolar gas exchange, and regulation of respiration. These changes may not affect a healthy elderly person. However, when stressed by coexisting diseases, surgery, or the effects of anesthesia, an elderly patient may become symptomatic due to a decreased pulmonary reserve.

Impaired mechanical ventilation is a result of multiple anatomic changes affecting lung parenchyma and thorax movement. Decreased lung elastin leads to loss of lung elastic recoil. Calcification of costochondral cartilage decreases chest wall compliance, making the thorax more rigid. Total lung capacity decreases approximately 10% by 70 years of age, secondary to loss of body height due to disintegrating intervertebral discs. However, if corrected for the change in height, total lung capacity is unchanged by aging. Progressive dorsal kyphosis increases the anteroposterior chest diameter, which further impairs chest expansion. The muscles of breathing, the intercostals and the diaphragm, have decreased strength and a lower fatigue threshold. There is an increase in abdominal musculature work to compensate for the decrease in rib cage compliance.

These changes alter lung volumes and flow rates. There is an increase in residual volume at the expense of expiratory reserve volume, leading to a decrease in vital capacity. Functional residual capacity (FRC) also increases. The forced exhaled volume in 1 s (FEV_1) and forced vital capacity (FVC) decrease with aging. The ratio FEV_1/FVC is normally greater than 80% in young adults but falls to less than 70% in persons over 70 years old. This decline is probably due to a combination of the loss of elasticity around the alveoli and alveolar ducts, an increased anteroposterior chest diameter, and weakening of the respiratory muscles. Maximum breathing capacity at 70 years old is only 50% of the value measured at 30 years old.

The parenchymal changes of the aging lung are similar to the changes associated with emphysema: loss of alveolar septal tissues with enlarged alveolar spaces. The physiologic dysfunction that follows is related to airway closure and loss of gas exchanging units. Normally, the alveolar septa keep the terminal bronchioles patent. However, with aging, this support is destroyed, and small airways close during exhalation. Closing capacity is the lung volume below which small airways close and alveoli are not ventilated. Because of the loss of lung elastic recoil, closing capacity increases with aging. For someone in their mid-thirties in the supine position, closing capacity exceeds FRC. By the mid-sixties, closing capacity exceeds FRC in the sitting position, encroaching on tidal volume and causing air trapping, atelectasis, and shunting. In addition, anatomic dead space increases because large airways increase in diameter while the small airways decrease.

The efficiency of gas exchange declines with aging, reflected by the declining arterial partial pressure of oxygen (Pa_{O_2}). The Pa_{O_2} decreases about 0.5 mmHg/year after the age of 20. The following equation estimates the Pa_{O_2} of room air as a function of age:

$$Pa_{O_2} = 100 - [0.3 \times age] mmHg \qquad (1)$$

The alveolar-to-arterial difference for oxygen tension increases with aging from a difference of 8 mmHg at 20 years old to greater than 20 mmHg at 70 years. This impaired arterial oxygenation is due to increased small airway closure, resulting in ventilation to perfusion mismatch; degenerative parenchymal changes and loss of alveolar septa also contribute by decreasing surface area for gas exchange. Pulmonary vasculature fibrosis that occurs with aging increases the ventilation of underperfused alveoli. The increase in physiologic dead space also increases the arterial to alveolar difference for carbon dioxide.

Central control of ventilation changes with aging. In the awake state, the response to hypoxia and hypercarbia is reduced. During sleep the elderly experience more irregular breathing patterns and more apneic periods, making them prone to apnea in the recovery room. In addition, premedication in the elderly requires carefully monitoring their respiration and arterial oxygen saturation.

Airway closure also interferes with intrinsic pulmonary toilet mechanisms. There are fewer cilia in the respiratory tract, further impeding mucociliary clearance. Coughing is also less effective. There is a decline in airway reactivity and protective reflexes in the elderly, putting them at risk for pulmonary aspiration. Considering all these factors, the elderly are predisposed to lung infections and postoperative pneumonia.

RENAL SYSTEM

The effects of aging on the renal system involve tissue atrophy, decreased renal blood flow, and decreased renal function. Approximately 30% of renal mass is lost by the eighth decade. Interstitial fibrosis and diffuse fat replace parenchymal and cortical losses. Glomeruli, the functional units of the kidney, also decrease with aging. In addition to a decline in the glomerular filtering function of the kidney, there is also a decrease in the tubular, or excretory, function of the kidney. Therefore, renal clearance is decreased.

Decreased renal blood flow is due to reductions in the size of the vascular bed as well as a possible age-related decrease in cardiac output. Renal blood flow is estimated to decrease 1 to 2% per year, resulting in a 40 to 50% decline between 25 to 65 years of age. Blood flow reduction is largely to the renal cortex, while flow to the renal medulla is maintained. This results in a reduced glomerular filtration rate (GFR) of about 1 mL/min/year, or approximately 1 to 1.5% per year. Therefore, the GFR decreases in parallel with renal blood flow. Despite the decrease in GFR, serum creatinine levels remain within normal limits. This results from the decrease in skeletal muscle mass relative to total body mass that creates a reduced creatinine load. Therefore, an elevated serum creatinine reflects renal dysfunction. Creatinine clearance is a more reliable predictor of renal function. This value remains steady until 35 years of age, when a linear decrease of 1 mL/min/year begins. The following formula estimates creatinine clearance for men based on age:

$$\text{Creatinine clearance} = \frac{[140 - \text{age (years)}] \times \text{weight (kg)}}{72 \times \text{serum creatinine}} \quad (2)$$

Multiply this formula by 0.85 for women to account for the difference in body composition.

The aging kidney also has a decreased urine concentrating capacity, another manifestation of degeneration of the renal cortical vasculature with sparing of the renal medullary vasculature. As a result, the proximal renal tubules remain intact, while function of the distal renal tubules is impaired. Geriatric patients are less able to concentrate urine if dehydrated and are less able to secrete an acid load and therefore compensate for respiratory or metabolic acidosis. In the elderly patient, the existing renal function can meet the basal requirements, but there is minimal reserve in the face of water and electrolyte imbalances.

The aging kidney is also less responsive to antidiuretic hormone (ADH) and has an impaired ability to conserve sodium; the threshold for serum glucose to produce glycosuria is also increased. Therefore, glycosuria in an elderly person indicates a higher serum glucose level than in a younger person. The plasma concentration of renin and aldosterone decreases approximately 30 to 50%, thereby increasing the susceptibility to developing hyperkalemia.

☐ NERVOUS SYSTEM

Aging produces structural and functional changes of the brain and the nervous system. Brain size decreases with aging, such that the average 80-year-old brain weighs 18% less than a 30-year-old brain. With a decrease in brain mass, there is a compensatory increase in cerebrospinal fluid. Most of the tissue wasting is due to a loss of neurons rather than of the supportive glial cells. Although neuronal loss is constant, it varies in different areas of the brain, and the rate of loss varies with age. The average rate of loss is 50,000 neurons per day. Since the initial neuron count approximates 10 billion, roughly 3% of neurons are lost during a lifetime. With the loss of neurons from specialized areas in the brain, there is also a decrease of neurotransmitters, including acetylcholine, dopamine, tyrosine, serotonin, and norepinephrine. In addition, there is an increase in concentration of catabolic enzymes, including monoamine oxidase and catechol-o-methyltransferase.

Cerebral blood flow decreases about 20% between ages 30 and 70 years in proportion to the decrease in neuronal tissue. The coupling of cerebral metabolic rate and cerebral blood flow remains intact with aging. Autoregulation of cerebrovascular resistance still responds to changes in arterial blood pressure. Hyperventilation continues to stimulate cerebral vasoconstriction in healthy elderly brain tissue. However, in patients with cerebrovascular disease there is decreased cerebral vasomotor activity, particularly in response to hypoxia. Glucose utilization by brain tissue also appears to be maintained.

Although aging is sometimes associated with a decline in mental function, recent studies suggest that retention of information, understanding, and long-term memory remain intact in healthy elderly patients well into their eighties. There is some decrease in short-term memory and reaction times, skills that demand rapid comprehension or information retrieval.

Sensory perception also declines with aging, involving all the special senses, including vision, hearing, touch, proprioception, smell, taste, temperature, and pain. This loss is due to a combination of central changes and degenerative changes at the specific sense organs. There are both a loss of afferent conduction pathways in the periphery and spinal cord and a decrease in velocity and amplitude of electrical impulses in the remaining pathways. In addition, there is a decline in electrical transmission along motor pathways. Skeletal muscle does not change significantly with aging; however, there is a decrease in the number of motor endplate units. To compensate, there is generation of extrajunctional cholinergic receptors.

As previously discussed, autonomic end-organ responsiveness decreases with aging. Despite elevated catecholamine levels (two to four times higher than normal) the elderly respond similarly to a patient on β blockers. Pharmacologic studies show that the aging β-adrenergic receptor has decreased affinity for both β agonists and antagonists. This suggests that a qualitative receptor change occurs rather than a quantitative change. The autonomic responses that support cardiovascular equilibrium are also decreased. The baroreflex, beat-to-beat heart variability after position changes, and the vasoconstrictor response to cold are all slower in onset, less intense in response, and less efficient in maintaining a stable blood pressure. Therefore, the aging autonomic nervous system is less effective in responding to stress.

☐ HEPATIC AND GASTROINTESTINAL SYSTEMS

Aging reduces liver size by as much as 40% by 80 years of age. Hepatic blood flow decreases in parallel with the decrease in cardiac output and the decreased tissue mass. The loss of functional hepatic tissue and decreased hepatic perfusion are significant factors contributing to decreased drug metabolism in the elderly. The bromosulphalein (BSP) retention test supports the concept that decreased hepatic mass impairs hepatic function. Healthy elderly patients without evidence of hepatic dysfunction have impaired BSP excretion. Albumin production also decreases with aging.

Aging produces qualitative but minimal quantitative changes in hepatocellular enzymes. Although the plasma concentrations remain stable, there is reduced activity of hepatic enzymes, especially the microsomal mixed-function oxidases. Hydroxylation and N-dealkylation of drugs are also reduced, therefore decreasing drug clearance and increasing plasma concentrations for a given dose of drug in elderly patients.

The function of the gastrointestinal tract also changes with aging. There is an approximately 35% decline in splanchnic perfusion and an equivalent decrease in surface area for mucosal absorption. The decrease in perfusion of the gastrointestinal tract can delay absorption of orally administered drugs. There appears to be no significant change in the transport time of intestinal contents with aging.

With aging there is decreased parietal cell activity, which results in impaired acid secretion and an increase in gastric fluid pH. However, gastric emptying is delayed with aging. Therefore, despite decreased gastric acid secretion, elderly patients are still at risk for aspiration, further compounded by the decrease in airway reflexes that occurs with aging.

☐ ENDOCRINE SYSTEM

Aging has minimal influence on the endocrine system. Aside from the hormonal changes of female menopause, the functional changes of the endocrine system are limited, involving the glands, hypothalamic releasing factors, and receptors in affected tissues.

The endocrine function of the pancreas declines with aging, and the incidence of diabetes mellitus increases with age, peaking at 60 to 70 years of age. Geriatric patients often have impaired glucose tolerance. The cause of this impairment is multifactorial, resulting from reduced insulin synthesis or secretion, insulin receptor insensitivity, impaired glucose utilization, changes in body composition, and changes in diet and activity. The elderly patient is more prone to developing a hyperosmolar, nonketotic state, rather than diabetic ketoacidosis. The onset of diabetes can be subtle in geriatric patients, who often remain asymptomatic until dehydration or ketosis occurs. Because of an elevated renal threshold for excreting glucose, urinary assessment alone may be unreliable.

Adrenal function is also altered with aging. There is a reduction in the plasma concentration of aldosterone due to the decrease in the plasma renin activity. Asymptomatic hypothyroidism is found in greater than 13% of the healthy geriatric population, especially women. The only sign of this condition is an elevated plasma concentration of thyroid-stimulating hormone.

☐ BODY COMPOSITION

Body composition changes with aging. Body weight increases up to 60 years of age; body weight in men is 25%

higher and in women is 18% higher than in developed young adults. After 60, body weight begins to decrease, leveling out at a weight equivalent to less than that of a young adult. Body tissues also change, and the ratio of fat content to water content increases in an elderly person. Total body fat content increases from 18 to 36% in men and from 33 to 48% in women. Total body water content decreases about 10 to 15%, reflecting a decrease in skeletal muscle mass. The decrease in total body water also occurs in parallel with the increase in fat content, which is anhydrous. There is no significant change in blood volume with aging. Because of all these changes, the volume of distribution changes for lipid- and water-soluble drugs.

☐ BASAL METABOLIC RATE AND THERMOREGULATION

After the age of 30, the basal metabolic rate decreases about 1% per year. Muscle mass and oxygen consumption also decrease, reflected in a reduced cardiac output with aging. This decrease in basal metabolic rate causes a reduction in basal heat production in the elderly person. The epidermis and subcutaneous tissue layers thin with aging, reducing intrinsic insulation.

Thermoregulation is impaired in the elderly due to effects in the afferent, hypothalamic, and efferent branches of the system. Thermoreceptors in the skin, the sensory or afferent component, become less sensitive to temperature changes. The central component of this system is intact in the majority of elderly patients, with the hypothalamic thermal set point remaining normal. Most of the dysfunction occurs in the motor or efferent limb. The autonomic reflex of cutaneous vessel vasoconstriction is less effective in the elderly patient. Therefore, core heat is released to the environment after it reaches the skin. There is also a slowing of the onset and effectiveness of shivering thermogenesis. Studies show that in comparison to younger patients, elderly patients have lower body temperatures during operative procedures and in the recovery room. The elderly are less able to maintain body temperature in a cold environment because of the combined effects of decreased body mass (and therefore decreased heat production) and dysfunctional thermogenesis mechanisms. Elderly patients also have difficulty dissipating excessive heat because impaired autonomic control affects cutaneous vasodilation, and sweat gland atrophy decreases sudomotor activity. Thus, the elderly person is more sensitive to both hypothermia and hyperthermia.

☐ PHARMACOKINETICS AND PHARMACODYNAMICS

Aging results in altered drug effects due to both pharmacokinetic and pharmacodynamic changes. The age-related changes in drug disposition probably reflect a combination of factors, including decreased cardiac output, increased body fat, decreased protein binding, and decreased renal and hepatic function.

Pharmacokinetic changes in the elderly are reflected by an increased elimination half-time ($T_{1/2}\beta$) of drugs, most often due to decreased clearance (Cl) or increases in volume of distribution (V_d), as expressed by the formula

$$T_{1/2}\beta = \frac{0.693 \times V_d}{Cl} \qquad (3)$$

Clearance is the volume of plasma cleared of drug over a unit of time, usually by the kidneys and/or liver. Reduced clearance, therefore, often reflects decreased renal excretion or decreased hepatic metabolism.

Renal blood flow decreases about 1% per year after age 30, and there is a simultaneous decrease in glomerular function, averaging 35% in elderly persons. The clearance of drugs dependent on renal excretion declines in proportion to the decreased GFR. Such drugs include digoxin, lithium, cimetidine, procainamide, and most of the commonly used antibiotics.

Reduced hepatic metabolism is a reflection of decreased hepatic blood flow and/or decreased hepatic microsomal enzyme activity. Decreased hepatic blood flow is due to a combination of decreased cardiac output and a decreased number of hepatocytes. There is an approximately 40 to 50% reduction in both liver size and liver perfusion in the elderly person. Decreased hepatic blood flow can reduce first-pass drug extraction, resulting in a higher drug concentration in the blood. This effect is seen with propranolol. The plasma concentration was found to be five times greater in geriatric patients than in younger patients after both groups received the same dose of propranolol.

Hepatic enzyme activity is responsible for biotransformation reactions that facilitate drug elimination. These reactions are defined as phase I and phase II reactions. Phase I reactions include oxidation, reduction, and hydrolysis. They result in minor configurational changes, making the compound more water-soluble, but with a pharmacologic activity similar to the parent drug. Phase II reactions involve the conjugation, or attachment, of a drug molecule to a moiety such as glucuronide, sulfate, or acetate. The conjugate becomes much more water-soluble than the parent drug and is usually excreted in the urine. Phase II metabolites usually have minimal or zero pharmacologic activity. Aging appears to have a significant effect on the function of the microsomal oxidase enzymes responsible for phase I reactions. However, aging has minimal effect on the phase II biotransformations. As a result, with aging, there is a decrease in total drug clearance and an increase in the steady-state plasma concentration of drugs.

Changes in body composition can affect drug distribution. In the elderly person, lean body mass decreases and adipose tissue mass increases. Volume of distribution is influenced by total body fat content, water content, and protein binding, all of which are modified with aging. Volume of distribution can be viewed as the amount of drug sequestered in the peripheral tissues relative to the concentration of drug in the plasma.

Elderly patients have an increase in total body fat content, which increases the fraction of total body mass acting as a depot for lipid-soluble drugs. In the elderly person, this increase in the volume of distribution for lipophilic drugs will prolong the elimination half-time of a drug from the plasma, thereby increasing the duration of action of the drug. Although elimination is lengthened, increased fat distribution of a drug can result in lessened systemic toxicity due to the decrease in plasma concentration of the drug. Thiopental, diazepam, and midazolam are examples of drugs with prolonged elimination half-times due to age-related increases in the volume of distribution. One study demonstrated recovery time from thiopental to be 28 min in young patients, compared to 45 min in elderly patients. In addition, the elimination half-life of diazepam in a 20-year-old is 20 h, versus approximately 70 h in a 70-year-old. Total body water decreases in parallel with the increase in fat content.

Total body water content decreases 10 to 15% in the elderly person, therefore decreasing the volume of distribution for water-soluble drugs that remain in the extracellular fluid. For example, plasma concentrations of nondepolarizing muscle relaxants are raised in part due to this mechanism.

The extent of protein binding of a drug contributes to its distribution and pharmacologic activity. The amount of drug that remains unbound and free in the plasma represents the active portion responsible for any drug effect. Several factors can influence binding of drugs to plasma proteins in elderly patients. Aging is associated with a decrease in the circulating level of many serum proteins, especially albumin. The decrease in albumin is due to decreased hepatic production. The majority of protein-bound drugs are bound partially or completely to albumin. Therefore, with aging there is a reduction in drug binding to serum protein, and this may contribute to an increase in drug effect in geriatric patients. Binding characteristics of the serum protein are unchanged with aging; therefore, the aging difference alone is based on quantitative, not qualitative, protein changes. Elderly patients often take multiple drugs, and one drug may influence the protein binding of another drug. The incidence of coexisting diseases increases in the elderly population, and these diseases may alter plasma protein binding by causing a structural change in plasma proteins. Therefore, the elderly patient may experience an increased effect from the usual dose of a highly protein-bound drug due to the decreased amount of circulating protein, a qualitative change in the proteins due to concomitant disease, and multiple drug interactions.

Pharmacodynamics is defined as the net clinical pharmacologic effects of receptor and drug interaction. This effect can be quantified, for instance, by measuring the minimal alveolar concentration (MAC) of volatile anesthetic or the median effective dose (ED_{50}) of an intravenous drug required to extinguish response to a stimulus in 50% of individuals. Pharmacodynamic changes occur with aging, as reflected by the change in anesthetic requirements for elderly patients where the MAC and ED_{50} decrease. The cause of the increased drug sensitivity is unknown; however, the consistent response to a variety of drugs implies a physiologic phenomenon, not pharmacologic. The decrease in requirements parallels the age-related decline in central nervous system function, including the loss of synaptic and neuronal density and decreases in cerebral metabolic rate and cerebral blood flow. However, changes in the neuromuscular junction do not occur with aging, as reflected by the unaltered plasma concentrations of the nondepolarizers necessary to produce twitch depression. It is accepted that elderly patients have reduced anesthetic requirements due to increased drug sensitivity. However, the pharmacodynamic and pharmacokinetic basis for this change are coextensive.

The dosing requirements of local anesthetics are influenced by aging. There is decreased clearance of local anesthetics; therefore, toxic levels may occur at lower doses of local anesthetics in the elderly patient. Anatomic changes that occur with aging may explain the decrease in the amount of local anesthetic used in various regional techniques. There is a decrease in quantity and a qualitative change as well in the myelinated fibers of the dorsal and ventral roots of the spinal cord. By the age of 90, approximately one-third of the original central nervous system neurons and peripheral nerve axons remain. Therefore, the change in the myelin sheath and reduced number of nerve fibers may account for the decrease in the local anesthetic requirements in elderly patients. In addition, the volume of epidural anesthetic required to produce a given sensory level decreases with aging. In the elderly patient, narrowing intervertebral spaces and osteophytic growth lead to progressive occlusion of the intervertebral foramina. Because of this anatomic change, less local anesthetic can leak out of the foramina, and there is increased spread of the drug upward in the epidural space, producing a higher sensory level for a given amount of local anesthetic.

The local anesthetic requirements for subarachnoid block remain the same for both the young and the geriatric populations. However, in the elderly patient, there appears to be a longer duration of effect after administration of subarachnoid local anesthetics. This prolongation may reflect decreased vascular uptake of the local anesthetic due to the decreased blood flow surrounding the subarachnoid space that occurs with aging. Although subarachnoid drug requirements are the same in the elderly and young adult populations, spinal anesthesia is less likely to result in a spinal headache in elderly patients than in younger patients. This phenomenon is attributed to aging changes of the intervertebral foramina which decreases the loss of cerebrospinal fluid through the dural defect produced by the spinal needle.

Medical advancement and lifestyle modifications have produced longer life expectancy. As a result, the geriatric population has increased, and more elderly patients are presenting for operative procedures. Aging is not a disease but, rather, a slow process that changes the composition and function of tissues and organs. For the healthy elderly individual, organ system function satisfies basal requirements but exhibits decreased functional reserve when exposed to stress. The elderly patient is at an increased risk of perioperative morbidity and mortality due to age-related coexisting diseases. Therefore, anesthetic management of the geriatric patient requires an understanding of the physiologic changes of aging and the altered pharmacokinetic and pharmacodynamic responses to drugs. An optimal technique includes a thorough preoperative evaluation, careful attention to intraoperative positioning, appropriate monitoring according to the patient's condition and the procedure, and drug dosage titration and adjustment as required. Past notions that age alone represents a significant risk factor are no longer an issue in the presence of a well-executed anesthetic plan.

BIBLIOGRAPHY

Brandstetter RD, Kazemi H. Aging and the respiratory system. *Med Clin.* North Am 1983;67(2):419–431.

Craig DB, McLeskey CH, Mitenko PA, et al. Geriatric anesthesia. *Can J Anaesth* 1987; 34:156–67.

Fleg JL. Alterations in cardiovascular structure and function with advancing age. *Am J Cardiol* 1986; 57:33c–44c.

Grenblatt DJ, Sellers EM, Shader RI. Drug disposition in old age. *N Engl J Med* 1982; 306:1081–1089.

Lakatta EG, Mitchell JH, Pomerance A, et al. Human aging: changes in structure and function. *J Am Coll Cardiol* 1987; 10:42A–47A.

McLeskey CH. Anesthesia for the geriatric patient. In: Stoelting RK, Barash PG, Gallagher TJ (eds). *Advances in Anesthesia.* Chicago. Year Book Medical Publishers 1985:31–68.

CHAPTER
19

Pain: Physiology and Pharmacology

Charles E. Laurito

Pain is defined as "an unpleasant sensory and emotional experience associated with actual or potential tissue damage, or described in terms of such damage." It is the most common condition that brings a patient to the attention of a physician. It is universally understood as a sign of disease and is commonly associated with intense levels of human suffering. Pain is ubiquitous following trauma, such as surgical intervention, and is seen both in patients with benign medical conditions and in those with malignancies. One aspect of the experience that is particularly frustrating for physicians caring for the patient is that pain is always a subjective phenomenon. Behaviors that can be observed and measured, such as limping and grimacing, may be helpful to confirm the complaints, but these behaviors can be absent in people who suffer. There is no objective test that can measure the presence or the intensity of a pain. The clinician is left with the patient's report of the experience as a data base.

☐ OVERVIEW

The function of the pain system is to detect, localize, and identify processes that cause tissue damage. The system provides an extremely valuable safeguard for the human organism. Without a visceral sensation, the punitive aspect of pain, people have no reason to avoid the experiences that cause tissue damage. Those rare individuals who are born with a congenital insensitivity to pain feel no anguish after injury and have no reason to avoid similar injuries in the future. They will sustain repeated traumas and, more often than not, live shortened life spans. An appreciation of pain and the emotional suffering that accompanies it force the person to take appropriate actions to decrease the experience and avoid future conditions that cause it.

Trauma and diseases cause characteristic patterns of pain. The onset, location, quality, duration, and intensity of a patient's complaint provide information for both diagnosis and treatment. In most patients, however, once the cause of pain is known, the sensation provides no further useful function. Instead, it is responsible for needless anguish.

The scope of the problem of unrelieved pain is immense. Approximately 25 million surgical procedures are performed in the United States each year. Without appropriate care, many patients will suffer postoperative pain and the medical complications associated with immobility and repetitive activation of the stress response. Moreover, cancer is newly diagnosed in more than a million Americans each year; approximately 1400 patients die from the disease daily. Although cancer pain can be controlled by simple means in approximately 90% of patients, many are undertreated and thus endure needless suffering. Once a cause for pain is established and all that can be learned from the patient's complaints is detailed, efforts should be directed toward complete pain relief.

UNDERTREATMENT OF PAIN

Many investigators feel that pain is the single most serious yet undertreated condition in medicine today. Despite advances in the understanding and knowledge of basic pain physiology, patients are commonly undertreated. This is in part because of the negative attitudes of patients and clinicians toward the use of drugs for pain relief and problems related to financial reimbursement for effective pain management. Studies have shown that a common reason for unrelieved pain in American hospitals is the failure of staff members to routinely assess pain and the degree of its relief. Many patients will silently tolerate extreme levels of pain if not specifically asked about it or made aware of the possibility for its relief. Most patients do not know what to expect postoperatively; they are unaware of the possibility of complete pain relief following surgery. This information is only gradually becoming more available.

CLINICAL PRACTICE GUIDELINES

Clinical practice guidelines are being established for more appropriate and compassionate patient care. Currently, guidelines for the care of patients with cancer pain mandate (1) a collaborative, interdisciplinary approach to the care of patients; (2) an individualized pain-control plan agreed upon by patients, their families, and physicians; (3) ongoing assessments of the patient's pain; (4) the use of both drug and nondrug therapies to control pain; and (5) explicit institutional policies on cancer pain management with clear lines of responsibility. The guidelines stress that the patient's report of pain should be the primary source of information, since it is more accurate than the observations made by others. Although the current guidelines focus on the treatment of cancer pain patients, algorithms are being devised for the care of patients with postoperative and chronic benign pains.

☐ ACUTE PAIN MECHANISMS AND PATHWAYS

In general, pain is divided into two broad categories: acute and chronic. Acute pain commonly follows injury to the body and generally disappears when the bodily injury heals. It is often, but not always, associated with objective physical signs of autonomic nervous system activity, such as tachycardia, hypertension, diaphoresis, mydriasis, and pallor. Surgical intervention is consistently painful for patients. Most of the work performed by anesthesiologists in the treatment of pain focuses on this group of patients. Understanding how the body is able to signal the occurrence of pain from the periphery to the cortex, the pathways these signals take, and how the process can be interrupted to produce analgesia provides a framework for postoperative pain relief.

FRAMEWORK FOR THE STUDY OF PAIN PERCEPTION

Four processes are identified in neural transmission from peripheral tissue trauma to the experience of pain: (1) Peripheral *transduction* of the energy to allow activation of the nerve endings, (2) *transmission* of the impulses centrally to the spinal cord and higher levels, (3) *modulation* of the neural electrical activity at various laminae of the spinal cord by concurrent input as well as by descending neural activity, and (4) eventual cognitive *perception* of the stimulus by the patient as both an emotional and a sensory experience (Fig. 19–1). Each process can be focused on independently to block or decrease the progression of impulses from the periphery to the central nervous system in an attempt to provide

analgesia. This framework can be used to provide specific approaches to pain relief.

Understanding the basic neuroanatomy of pain perception forms the foundation for any approach to treatment. Although the neural pathways for pain sensation can be seen as cables leading from the periphery to the higher neural areas, this analogy is much too simple. In reality, nociception is a highly dynamic and fluid process capable of modification and modulation at many levels. The perception of pain is altered by the setting in which the stimulus occurs, the presence of additional impulses arriving at the spinal cord, and higher-level neural activity that descends in the spinal cord to the dorsal horn. The pathways are complicated and confusing. Study is made more difficult by the innumerable interconnections of individual nerves. Neural impulses activate, or have the potential to activate, many other nerves.

TRANSDUCTION AT PERIPHERAL RECEPTORS

Specific kinds of nociceptors are responsive to specific kinds of stimuli. There are three major classes of nociceptors, and the role played by each in pain transduction and eventual perception has been analyzed by stimulation at the skin followed by measurements of electrical activity of the nerves. The three receptor classes are:

Aδ mechanoreceptors, high-threshold mechanoreceptors (HTMs) which respond to mechanical stimulation
Aδ mechanothermal nociceptors, which respond to mechanical and thermal stimuli
C polymodal nociceptors (C-PMNs), which respond to a wide range of stimuli: chemical, mechanical, and thermal

Most of the evidence identifying the nociceptors comes from studies performed on cutaneous nerves. When painful stimuli are applied peripherally, there is no change in the number of impulses that travel along the large-diameter, myelinated afferents. Therefore, these nerves are not thought to be involved in the conveyance of impulses that eventually result in the perception of pain. Furthermore, direct stimulation of these afferent fibers in humans does not cause the subjects to complain of pain. In contrast, small myelinated and unmyelinated afferents respond maximally to noxious stimulation. When these fibers are activated experimentally, volunteers consistently complain of cutaneous pain.

When stimulation to the skin is increased slowly, low-intensity energy input will, at first, activate the largest nerve fibers only. This is consistent with the fact that touch is perceived by external stimulation that is less intense than that which would cause pain. The Aβ fibers (which carry the impulses eventually perceived as touch) are well myelinated and therefore more efficient in the transmission of faint stimuli. As the stimulation is increased, the energy activates more receptors and increases firing along the smaller afferent nerves. Activity along these fibers is associated with the perception of pain. The basic unit for pain sensation consists of

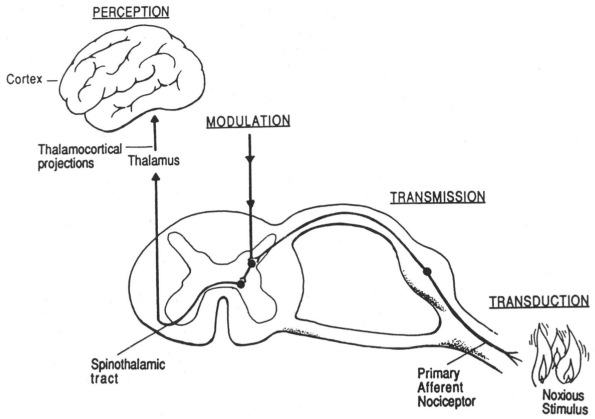

Figure 19-1 Gate control theory of pain. The physiologic process underlying nociception (transduction, transmission, and modulation) all converge on and impact on the discharge of nociceptive neurons in laminae I, II, and V of the dorsal horn. Thus, the dorsal horn is the focal point or *gate* for the integration and modulation of nociception. The pharmacologic manipulation of the processes of transduction, transmission, and modulation with highly specific agents can effectively "close the gate." This key concept forms the philosophic underpinning of the effective management of postoperative pain. (Reproduced with permission from Ferrante and VadeBoncouer, 1993.)

nociceptive and mechanoreceptive endings of small myelinated (Aδ) and unmyelinated (type C) fibers.

Within certain experimental conditions and limits, various fiber types can be preferentially blocked to better understand how activation and transmission are involved in pain perception. At very dilute concentrations, local anesthetics block small, unmyelinated fibers exclusively; there is no change in conduction along the Aβ fibers. In contrast, application of a steady external pressure will block conduction along myelinated nerve fibers but not affect conduction along C fibers. As expected, pain perception is transmitted during the external application of pressure, since this correlates with the preservation of C-fiber activity toward the spinal cord.

Stimulation of the skin causes transduction of the energy into discrete electrical activities at the nerve endings. Depending on the intensity of the stimulation, various information is propagated along the various-sized nerves toward the spinal cord (Table 19-1).

When the peripheral stimulation is gentle (i.e., touch), only pressure-sensitive receptors are activated, and the conveyance occurs along Aβ fibers to the central nervous system (CNS) at a characteristic rate and with a specific pattern.

Table 19-1
CLASSIFICATION OF FIBERS IN PERIPHERAL NERVES

Fiber Group	Innervation	Mean Diameter (Range), μm	Mean Conduction Velocity (Range), m/s
A α	Primary muscle spindle motor to skeletal muscles (myelinated)	15 (12–20)	100 (70–120)
β	Cutaneous touch and pressure afferents (myelinated)	8 (5–15)	50 (30–70)
γ	Motor to muscle spindle (myelinated)	6 (6–8)	20 (15–30)
δ	Mechanoreceptors, nociceptors (myelinated)	<3 (1–4)	15 (12–30)
B	Sympathetic preganglionic (myelinated)	3 (1–3)	7 (3–15)
C	Mechanoreceptors, nociceptors, sympathetic postganglionic (unmyelinated)	1 (0.5–1.5)	1 (0.5–2)

Table 19-2
ALGOGENIC SUBSTANCES INVOLVED IN TRANSDUCTION

Substance	Source	Enzyme	Effect on Primary Afferent
Potassium	Damaged cells	———	Active
Serotonin	Platelets	———	Active
Bradykinin	Plasma kininogen	Kallikrein	Active
Histamine	Mast cells	———	Active
Prostaglandins	Arachidonic acid-damaged cells	Cyclooxygenase	Sensitize
Leukotrienes	Arachidonic acid-damaged cells	Lipoxygenase	Sensitize
Substance P	Primary afferent	———	Sensitize

When touch receptors are activated, impulses travel at a rate of approximately 50 m/s to the spinal cord. There, the impulses are modified at the dorsal horn before eventual transmission to higher levels of the CNS. By this mechanism, the initial stimulus is localized to a specific body site, is characterized as touch instead of cold or pain, and is responsible for the response of awareness of touch.

Sensitization   After local injury, nociceptors can become hypersensitive to noxious stimuli through a process called sensitization. In this instance, the HTMs, which usually do not respond to nonnoxious stimuli, begin to respond. After repeated thermal stimulation, for example, HTMs change firing characteristics such that a less noxious or even a mild stimulus will cause an increased frequency of firing. With repetitive application of heat to an area of skin, additional receptors are recruited to convey information to the spinal cord and higher levels. When this occurs, the threshold for other types of stimulation (mechanical) is unchanged. This response is thought to be mediated by the release of algogenic substances in the periphery from the previous stimulation. Several of these substances are listed in Table 19-2.

TRANSMISSION ALONG PERIPHERAL NERVES

Peripheral nerves are classified according to their size, degree of myelination, and rates of conduction. Within this schema, classes of nerves have specific properties. Nerves that enable motor activity to be signaled (Aα) are larger and better myelinated than are nerves that enable touch to be perceived (Aβ). Nerves that convey the impulses eventually perceived as pain have little or no myelin, and therefore impulses travel at slower rates of conduction (Aδ and C fibers).

First and Second Pains   Transmission from nociceptive endings appears to be interpreted exclusively as pain. When a brief, intense stimulus is applied to the skin, such as a burn, a characteristic phenomenon is noted. The subject perceives a brief, sharp pain (first pain), which is then followed by a more prolonged, dull sensation (second pain). In this instance, the physiology of the conduction along the nerves of different diameters corresponds with the perception.

Measurement of the latencies between the application of the noxious stimulus and detection of the first pain correlates with a conduction velocity in the Aδ range. The first pain is usually described as distinct in nature. The person can easily determine its site and specific characteristics. First pain is carried by Aδ fibers. In contrast, the second pain is more emotional and punitive. This is the pain that causes suffering. It is less distinct and harder to localize than is the first. Second pain is carried by C fibers.

This particular phenomenon mirrors the overall organization of the nervous system involved in pain perception. The unmyelinated C fibers can be seen as a part of the older or paleospinothalamic system, and the Aδ fibers tend to serve the evolutionary newer, neospinothalamic system. As fibers within the anterior lateral quadrant of the spinal cord ascend toward the brain, they are organized into two distinct pathways as the spinothalamic tract (STT) approaches the thalamus. The lateral STT (neospinothalamic) synapses in the lateral thalamus and subsequently projects to the somatosensory cortex. The lateral STT indicates the sensory and discriminative aspects of pain perception. It enables the person to know what site is being stimulated and certain basic characteristics of the stimulation. The medial STT (paleospinothalamic), on the other hand, has multiple synapses in the brainstem, the medial thalamus, and the hypothalamus. The subsequent projections from this area are to diffuse areas of the cortex and limbic system. The medial STT provides information that results in the more primitive (thalamic) aspects of pain perception. These projections to the brainstem provide the basis for the emotional aspect of pain; projections to the cerebral cortex provide the basis for the sense of pain quality and location. This is consistent with the observation that pain is not just a perception; it is also an emotion best described as suffering. This phenomenon of suffering seems to lie in neural links between ascending pain pathways and the limbic system.

MODULATION IN THE SPINAL CORD AND HIGHER CENTRAL NERVOUS SYSTEM

Modulation of the incoming information occurs as the impulses arrive at the spinal cord on various nerve fibers and are modified by synaptic connections (Figs. 19-2 and 19-3). In addition, descending pathways within the CNS op-

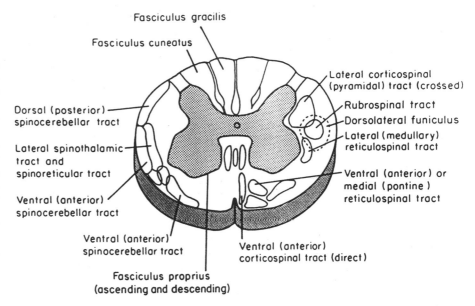

Figure 19–2 Transverse section of the spinal cord. Major ascending tracts are illustrated on the left: the dorsal columns (the fasciculus gracilis and the fasciculus cuneatus), the spinocerebellar tracts, the spinoreticular tract, and the spinothalamic tract. The major descending tracts are illustrated on the right: the lateral and ventral corticospinal tracts, the rubrospinal tract, and the reticulospinal tracts. The dorsolateral funiculus *(broken lines in diagram)* is extremely important with respect to descending antinociceptive pathways. The gray matter is surrounded by the fasciculus proprius, which consists of short ascending and descending fibers. (Reproduced with permission from Ferrante and VadeBoncouer, 1993.)

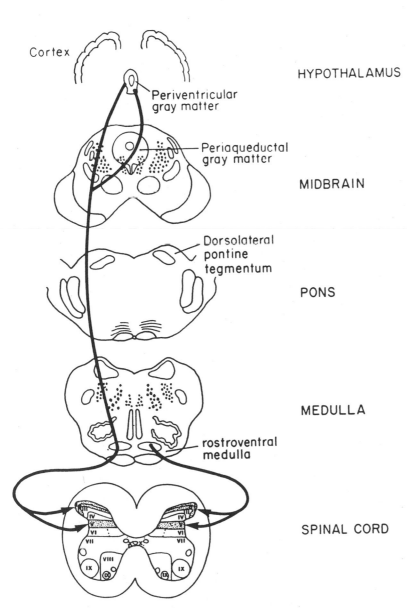

Figure 19–3 Descending modulating pathways. The periventricular gray matter lateral to the hypothalamus and the periaqueductal gray matter of the midbrain are anatomically interconnected. They give rise to a descending projection that passes through the rostroventral medulla and descends in the dorsolateral funiculus of the spinal cord to synapse with nociceptive neurons in laminae I, II, and V. As there is only a minor direct projection from the periaqueductal gray matter to the spinal cord, the rostroventral medulla acts as a relay to the spinal cord for more rostral centers. Separate from this projection pathway, noradrenergic neurons in the dorsolateral pontine tegmentum and serotonergic neurons of the rostroventral medulla also discretely project to the dorsolateral funiculus and then to laminae I, II, and V. (Reproduced with permission from Ferrante and VadeBoncouer, 1993.)

pose this input within the spinal cord and decrease the perception of pain. Important centers of this descending system originate at the periventricular and periaqueductal gray areas of the brain. Various biogenic amines (e.g., serotonin and norepinephrine), as well as endogenous opioids, act as neurotransmitters for these descending pathways. The final descending projection is to the dorsal laminae of the spinal cord.

Descending pathways that block the perception of pain are activated by electric stimulation, systemic or neuraxial injection of opioids, and neuraxial injection of α_2 agonists. In addition, these pathways can be activated by stimuli as subtle as verbal suggestion. In this respect, interventions as basic as reassuring a patient and providing emotional support will significantly decrease the perception of pain.

Gate Control Theory   Gate control is a theoretical construct to explain why pain is felt in some situations but not in others when the stimulus to the person is similar. It is thought to provide an example of the modulation that occurs within the spinal cord before the impulses ascend to cause perception. The idea is that a combination of impulses from the periphery or descending impulses from higher levels of the CNS act to block nociceptive impulses from reaching the higher brain centers, where they are converted to the perception of pain. Concurrent impulses that are carried on larger nerve fibers ($A\beta$) are thought to decrease or completely block the impulses carried by smaller fibers ($A\delta$). In this way the gate is closed.

In this manner, the use of transcutaneous electrical nerve stimulator (TENS) units, mustard poultices, and compresses is thought to decrease the perception of pain. In more sophisticated examples of the theory, impulses from cortical centers influence the activity of neurons as they synapse at the spinal cord level. The theory of gate control helps explain the relationship of input from the nociceptors to the eventual perception of pain. The anatomic location of the system is thought to be at the dorsal laminae of the spinal cord. This site is the focal point, or gate, for much of the integration and modulation of incoming and descending impulses (Fig. 19–1).

Substance P   Substance P (sP) is an 11 amino acid peptide that was first isolated in the 1930s and found to be involved with both sensory transmission and vasodilation. Recent laboratory work has shown a strong relationship between the sP level found in the dorsal horn region of the spinal cord and the perception of pain. The sP is synthesized in neuronal cell bodies and transported to the peripheral and central terminals, where it is stored in vesicles. It produces depolarization of second-order neurons in the dorsal horn when algogenic stimuli are applied at the periphery. Since substance P is present in only 25% of the dorsal root ganglion cells, it probably is not the only neurotransmitter of painful stimuli. Other neurotransmitters include dynorphin, bombesin, and cholecystokinin. Furthermore, nociception can take place in the absence of sP. When vesicles are depleted with the use of capsaicin, some painful stimuli are still

transmitted centrally. Several lines of reasoning have shown that the excitatory neurotransmitters are the primary afferent transmitters: aspartate and glutamate. These are also shown to provide a rapid response to algogenic stimuli.

We have seen that slower responses follow after a single brief stimulus. These slower depolarizations at the second-order neurons are thought to result from the release of sP from C afferents when they are stimulated. This release in turn, causes depolarization of second-order neurons.

Substance P mediates release of histamine from mast cells and is involved with neurogenic inflammation. Most tissue injuries result in the release of this and other inflammatory mediators. Therefore, sP has several actions. At the periphery and at the dorsal horn, it acts as a neurotransmitter. It also functions as a neuromodulator, in that it stimulates the release of growth hormone and prolactin from the cells of the anterior pituitary. It also modulates interleukin release from white blood cells. Peripheral release of sP can modify exocrine and endocrine pancreatic function. The local release of sP at the periphery can initiate and sustain a systemic stress response.

PERCEPTION AT THE HIGHEST LEVELS OF THE CENTRAL NERVOUS SYSTEM

Injuries of similar severity give rise to highly varying degrees of pain perception in various people and in various settings. The reactions and complaints of pain are integrated with the situations in which the stimulation occurs. This is why soldiers in battle and players in the midst of a game have significant injuries yet complain of no pain, while others with less dramatic examples of trauma complain of severe pain. More than the simple reflex arc of afferent impulses to the spinal cord and its conveyance to the brain is involved in perception. The brain and spinal cord are actively involved in shaping the type of experience a person perceives. The CNS is well able to modulate pain perception. The specific mechanisms, however, are not clearly understood. Experimental evidence shows that several areas of the brain, when stimulated, are able to evoke analgesia in both animals and humans. Injection of minute quantities of morphine into these sites causes a dense analgesia. This analgesia is also attenuated by opioid antagonists, such as naloxone. These regions in the brain contain or overlap with brain areas that contain a high concentration of endogenous opioids. Previous experiences, ongoing stimuli, and situational factors stimulate the release of these substances within the brain spontaneously. Specific levels of endogenous opioids here profoundly alter an individual's perception of pain.

As we have seen, the perception of pain is more than just a chain from the periphery to the CNS. The entire nervous system is plastic and redundant. Many factors come into play. An effective interruption in the chain leading from transduction through perception blocks input to the higher levels of the CNS. However, the local tissue injury created by a surgical incision sets many other reactions in motion.

Central Hypersensitization or Wind-Up When a volley of repetitive nerve impulses along C fibers arrive at the spinal cord, cells of the dorsal horn enter a state of increased sensitivity. These cells, which previously responded only to intense stimuli, now respond to fainter stimuli. In addition, their receptive field size (the peripheral area that corresponds to their innervation) expands to a wider area. Ongoing pain and tenderness following injury, disease, and surgery are a function of this process of sensitization. Sensitization is diminished if opioids are administered before an injury is sustained. Much higher doses of opioids can only occasionally suppress the process if they are given after the injury has occurred. The effects from sensitization are similar to those caused by the excitatory amino acids that act at the N-methyl-D-aspartate (NMDA) receptors of the dorsal horn. Enhanced sensitivity is triggered by the afferent nerve impulses because of the peptides that are released locally and also by a generalized activation of the specific receptors involved. Sensitization can be prevented by the use of NMDA antagonists, such as ketamine, if they are given before the tissue trauma is sustained.

☐ TREATMENT OF PAIN STATES

The most common error made by physicians in managing severe pain is to prescribe an inadequate dose of opioid. This practice leads to needless suffering. In the absence of sedation at the time of peak effect, a physician should continue dosing until satisfactory relief is obtained.

Opioids act at specific receptors. They are grouped into five categories according to the changes seen following use. In general, the effects of specific receptor activation are as follows:

μ_1: CNS analgesia, miosis, and euphoria
μ_2: respiratory depression, sedation, and bradycardia
δ: supraspinal analgesia and modulation of μ activity
κ: spinal analgesia, miosis, sedation, and respiratory depression
σ: dysphoria, hallucinations, tachypnea, and tachycardia

An ideal opioid provides intense analgesia with no unwanted side effects. Since no currently available agent meets this ideal, several investigators have tried combinations of opioids and opioid antagonists to maximize analgesia while decreasing unwanted actions.

USE OF PARENTERAL OPIOIDS

Opiates are a mainstay in the treatment of immediate postsurgical pain. They are extremely effective analgesics. They work quickly and are easy to administer. Psychological drug dependency is rarely, if ever, seen in patients suffering from pain. Patients in pain need an adequate dose of medication to relieve the suffering. Rough guideline doses for pain relief in postsurgical patients are shown in Table 19–3.

Opioid Side Effects Opioids have predictable side effects. Many of them are rarely seen with brief administrations of the agents yet become more significant with chronic use of the medication. The most common side effects are:

1. Constipation. This nearly universal complaint does not abate with chronic administration. Untreated constipation will lead to abdominal distention, pain, and, ultimately, colonic obstruction. Constipation is best treated prophylactically by the daily administration of bulk-forming agents and good hydration.
2. Nausea. Tolerance to nausea will usually develop with repeated doses. Antiemetic therapy is often helpful, as is eventual change to an alternative opioid.
3. Sedation. This is a common complaint after large doses or from accumulation of long-acting opioids. In patients who suffer from chronic pain states, amphetamines and caffeine are sometimes helpful to counteract the sedating effects that accompany adequate pain relief.
4. Respiratory depression. This is the most dangerous side effect of opioid use. Frequent monitoring of vital signs are necessary if large doses are administered to patients with little past opioid exposure. Significant depression can be treated by the slow infusion of dilute naloxone. A constant, slow infusion allows the mainte-

Table 19–3
SYSTEMIC OPIOID DOSAGES FOR THE TREATMENT OF ACUTE PAIN

Drug	Route of Administration	Front Load, mg/kg	Maintenance Dose, mg/kg	Frequency
Morphine	IV	0.15	0.01–0.04/h	Continuous
Meperidine	IV	1.5–2.0	0.3–0.6/h	Continuous
Hydromorphone	IV	0.02	0.01/h	Continuous
Fentanyl	IV	0.0008–0.0016	0.0003–0.0016/h	Continuous
Alfentanil	IV	0.03–0.05	0.06–0.09/h	Continuous

nance of analgesia while preventing episodes of respiratory depression.

5. Pruritis. Like nausea, pruritis usually subsides with repetitive doses. The cause is unknown, but histamine release seems to play a role. Many patients will achieve relief with the use of small doses of agonist-antagonist agents (nalbuphine 5 mg IV), as well as the slow infusion of naloxone, which antagonizes the itchiness while preserving analgesia.

Other side effects include confusion, dizziness, and urinary retention, which commonly resolve after repeated administrations. Side effects should be anticipated and appropriate medications ordered as part of the therapy. Agents that address nausea include droperidol, metoclopramide, nalbuphine, scopolamine, and naloxone. Pruritis can be treated with benadryl, nalbuphine, and naloxone (at higher rates, the analgesic properties of the opioid are reversed). Urinary retention is a problem that affects few patients because many patients who receive postoperative pain relief also have catheters in their bladders. In those without catheters, this side effect can be treated with the use of bethanechol 15 to 30 mg subcutaneously, small doses of naloxone, or if needed, the use of straight catheterization.

Patient-Controlled Analgesia Physicians treating postoperative patients have new modalities available to provide pain relief. Patient-controlled analgesia (PCA) has become a more common technique for pain relief during the last few years. The basic idea is intermittent dosing of opioids by the patient. The patient decides the timing of the analgesic dose. Since pain relief is obtained when the opioid concentration reaches a particular blood level in the patient, it is the individual patient who can best decide when the next dose should be given. The blood opioid levels at which pain relief is obtained differ greatly from patient to patient. Some investigators have shown this difference can be as high as tenfold.

The technique of PCA is elegant in that it allows the patient to titrate the dose and, therefore, maintain a relatively constant blood level of the agent. This, in turn, provides more personalized pain relief. In most hospitals, PCA is offered to treat postoperative and some more chronic medical conditions (e.g., sickle cell crisis and cancer pain). The machinery uses a microprocessor and infusion pump. The technique is most commonly used for the intravenous administration of opioid but is available for subcutaneous and epidural administration of the agent as well.

The PCA technique allows for variation in the delivery of pain medication and gives the patient considerable control over dosage. The system acts as a negative feedback loop. As the patient uses the analgesic, the pain level decreases. In turn, the patient feels less pain and demands less of the medication. Most studies report that compared to prn intramuscular injections, PCA produces an overall improvement in analgesia with no increase in sedation. When a patient begins to feel pain, he or she activates a demand switch, which delivers a preset dose of opioid into the intravenous line and, subsequently, the bloodstream. A lockout interval prevents the next dose from being administered before effects of the first are perceived. A maximum safe dose is programmed into the system to guarantee that an upper limit is not exceeded. This lockout can be bypassed when the demand for opioid is large. Many feel that the lockout feature is useful in that it provides an additional safety feature against accidental programming errors. Common doses of medications used for PCA are shown in Table 19–4.

A part of the PCA opioid dose may be given as a continuous infusion. Using the continuous mode in addition to PCA has the advantage of letting the patient sleep for longer periods of time before being awakened by the onset of pain. The background infusion should generally be less than one-half of the projected hourly requirement for opioid. As the patient's need for opioid decreases with time, the use of PCA is tapered by reducing the bolus size, increasing the lockout period, and lowering the maximal upper limit that can be given over a set time interval. As time passes and the patient is able to tolerate food, conversion to oral medication can then be made.

Conversion from Parenteral to Oral Opioids Anesthesiologists are called upon to help formulate a plan for converting a parenteral dose to an oral dose of opioid in those patients who suffer from intense, chronic pain. Knowing how to make this change provides uninterrupted pain relief and is based on an understanding of the enteric absorption of oral medications and their respective half-lives. The following is a reliable method:

1. Measure the 24-h IV dose that provided adequate analgesia.

Table 19–4
GUIDELINES FOR NARCOTIC INTRAVENOUS PATIENT-CONTROLLED ANALGESIA

Drug Concentration	Size of Bolus, mg	Lockout Interval, min
Morphine (1 mg/mL)	0.5–2.5	5–10
Meperidine (10 mg/mL)	5–25	5–10
Hydromorphone (0.2 mg/mL)	0.05–0.25	5–10
Methadone (1 mg/mL)	0.5–2.5	8–20
Fentanyl (0.01 mg/mL)	0.010–0.020	3–10

Table 19–5
CONVERSION TO ORAL DOSING

Drug	Parenteral Dose Equivalent to 1 mg IV Morphine	Bioavailability of Oral Dose	Oral Dosing Interval Based on Half-Life, h
Morphine	1	0.3	3–4
Meperidine	8	0.3	3
Hydromorphone	0.15	0.6	3–4
Codeine	10	0.3	3
Oxycodone	1	0.8	2–3
Methadone	1	0.8	8–12
Sustained-Release Morphine (MS-Contin)	No parenteral formulation	0.5	8–12

2. Use Table 19–5 (dose equivalents and bioavailability) to convert this amount to an equivalent dose of an oral agent.
3. Note the half-life of the oral opioid to be used.
4. Administer the 24-h oral dose in increments based on the half-life of the agent.

For example, a patient is comfortable while receiving an IV infusion of morphine at a rate of 2 mg/h. What is an appropriate dose of oral oxycodone?

1. Morphine 2 mg/h = 48 mg/24 h
2. 48 mg morphine = 60 mg oxycodone (48/0.8)
3. Half-life of oral oxycodone ~3 h
4. Rx: 7.5 mg oxycodone q 3 h

USE OF NONOPIOID AGENTS

After the patient recovers from the intense pain of surgery, it is appropriate to use nonopioid analgesics for the treatment of residual pain. Many of these agents and their doses are listed in Table 19–6.

Aspirin, acetaminophen, and nonsteroidal anti-inflammatory drugs (NSAIDs) are useful in a variety of patients. They differ from morphinelike analgesics in that (1) there is a ceiling effect to the analgesia they can provide; (2) they do not produce tolerance or physical or psychological dependence; (3) they are antipyretic; and (4) their primary mechanism of action is inhibition of the enzyme cyclooxygenase, which in turn inhibits prostaglandin synthesis. This inhibition decreases peripheral nerve impulse formation and decreases pain perception.

Aspirin is one of the oldest nonnarcotic analgesics. It is generally a safe agent but is not without complications. Gastric disturbances and bleeding are the most common complications following its use. Hypersensitivity can present with two different clinical pictures. One group of patients develops a respiratory reaction with rhinitis and asthma. The other subset develops urticaria, wheals, symptoms of angioedema, and hypotension within minutes of ingestion. Many patients who are sensitive to aspirin may experience cross-reactivity to the NSAIDs.

Acetaminophen is a nonsalicylate that is similar to aspirin in its analgesic and antipyretic potency but has no antiplatelet effects and relatively few anti-inflammatory properties. Its mechanism of action is unknown. At therapeutic doses, acetaminophen is well-tolerated and does not affect the gastric mucosa. Patients with chronic alcoholism and liver disease can develop severe hepatotoxicity, usually with jaundice, when the agent is taken in usual therapeutic doses.

Many NSAIDs are available for clinical use. Some are equivalent to aspirin, while others are more efficacious. Ketorolac is the only one of the NSAIDs available for parenteral use. Patients vary in their responses to the various agents. If a patient with persistent pain does not respond to a particular drug at its maximal therapeutic dose, an alternative NSAID should be tried.

All NSAIDs cause side effects at three sites—hematologic, gastrointestinal, and renal—which may limit their usefulness. All NSAIDs inhibit platelet aggregation by reversibly inhibiting prostaglandin synthetase. In contrast to aspirin, this inhibition lasts only as long as there is an effective serum drug concentration. The inhibition is usually gone after five half-lives of the drug have passed. Anticoagulation, coagulopathy, and thrombocytopenia are relative contraindications for the use of the agents. NSAIDs will interact with oral anticoagulants to prolong prothrombin times and cause bleeding. Minor gastrointestinal complaints, such as dyspepsia, can be seen early in therapy. Serious events, such as gastric ulceration, bleeding, and perforation, can occur with or without warning symptoms. Patients receiving pharmacological doses of steroids and those with previous gastric ulcers, debilitating diseases, and advanced age seem to be the most susceptible to these complications. In these patients, the lowest possible doses that will provide adequate analgesia should be used, and all alcohol ingestion should be stopped. The addition of ranitidine or misoprostol can provide partial protection against ulcer formation.

Acetaminophen use is relatively contraindicated in patients with hepatic disease. The agent is known to cause hepatic disorders when given in high doses. NSAIDs can cause renal insufficiency. The agent decreases the synthesis of prostaglandins within the kidney. Adequate

Table 19–6
NONOPIOID ANALGESICS FOR THE TREATMENT OF ACUTE PAIN

Agent	Adult Dose, mg po	Interval, h	Maximum Dose per Day, mg	Comments
Salicylates				
Aspirin	500–1000	4–6	6000	Gastrointestinal upset and bleeding, irreversible reduction in platelet aggregation
Diflunisal (Dolobid)	1000 initial, 500 subsequent	8–12	1500	No antiplatelet effect at lower doses
Choline magnesium trisalicylate (Trilisate)	1000–1500	12	4000	No antiplatelet effect
Acetaminophen	500–1000	4–6	4000	Hepatotoxic with sustained high doses
NSAIDs				
Ibuprofen (Motrin, Nuprin, Advil, Mediprin)	200–400	4–6	3200	All NSAIDs reversibly reduce platelet aggregation, can produce gastrointestinal effects, can cause renal insufficiency, and can cause CNS impairment
Naproxen (Naprosyn)	500 initial, 250 subsequent	12	1250	
Fenoprofen (Nalfon)	300–600	6–8	3000	
Indomethacin (Indocin)	25	8–12	150	
Sulindac (Clinoril)	150–200	12	400	
Mefenamic acid (Ponstel)	500 initial, 250 subsequent	6	1000	Do not use longer than 7 days
Meclofenamate (Meclomen)	50	6	400	
Tolmetin (Tolectin)	400	8	2000	
Piroxicam (Feldene)	10	12	30	
Ketoprofen	50	6–8	300	
Diclofenac	50–100	6–12	200	
Ketorolac (Toradol)	30–60	6	150	
Tenoxicam	20	24	20	

prostaglandin levels are essential to maintain high levels of blood flow to this region. Those at increased risk suffer from preexisting renal failure, congestive heart failure, or intravascular volume depletion. Patients who receive ketorolac should be carefully monitored for renal impairment. Affected patients will develop oliguria with sodium and water retention.

NSAIDs are useful analgesics in postoperative pain states, particularly those involving inflammation. Unless there is a specific contraindication, they can be routinely used in postoperative patients.

USE OF INTRATHECAL AND EPIDURAL MEDICATIONS

Opioids exert a powerful effect at the level of the spinal cord. Small doses of the agent can provide dense analgesia. The quality of pain relief is usually more intense than that which can be attained by parenteral medication. Epidural opioids have been used to control pain following a variety of surgical procedures as well as in patients suffering from cancer.

Although the data have not been substantiated in all patients recovering from operative procedures, there is growing evidence to indicate that patients with good pain relief have a lowered incidence of morbidity. Improvement in the ability to breathe deeply and cough after thoracic and upper abdominal surgery is readily apparent when epidural analgesia is used. Similarly, patients are better able to ambulate and tolerate the use of continuous passive movement equipment after joint replacement. Patients treated with neuraxial opioids have less central nervous system depression and a reduction in the incidence of ileus.

Postsurgical analgesia can be maintained for long periods of time by repeat doses or infusions of local anesthetics through an indwelling epidural catheter. The technique offers a profound level of analgesia but is capable of producing unwanted side effects, such as hypotension and weakness. Bupivacaine is often used because it has a long duration of action. The results are most satisfactory when the tip of the catheter is placed close to the midpoint of the surgical incision. This placement allows use of only minimal volumes of local anesthetics while maintaining pain relief. Although there are still problems with the technique (tachyphylaxis, risk of infection, or catheter migration), the use of the epidural catheter with infusion of local anesthetics provides a dense relief from postoperative pain.

Table 19–7
COMMONLY USED EPIDURAL OPIOIDS

Drug	Lipid Solubility	Bolus Dose	Onset, min	Duration, h	Comments
Morphine	1	2–5 mg	30–60	6–24	Because of spread in CSF, preferred for extensive incisions and when injection site is distant from cord segments mediating nociception
Meperidine	30	50–100 mg	5–10	6–8	
Fentanyl	800	50–100 μg	5	4–6	Not recommended when incision is extensive or injection site is distant from cord segments mediating nociception
Sufentanil	1500	10–60 μg	5	2–4	Higher doses may produce excessive sedation or respiratory depression, presumably because of vascular uptake

Opioid Injections into the Epidural Space Opioid drugs applied to the dorsal horn of the spinal cord cause profound analgesia. The analgesia is associated with few, if any, motor, sensory, or autonomic changes. Since the agents act at a highly specific site, only a small dose will provide dense analgesia, while the identical dose administered systemically would have almost no effect. The characteristic that best predicts how the individual opioid will act is its lipid solubility. The two most commonly used drugs, morphine and fentanyl, differ greatly in their uptake and distribution after epidural injection, producing quite different time profiles of analgesia and side effects. Fentanyl, which is more highly lipid-soluble, penetrates the dura and binds at the dorsal horn to provide a short onset time. Morphine, which is much more water-soluble, binds at the dorsal horn more slowly and provides a slower onset of analgesia. Lipid-soluble drugs are rapidly absorbed by spinal cord tissue. Since lipid-soluble opioids are taken up quickly after injection, they have a limited ability to migrate within the cerebrospinal fluid (CSF) to cause respiratory depression. Delivery of these drugs should be as close as possible to the nerve roots and spinal cord subserving the injured area. Specific guidelines for the bolus dosing of epidural opioids are given in Table 19–7.

Opioids injected into the epidural space are effective for severe postsurgical pain. The site of the wound, the location of the catheter tip, and the desired duration of analgesia are the important clinical considerations for treatment. If the catheter tip is not positioned at the midpoint of the incision, a more water-soluble opioid should be used. Morphine will spread within the CSF to affect activity at the higher spinal cord levels; morphine is less dependent on exact catheter tip placement.

Epidural opioids have been used effectively as either bolus doses or continuous infusions. With either method, the use of an indwelling catheter permits titration of the analgesic to the individual patient. With continuous infusions, guidelines are as shown in Table 19–8.

The usual opioid side effects are to be anticipated with an increased concern for respiratory depression. The depression that occurs after epidural injections of the opioid is biphasic. Both early and late phases of compromise are documented. The early depression is due to elevated blood levels of opioid following absorption via the epidural veins. This is usually seen within the first hour following injection. The delayed depression is more commonly seen with water-soluble agents, such as morphine. The time course of the delayed respiratory depression corresponds to the cephalad migration of morphine within the CSF to the higher centers of the CNS. The delayed respiratory depression has been documented to occur as long as 24 h after injection. Therefore, vigilance is required well after the injection has been made. The usual signs and symptoms of respiratory depression are subtle in most patients; the onset of ventilatory insufficiency

Table 19–8
COMMONLY USED EPIDURAL OPIOID INFUSIONS

Drug	Usual Infusion Rate, mg/h	Comments
Morphine	0.2–1.0	May produce excessive CSF levels; lowest effective rates should be used after a loading injection.
Meperidine	10–25	Rates greater than 20 mg/h may produce significant systemic levels in accumulation of normeperidine with risk of myoclonus and seizures.
Fentanyl	0.03–0.1	Rates greater than 0.1 mg/h may produce significant systemic levels; contribution of systemic level to analgesia may be significant; requires catheter site close to cord segments mediating nociception.

is gradual. Often it is accompanied by somnolence. Factors that increase the chances of the complication include concomitant parenteral opioid or sedative use, advanced age, and the use of large doses in opioid-naive patients. The patients who are kept in a supine, as opposed to the head-up, position are also at a higher risk.

If severe respiratory depression occurs, naloxone IV 0.2 to 0.4 mg, should be administered immediately to restore the ventilatory drive. Patients must be monitored closely after the use of naloxone, since respiratory depression may recur. The epidural opioid is almost always longer-acting than is a single IV dose of naloxone.

Respiratory depression, although potentially life-threatening, is very rare and can be prevented by having the patient's level of consciousness and rate and depth of ventilation checked regularly throughout therapy. Widespread experience has shown that epidural opioids can be given safely on conventional hospital wards if treatment specialists are involved in the patient's care. Key issues are appropriate selection of patients, ongoing in-service education for the nurses, protocols for treatment of complications, and readily available support by physicians.

Incident pain, which may occur when the patient is moved from the bed to a chair, can be treated with the concurrent use of NSAIDs or agonist-antagonist medications or the use of additional epidural opioids. As always, there are many more options for care when good nursing is available.

Both morphine and fentanyl have been administered by a variety of techniques (bolus, infusion, and PCA on demand). Typical opioid doses are shown in Table 19–9. The superiority in analgesia of one epidural opioid over another or the use of opioids alone as opposed to a combination with local anesthetics is unclear. Continuous infusion techniques, requiring an indwelling catheter are favored in cases in which intense analgesia is likely to be needed for a time period longer than the duration of a single epidural dose. The combination of local anesthetic with opioid appears to produce analgesia at dosage levels of each individual drug that would be ineffective if used separately. Many practitioners reserve the use of the combination of opioids and local anesthetic mixtures to operative procedures known to be unusually painful (e.g., thoracotomy) or that require use of a continuous passive motion machine to maintain movement of the joint during recovery.

Although it is more difficult to measure, aggressive pain relief in those suffering from chronic pain conditions also improves the quality of life and reduces suffering. As always, general principles focus on (1) basing the analgesic and its dose on the patient's report of pain; (2) administering drugs intravenously, neuraxially, or orally and avoiding intramuscular injections; (3) administering analgesics around the clock instead of only after the patient is already experiencing severe pain; and (4) anticipating and aggressively treating the side effects that accompany the use of analgesics.

CONCLUSION

Acute and chronic pain are major health problems in the United States. Suffering can usually be relieved with compassionate care of patients. To achieve this care, however, physicians and patients must know that complete pain relief is often possible. The medications and techniques are already available and in clinical use. Several measures have indicated dramatic improvement in the clinical outcome of postsurgical patients, including a decreased duration of mechanical ventilation, fewer cardiovascular and pulmonary complications, lowered incidence of vascular graft thrombosis, lower incidence of major infections, decreased perioperative blood loss, decreased hospital stay, and lower hospital costs. Many of the studies are confounded by other factors, yet the overall conclusions, coupled with the marked reduction in the degree of anguish, overwhelmingly support the need for aggressive pain management for this subset of patients.

Table 19–9
PREPARATION OF SELECTED EPIDURAL INFUSIONS

Preparation	Amount, mL	Preparation	Amount, mL
B 1/8 D2.5		D2.5	
0.25% bupivacaine	100		
PF meperidine	10 (500 mg)	PF meperidine	10 (500 mg)
PFNS	90	PFNS	190
B 1/8 F5		F5	
0.25% bupivacaine	100		
Fentanyl	20 (1 mg)	Fentanyl	20 (1 mg)
PFNS	80	PFNS	180
B 1/8 M0.05		M0.05	
0.25% bupivacaine	100		
PF morphine	10 (10 mg)	PF morphine	10 (10 mg)
PFNS	90	PFNS	190

NOTE: Epidural solutions may be abbreviated by listing the local anesthetic and/or opioid followed by the respective concentration after each letter. For example, B 1/8 D2.5 = 0.25% bupivacaine with 2.5 mg demerol/mL, F5 = 5 μg fentanyl/mL, and M0.05 = 0.05 mg morphine/mL.
ABBREVIATIONS: PF, preservative-free; PFNS, preservative-free normal saline solution.
SOURCE: Reproduced with permission from Ferrante and VadeBoncouer, 1993.

BIBLIOGRAPHY

Abram SE: Advances in chronic pain management since gate control. *Reg Anesth* 18:66–81, 1993.

American Pain Society: *Principles of Analgesic Use in the Treatment of Acute Pain and Cancer Pain*, 3d ed. Glenview, IL, 1992.

Cohen SE, Ratner EF, Kreitzman TR, et al: Nalbuphine is better than naloxone for treatment of side effects after epidural morphine. *Anesth Analg* 75:747–752, 1992.

Collin E, Povlain P, Galvain-Piquard A, et al: Is disease progression the major factor in morphine "tolerance" in cancer pain treatment? *Pain* 55:319–326, 1993.

Ferrante FM, VadeBoncouer TR (eds): *Postoperative Pain Management*. New York, Churchill Livingstone, 1993.

International Association for the Study of Pain, in Ready LB, Edwards WT (eds): *Management of Acute Pain: A Practical Guide*. Seattle, IASP Publications, 1992.

Jayr C, Thomas H, Rey A, et al: Postoperative pulmonary complications: Epidural analgesia using bupivacaine and opioids versus parenteral opioids. *Anesthesiology* 78:666–676, 1993.

Portenoy RK: Cancer pain management. *Semin Oncol* 20:19–35, 1993.

Rawal N, Sjöstrand V, Christoffersson E, et al: Comparison of intramuscular and epidural morphine for postoperative analgesia in the grossly obese: Influence on postoperative ambulation and pulmonary function. *Anesth Analg* 63:583–592, 1984.

Ready LB, Loper KA, Nessly M, Wild L: Postoperative epidural morphine is safe on surgical wards. *Anesthesiology* 75:452–456, 1991.

Sandler AN, Stringer D, Panos L, et al: A randomized double-blind comparison of lumbar epidural and intravenous fentanyl infusions for postthoracotomy pain relief. *Anesthesiology* 77:626–634, 1992.

Tuman KJ, McCarthy RJ, March RJ, et al: Effects of epidural anesthesia and analgesia on coagulation and outcome after major vascular surgery. *Anesth Analg* 73:696–704, 1991.

Yeager MP, Glass DD, Neff RK, Brinck-Johnson T: Epidural anesthesia and analgesia in high-risk surgical patients. *Anesthesiology* 66:729–736, 1987.

Peripheral Neuroanatomy

Timothy VadeBoncouer

A sound knowledge of peripheral neuroanatomy is essential for the performance of regional anesthesia and for avoiding the complications of neural injury from positioning of the patient. This chapter outlines the pertinent anatomy of the nerves of the upper and lower extremities, the trunk, and the head and neck. Necessary landmarks for the blockade of each neural structure are presented, and the risk of injury to these structures during positioning for surgery is discussed.

☐ THE UPPER EXTREMITY

BRACHIAL PLEXUS

Anatomy The upper extremity is innervated by the brachial plexus, which is formed from the fifth, sixth, seventh, and eighth cervical nerves and the first thoracic nerve (C5, 6, 7, and 8 and T1). These nerve roots exit from their respective intervertebral foramina and undergo a series of combinations and divisions before emerging in the axilla as the terminal nerve branches of the arm. The proximity of the neural elements to bony and vascular landmarks permits reliable neural blockade at distinct locations between the cervical vertebrae and the axilla.

Following their emergence from the intervertebral foramina, the five roots of the brachial plexus unite to form the three plexus trunks. The superior trunk is formed by a union of C5 and C6, the middle trunk is a continuation of C7, and the inferior trunk is formed by a union of C8 and T1 (Fig. 20–1). These three trunks pass over the first rib just posterior to the midpoint of the clavicle. The trunks continue toward the axilla above the first rib and underneath the clavicle, where they divide into six divisions (three anterior and three

posterior). The posterior divisions are responsible for innervation of the posterior surface of the arm, while the anterior divisions innervate the anterior (volar) surface. The anterior divisions of the superior and middle trunk form the lateral cord of the plexus; the anterior division of the inferior trunk continues on as the medial cord; and all three posterior divisions (one from each trunk) unite to form the posterior cord. Prior to emerging in the axilla, each cord gives off a major branch and continues on as a major terminal nerve of the arm. Thus, the lateral cord gives off the musculocutaneous nerve before continuing on as the lateral head of the median nerve; the posterior cord gives off the axillary nerve and continues as the radial nerve; and the medial cord gives off the ulnar nerve and the medial cutaneous nerve before contributing the medial head of the median nerve (Fig. 20–1).

Besides the first rib and clavicle, muscular and vascular structures also provide useful landmarks for locating the brachial plexus for nerve blockade. Above the first rib and clavicle, the plexus is enveloped by the anterior and middle scalene muscles. These muscles arise from the respective anterior and posterior tubercles of the transverse processes of the upper two to four cervical vertebrae. They travel parallel together, with the brachial plexus between them, and insert onto the first rib. Just behind the anterior scalene muscle and just anterior to the plexus is the subclavian artery, which continues with the plexus into the axilla as the axillary artery. With the upper extremity abducted and supinated, the usual orientation of the axillary artery is lateral to the ulnar nerve, medial to the median nerve, and ventral to the radial nerve (Fig. 20–2). Since the brachial plexus passes between the scalene muscles, it is surrounded by the posterior fascia of the anterior scalene and the anterior fascia of the middle scalene. Where the scalenes terminate on the first rib, the plexus invaginates their fascia, which continues into the axilla as a

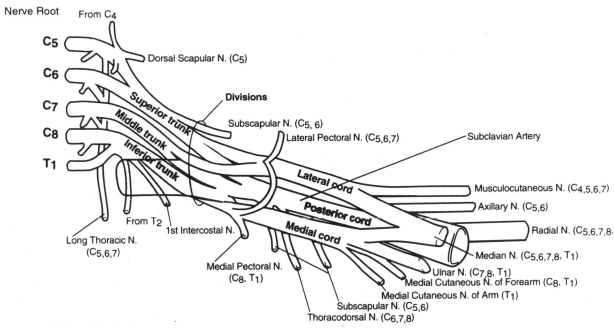

Figure 20–1   Organization of brachial plexus into roots, trunks, divisions, cords, and terminal branches.

tubular sheath containing the axillary artery and the plexus elements. Two notable branches of the plexus exit the tubular sheath proximal to the axilla. The musculocutaneous nerve exits the sheath high in the axilla and enters the substance of the coracobrachialis muscle. The axillary nerve exits the sheath at a similar point (Fig. 20–2). The early exit of these nerves has implications for neural blockade of the brachial plexus (see below).

Neural Blockade   Bony, muscular, and vascular landmarks provide the basis for blockade of the brachial plexus at various anatomic sites. The interscalene approach, which blocks the plexus at the level of the roots, requires palpation of the groove between the anterior and middle scalene muscles, where the plexus is situated. This is usually done at the level of the cricoid cartilage and the lateral border of the clavicular head of the sternocleidomastoid muscle. The ex-

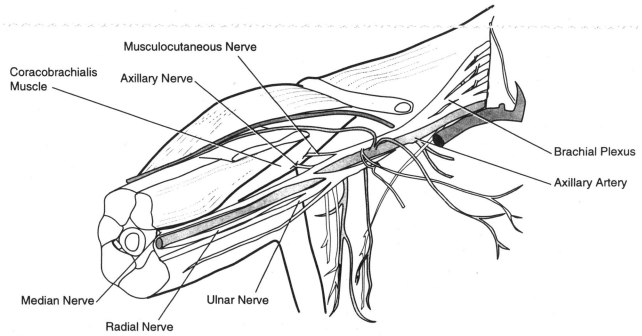

Figure 20–2   Brachial plexus anatomy in the axilla. Note the early exit from the plexus of the axillary and musculocutaneous nerves and the close relationship of the axillary artery to the radial, median, and ulnar nerves.

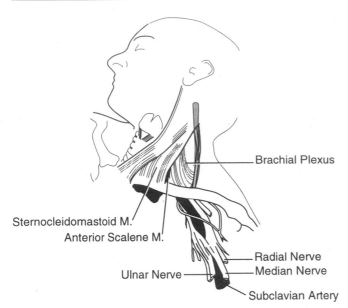

Figure 20–3 Relationship of brachial plexus to the junction of the clavicle and the lateral head of the sternocleidomastoid muscle.

ternal jugular vein frequently crosses over the sternocleidomastoid muscle at this point. The supraclavicular approaches to the brachial plexus use several different landmarks. As with the interscalene technique, a groove may be palpable just lateral to the clavicular head of the sternocleidomastoid and just superior and posterior to the clavicle. Alternatively, the subclavian artery pulse may be palpated, and neural blockade attempted just posterior to this, since the trunks of the plexus are located just behind the subclavian artery. A recently described technique of plexus blockade utilizes the reliable emergence of the plexus immediately lateral to the clavicular head of the sternocleidomastoid and immediately above the clavicle. A needle placed at this point and ad-

vanced perpendicular to the horizontal plane with the patient supine should reliably contact the plexus (Fig. 20–3).

The axillary approach to the brachial plexus uses the proximity of the axillary artery to the plexus elements. The arterial pulse is felt as high in the axilla as possible, usually as it emerges from under the pectoralis major muscle. A needle placed over the pulse and advanced should contact the plexus elements (Fig. 20–2).

The presence of a fascial tubular sheath around the brachial plexus explains the reliability of single injection techniques in producing brachial plexus anesthesia. The early emergence of the axillary and musculocutaneous nerves from this sheath accounts for the occasional failure to block these nerves during axillary approaches to the plexus.

Nerve Injury   Shoulder braces placed too tightly against the base of the neck might injure brachial plexus roots. Extreme lateral head displacement may stretch the plexus elements, particularly if the upper extremity position is fixed.

Brachial plexus compression between the first rib and clavicle can occur if the supine patient shifts cephalad while the arm is immobilized. Compression of the plexus in this manner may also occur during excessive sternal retraction in patients undergoing sternotomy procedures.

Excessive arm abduction may force the head of the humerus into the axillary brachial plexus. Stretch injury to the plexus may result. Arm abduction greater than 90° should be avoided.

MEDIAN NERVE

Anatomy   The median nerve innervates the palmar aspect of the hand from the thumb to the midpoint of the ring, or fourth, finger (Fig. 20–4). It also supplies sensation to the

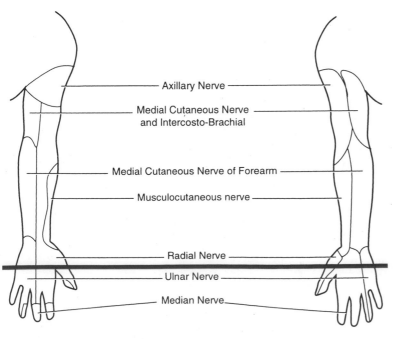

Dorsal   **Palmar**

Figure 20–4   Sensory dermatomes of the upper extremity.

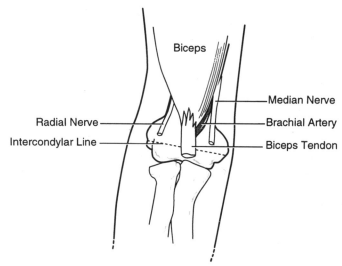

Figure 20–5   Anatomy of the median and radial nerves at the right elbow.

dorsal tips of the same digits. The nerve is conveniently blocked at either the elbow or the wrist. At the elbow, with the arm abducted and forearm supinated, the median nerve lies just medial to the pulsation of the brachial artery, which itself is just medial to the tendon of the biceps (Fig. 20–5). At the wrist, with the forearm again supinated, the median nerve is situated between the tendons of the flexor carpi radialis and palmaris longus. It lies under the deep fascia, usually no deeper than 1 cm below the skin, and may be blocked at a level 2 cm proximal to the distal skin crease (Fig. 20–6).

Neural Blockade   Median nerve block alone can be used for repair of some palmar lacerations and for reduction of metacarpal fractures (usually the first metacarpal). Most surgical procedures of the hand and fingers necessitate multiple nerve blocks. For these procedures, radial and ulnar nerve blocks are performed in addition to the median nerve blockade.

Nerve Injury   Median nerve injury from improper positioning of the patient is unusual. The nerve can be injured by indiscriminate probing in the antecubital fossa during attempted venipuncture.

MUSCULOCUTANEOUS NERVE

Anatomy   The musculocutaneous nerve provides motor innervation to the biceps, and sensory innervation to the skin of the lateral aspect of the volar forearm (Fig. 20–4). After leaving the plexus sheath high in the axilla, it immediately enters the coracobrachialis muscle. Just proximal to the elbow, it leaves the coracobrachialis and runs between the brachialis and biceps muscles. The nerve then travels lateral to the biceps tendon at the level of the intercondylar line and ramifies subcutaneously to innervate the skin of the volar aspect of the forearm.

Neural Blockade   Isolated musculocutaneous nerve block is rarely used for surgical anesthesia, since it innervates a small portion of the skin of the forearm. However, it is often blocked as a supplement to axillary brachial plexus block, which frequently misses the musculocutaneous nerve. It can be blocked through the same skin puncture as the axillary brachial plexus approach, by redirecting the needle laterally over the axillary artery and into the substance of the coracobrachialis (Fig. 20–7).

The musculocutaneous nerve can also be easily blocked at the elbow, either under the deep fascia just lateral to the biceps tendon at the flexor crease of the elbow or subcutaneously just distal to the crease and over the lateral volar aspect of the forearm (Fig. 20–8). It should be noted that

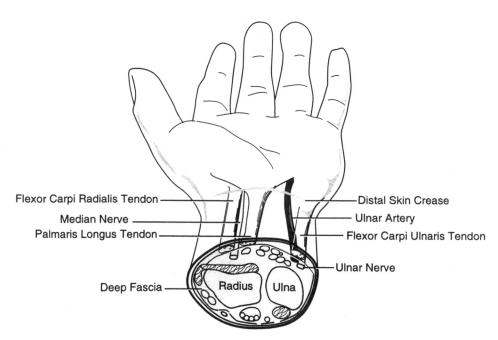

Figure 20–6   Anatomy of the median nerve at the wrist.

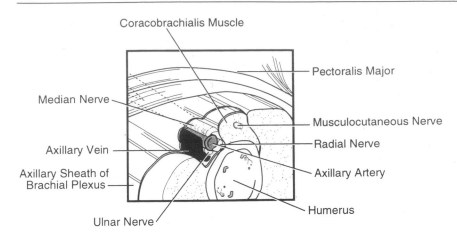

Figure 20-7 Relationship of musculocutaneous nerve, coracobrachialis muscle, and brachial plexus in the axillary approach to brachial plexus blockade.

blockade at the elbow spares motor function of the biceps, whereas the coracobrachialis infiltration in the axilla does not.

Nerve Injury Musculocutaneous nerve injury from positioning of the patient is rare, probably owing to the deep location of the nerve through most of the upper arm.

RADIAL NERVE

Anatomy The radial nerve crosses the volar aspect of the elbow joint. It is located approximately 2 cm lateral to the biceps tendon along a line connecting the lateral and medial epicondyles of the humerus (see Fig. 20-5). The nerve is quite deep under the skin surface, just superficial to the bone.

At the wrist, the radial nerve is much more superficial. Af-

ter passing dorsal and lateral to the radial artery, it emerges superficially on the dorsum of the hand to innervate the dorsoradial hand and proximal first three and one-half digits. It ramifies into terminal branches near the anatomic "snuffbox," formed by the extensor pollicis brevis and longus tendons (Fig. 20-9). These terminal branches continue superficially to the aforementioned dorsal three and one-half digits.

Neural Blockade Radial nerve block is rarely used in isolation. It is usually combined with median and/or ulnar block for procedures on the hand or digits, or used to supplement inadequate brachial plexus block.

Nerve Injury The radial nerve is vulnerable to injury proximal to the elbow. The nerve passes dorsal and lateral through the middle and distal aspects of the upper arm. Three to four centimeters proximal to the lateral epicondyle, it can be compressed against the underlying humerus. This may oc-

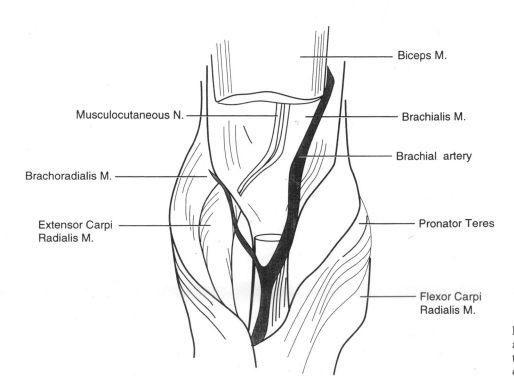

Figure 20-8 Musculocutaneous nerve anatomy at the right elbow (biceps insertion has been cut away to reveal the course of the nerve).

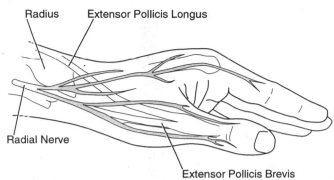

Figure 20–9 Location of the radial nerve at the wrist in the anatomic "snuffbox."

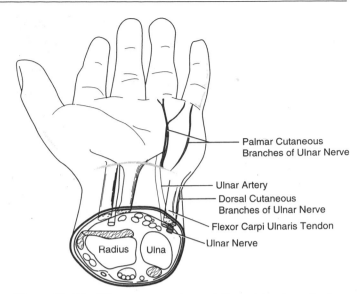

Figure 20–11 Ulnar nerve anatomy at the wrist, where it gives off palmar and dorsal cutaneous branches.

cur whenever the lateral upper arm is compressed against a bed side rail or components of an operating room table. Radial nerve injury presents as inability to extend the wrist and thumb.

ULNAR NERVE

Anatomy The ulnar nerve is located at the dorsomedial aspect of the elbow. It runs in the ulnar groove, formed by the medial humeral epicondyle and the ulnar olecranon (Fig. 20–10).

At the wrist, the ulnar nerve lies beneath the flexor carpi ulnaris tendon, below and medial (on the ulnar side) to the ulnar artery. Just proximal to this, the nerve has given off palmar and dorsal cutaneous branches (Fig. 20–11).

Neural Blockade Ulnar nerve block may be used in isolation for surgery on the ulnar side of the hand or procedures on the ulnar-most one and one-half digits. It is also used in conjunction with radial and/or median nerve block for hand and digit procedures and as a supplement for inadequate brachial plexus blockade.

Nerve Injury Ulnar nerve injury is not uncommon at the elbow. It can occur whenever the medial humeral epicondyle supports most of the weight of the arm. This most often occurs under anesthesia when the abducted arm is allowed to pronate, compressing the ulnar nerve between the arm board and the bones bordering the ulnar groove. It may also occur in a sleeping patient or a patient with residual brachial plexus anesthesia if the forearm is allowed to rest on the trunk while the flexed elbow rests on the bed. Ulnar nerve injury is usually detected by sensory loss of the fifth digit.

MEDIAL CUTANEOUS NERVE

Anatomy The medial cutaneous nerve is derived from the medial cord of the brachial plexus (Fig. 20–1). It courses with the basilic vein and bifurcates at the elbow into volar and posterior branches. The volar branch passes over the front of the cubital fossa medial to the tendon of the biceps. It supplies sensation to the medial volar aspect of the forearm. The posterior branch courses more medially and downward near the medial epicondyle. It supplies sensation to the dorsal medial aspect of the forearm.

Neural Blockade Neural blockade of the medial cutaneous nerve is rarely used in isolation but may be useful for supplementing incomplete brachial plexus blockade when cutaneous sensation of the medial forearm is still present.

Nerve Injury Compression of the medial cutaneous nerve at the cubital fossa may result in loss of sensation over the medial forearm.

INTERCOSTOBRACHIAL NERVE

Anatomy The intercostobrachial nerve is a branch of the second intercostal nerve and supplies cutaneous sensation to

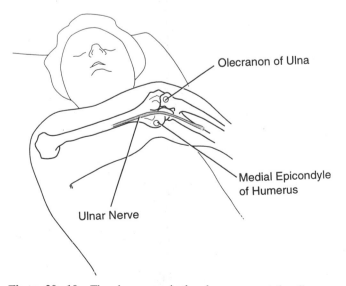

Figure 20–10 The ulnar nerve in the ulnar groove at the elbow.

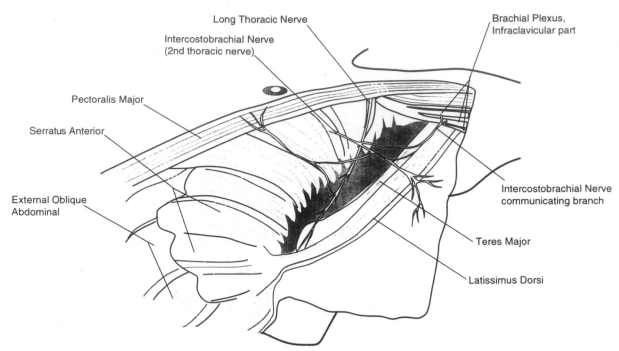

Figure 20–12   Anatomy of the intercostobrachial nerve in the axilla.

the upper inner arm. It is not part of the brachial plexus proper and must be blocked separately if the surgical incision involves this skin distribution or if a pneumatic tourniquet is to be used on the upper arm. The nerve emerges from the axilla subcutaneously and medial to the axillary artery pulse (Fig. 20–12).

Neural Blockade   As described above, intercostobrachial nerve block is used whenever a tourniquet is necessary for upper extremity surgery or when the incision involves the upper, inner arm.

Nerve Injury   The intercostobrachial nerve may be injured during surgical procedures in the axilla (e.g., mastectomy). It presents as numbness or dysesthesia of the upper, inner arm.

☐ THE LOWER EXTREMITY

The lower extremities are innervated by the lumbar plexus and sacral plexus. Although they have similarities to the brachial plexus, single injection techniques for nerve blockade of the entire lower extremity are less reliable. Because of this, the lumbar plexus and sacral plexus are usually anesthetized separately, and often quite distal to their origin from the lumbar and sacral vertebral foramina.

LUMBAR PLEXUS: FEMORAL, LATERAL FEMORAL CUTANEOUS, AND OBTURATOR NERVES

Anatomy   The lumbar plexus is formed from the anterior rami of the first, second, third, and fourth lumbar nerve roots.

Occasionally, the fifth lumbar root and twelfth thoracic root also contribute. Much in the manner of the brachial plexus, these roots exit their respective foramina and pass between the fascia of two muscles. The fascia of the psoas muscle forms the anterior border, and the fascia of the quadratus lumborum, the posterior border of the lumbar plexus prior to formation of the terminal nerves to the leg.

The three terminal nerves of the lumbar plexus—lateral femoral cutaneous, femoral, and obturator—are formed soon after the plexus emerges from the vertebral foramina. All three nerves pass anterolaterally in the pelvis and emerge in the groin (Fig. 20–13). The lateral femoral cutaneous nerve passes laterally early in the pelvis and emerges under the inguinal ligament near the anterior superior iliac spine. The obturator nerve passes medially and posteriorly in the pelvis and emerges beneath the superior ramus of the pubis. The femoral nerve travels in the groove between the psoas and iliacus muscles and emerges in the groin under the inguinal ligament, where it passes lateral to, and in conjunction with, the femoral artery.

The three terminal nerves of the lumbar plexus innervate the anterior, medial, and lateral aspects of the thigh. The lateral femoral cutaneous nerve (L2-3) provides sensory innervation only to the skin of the lateral thigh. The femoral nerve (L2-4) gives rise to an anterior and posterior bundle. The anterior bundle innervates the skin of the anterior thigh and the sartorius muscle. The posterior bundle innervates the quadriceps muscle, the knee, and the skin of the medial calf (through the distal extension of the femoral nerve called the saphenous nerve). The obturator nerve (L2-4) supplies motor and sensory function to the medial thigh and medial knee.

Neural Blockade   Blockade of the lumbar plexus is rarely used in isolation for anesthesia. It is usually combined

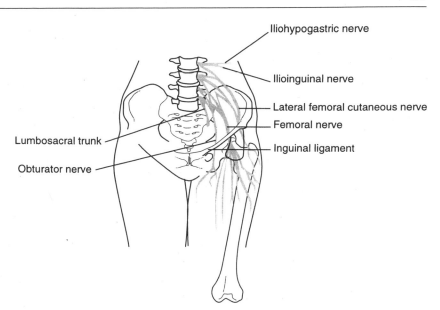

Figure 20–13   Lumbar plexus anatomy and the relationship of the lateral femoral cutaneous, femoral, and obturator nerves in the inguinal region.

with sciatic nerve block to achieve complete anesthesia of the leg when spinal or epidural anesthesia is contraindicated. Similarly, the component peripheral nerves described below are usually blocked together to achieve anesthesia of the lumbar plexus distribution.

The femoral nerve may be blocked to achieve anesthesia for operations of the anterior thigh, including muscle biopsy for the diagnosis of suspected malignant hyperthermia. Femoral nerve blockade is also useful for analgesia after femoral fracture.

Lateral femoral cutaneous nerve block is useful for anesthetizing the donor site for skin grafting procedures. It may also be used for treatment of the painful condition meralgia paresthetica, which results from trauma to the lateral femoral cutaneous nerve.

Obturator nerve blockade is also rarely used in isolation, except to relieve adductor spasm of the hip.

Nerve Injury   Injury to the lateral femoral cutaneous nerve may result in pain and dysesthesia over the lateral thigh, a syndrome known as meralgia paresthetica. It results from nerve entrapment at the inguinal ligament, often secondary to an expanding abdominal girth (e.g., pregnancy, morbid obesity, ascites, etc.)

SCIATIC NERVE

Anatomy   The sciatic nerve is formed from the first three sacral nerves and a contribution from the anterior rami of the fourth and fifth lumbar nerves. These components pass laterally in the pelvis and exit posteriorly through the sciatic notch. At this level, the lower border of the piriformis muscle is just above the nerve (Fig. 20–14). As it exits the sciatic notch, the posterior cutaneous nerve of the thigh leaves the larger sciatic nerve proper. The sciatic nerve continues on its course between the ischial tuberosity and the greater trochanter of the femur; it lies anterior and inferior to the piriformis muscle at this point. The nerve continues down the posterior aspect of the thigh behind the femur and into the

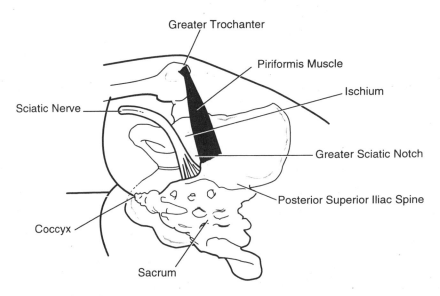

Figure 20–14   Anatomy of the sciatic nerve as it exits the pelvis through the sciatic notch.

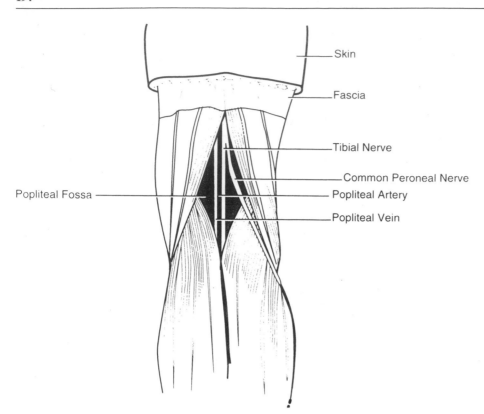

Skin

Fascia

Tibial Nerve

Common Peroneal Nerve

Popliteal Artery

Popliteal Vein

Popliteal Fossa

Figure 20–15 Anatomy of the sciatic nerve in the popliteal fossa as it divides into tibial and common peroneal branches.

popliteal fossa (Fig. 20–15). Here it divides into (1) the common peroneal nerve, which courses laterally, winding around the head of the fibula and supplying motor and sensory innervation to the anterior calf and dorsum of the foot; and (2) the tibial nerve, which continues posteriorly into the calf, providing motor and sensory innervation to the back of the calf and sole of the foot.

At the ankle, the tibial and common peroneal nerves contribute to four of the five nerves making up nerve block at the ankle: the posterior tibial, sural, deep peroneal, and superficial peroneal nerves. The fifth nerve, the saphenous, is derived from the femoral nerve and was described previously; it provides cutaneous innervation to the medial aspect of the foot.

The tibial nerve arrives in the ankle region medially and becomes the posterior tibial nerve (Fig. 20–16). It is located deep and medial to the Achilles tendon and the posterior tibial artery. It sends off a branch to the inner heel and then divides into medial and lateral plantar branches, which provide innervation to the medial and lateral sole, respectively. The tibial nerve also contributes a branch, along with a branch from the common peroneal nerve, to the sural nerve. This cutaneous nerve runs posteroinferiorly to the lateral malleolus to supply sensation to the posterolateral surface of the lower leg, the lateral foot, and occasionally the lateral aspect of the fifth toe.

The common peroneal nerve divides into the superficial and deep peroneal nerves in the proximal lower leg. The superficial peroneal nerve emerges subcutaneously at the middle third of the anterior calf to innervate the dorsum of the foot and toes. The deep peroneal nerve runs deeper than the superficial peroneal and enters the foot between the tendons

of the anterior tibialis (foot extensor) and extensor hallucis longus (great toe extensor) muscles at the level of the malleoli (Fig. 20–16). The deep peroneal nerve innervates the short extensor muscles of the toes and the skin of the web space formed by the first and second toes.

The cutaneous distribution of the nerves of the leg is summarized in Fig. 20–17.

Neural Blockade For certain lower extremity operations, the component nerves may be blocked in isolation to provide anesthesia. When surgery involves both lumbar plexus and sciatic distributions or when a pneumatic thigh tourniquet is utilized, the entire lumbar plexus and sciatic nerve must usually be blocked.

Sciatic nerve blockade may be used alone for operations on the foot or lower leg. It is easily blocked at the level of the sciatic notch or the popliteal fossa, where the nerve is accessible to commonly used regional anesthesia needles. Saphenous nerve blockade may need to accompany sciatic block if the surgical field (or tourniquet) includes the medial calf or foot. When used with lumbar plexus blockade, sciatic nerve block produces complete anesthesia of the leg.

Blockade of the five nerves at the ankle may be used for most foot operations. If a calf tourniquet must be used, popliteal fossa sciatic blockade with saphenous nerve block may be utilized as an alternative. Obviously, operations requiring a thigh tourniquet necessitate the more proximal sciatic nerve block at the sciatic notch, as well as lumbar plexus block, to ensure anesthesia of the anterior, medial, and lateral thigh.

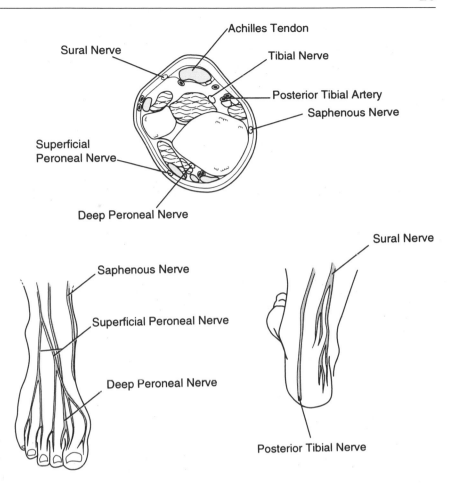

Figure 20–16 Posterior tibial, saphenous, sural, deep peroneal, and common peroneal nerve anatomy at the level of the ankle and foot (cross-sectional view is from above the right ankle).

Nerve Injury   Injury to the sciatic nerve can occur with excessive hip flexion, resulting in severe nerve stretch. This may present as foot drop or pain and/or numbness of the lower leg, posterior thigh, or foot. Foot drop may also result from common peroneal nerve injury, which is vulnerable to pressure injury as it passes around the head of the fibula. This can affect the dependent leg in the lateral decubitus position and either leg in the lithotomy position, where the common peroneal nerve can be compressed against leg stirrups.

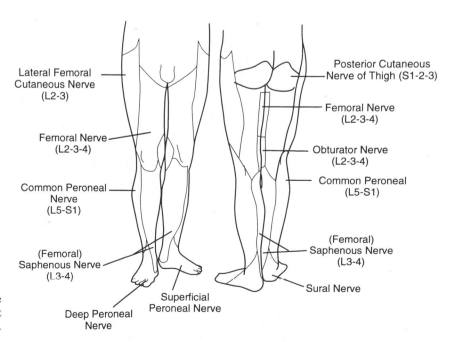

Figure 20–17 Sensory dermatomes of the lower extremity. The posterior tibial nerve is not shown; it innervates the plantar aspect of the foot.

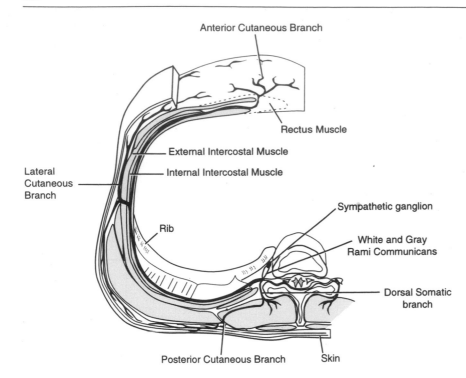

Figure 20–18 Intercostal nerve anatomy. Note sympathetic ganglion and connections to intercostal nerve via gray and white rami communicans in paravertebral space.

☐ THE TRUNK

The neural anatomy of the chest and abdomen consists of a somatic component, responsible for sensation to the skin and musculoskeletal structures, and an autonomic component, responsible for innervating the viscera and their associated mesenteries. Only the somatic components are discussed here.

INTERCOSTAL NERVES

Anatomy Each intercostal nerve (first thoracic through twelfth thoracic somatic nerves) emerges from an intervertebral foramen and enters the paravertebral space. Early in their course through the foramina, each nerve gives off a sympathetic branch (white rami communicans), which merges with the sympathetic chain of ganglia at the ventrolateral aspect of the vertebral column (Fig. 20–18). A dorsal somatic branch also leaves the somatic nerve proper early in its course to provide sensation to the midline back structures. The major portion of the intercostal nerve then passes into the intercostal groove, which lies below and just ventral to the corresponding rib (Fig. 20–19). A neurovascular bundle is formed by each intercostal nerve and an accompanying intercostal artery and vein. The fascia of the external and internal intercostal muscles forms a sheath that envelops each neurovascular bundle. At the level of the midaxillary line, the intercostal nerve gives off a lateral sensory branch and then continues on to innervate the ventral trunk and abdominal somatic structures.

The 12 intercostal nerves provide sensation to the entire chest and abdominal wall from just above the nipple line down to the level of the pelvis. Segmental sympathetic inner-

vation (i.e., vasomotor tone, sweat glands, etc.) is provided by the gray rami communicantes, postganglionic fibers that leave the sympathetic chain and merge with the individual intercostal nerves early in their course (Fig. 20–18).

Neural Blockade Blockade of the intercostal nerves is rarely used in isolation for surgical anesthesia except for superficial chest or abdominal wall procedures. When combined with celiac plexus blockade, intercostal nerve blockade can produce complete anesthesia for some intraabdominal procedures.

A major use of intercostal nerve blockade alone is for pain management of rib fractures.

Blockade of the intercostal nerves is usually performed at the level of the posterior angle of the rib. The rib is easily palpable here, even in the most generously sized patients. More lateral approaches may miss the lateral sensory branch. It should be noted that the traditional approach to intercostal

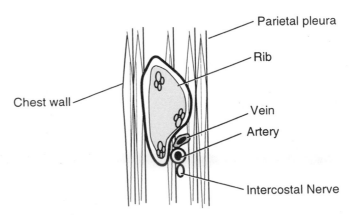

Figure 20–19 Relationship of intercostal nerve to rib, shown in cross section.

nerve blockade spares the dorsal branch, and therefore anesthesia and analgesia will not be attained for the midline back somatic structures.

The first five intercostal nerves are difficult to block with the traditional approach, since the angle of the rib is obscured by the overlying scapula. For blockade of these nerves, a paravertebral approach, utilizing the vertebral transverse processes as landmarks, is preferred.

Nerve Injury Intercostal nerve injury may occur during intrathoracic surgical procedures as a result of cutting, crushing, or stretching the nerves during surgery. Intercostal nerve injury usually presents as pain or dysesthesia through the affected dermatome.

ILIOINGUINAL AND ILIOHYPOGASTRIC NERVES

Anatomy The ilioinguinal and iliohypogastric nerves are branches of the lumbar plexus, originating from the twelfth thoracic and first lumbar nerves. These nerves sweep around anteriorly at the level of the anterior superior iliac spine of the pelvis (Fig. 20–20). The iliohypogastric nerve courses between the external and internal oblique muscles, while the ilioinguinal nerve initially runs between the transversus abdominus and the internal oblique muscles before penetrating the latter medial to the anterior superior iliac spine. These nerves innervate skin and muscle of the inguinal region.

Neural Blockade Ilioinguinal and iliohypogastric nerve blockade are two of the series of blocks needed to produce anesthesia for inguinal herniorrhaphy. It is inadequate as the

sole anesthetic for this operation. The block is frequently used as a means of postoperative pain control following herniorrhaphy in infants and children.

Nerve Injury Both of these nerves may be injured directly or become entrapped in scar during herniorrhaphy. Presentation is of pain and dysesthesia in the inguinal region.

☐ THE HEAD AND NECK

CERVICAL PLEXUS

Anatomy The cervical plexus is formed from the second, third, and fourth cervical nerves. These three nerves emerge from their respective intervertebral foramina and course through the troughlike cervical transverse processes (Fig. 20–21). Anterior and posterior tubercles are formed at the end of these processes and serve as attachments for the anterior and middle scalene muscles. As the cervical nerves emerge from the processes, they give off anterior and posterior branches. The anterior branches wind around the anterior scalene muscle and provide motor innervation to the muscles of the neck. These fibers also give rise to the phrenic nerve, which descends to provide innervation to the diaphragm. Sensory fibers separate from the motor fibers at the level of the tubercles and emerge at the posterolateral border of the sternocleidomastoid muscle near the midpoint of its length (Fig. 20–22). This so-called superficial cervical plexus gives off four branches. The lesser occipital nerve innervates the posterior upper ear and skin behind the ear. The great auricular nerve provides sensation to the remainder of the posterior ear surface as well as the lower anterior ear and the skin over

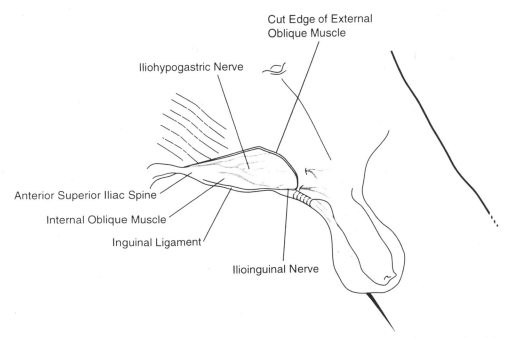

Figure 20–20 Relationship of the ilioinguinal and iliohypogastric nerves to the external and internal oblique muscles in the lower anterior abdominal wall.

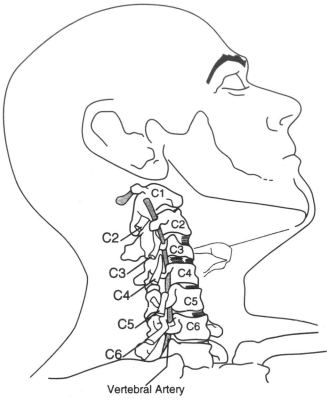

Figure 20–21 The cervical plexus is formed by the union of the second through fourth cervical nerves (C2–4) after they emerge from their respective intervertebral foramina.

the angle of the mandible. The anterior cervical nerve provides sensation to the skin from the chin to the sternal notch. Finally, the supraclavicular nerve innervates the skin over the caudal aspect of the neck, the skin over the deltoid muscle, the skin below the clavicle to the level of the second rib, and the skin over the posterior shoulder down to the scapula.

Neural Blockade   Cervical plexus anesthesia is rarely used in isolation for surgery. It may be useful for such operations as carotid endarterectomy and tracheostomy. Either superficial cervical plexus blockade or a deeper block of the cervical plexus where the motor and sensory fibers divide can be used, although the latter may provide more satisfactory operating conditions. Cervical plexus blockade may also be used as an adjunct to interscalene brachial plexus blockade for shoulder surgery. However, the cervical plexus is usually blocked incidentally by proximal spread of local anesthetic when the interscalene approach is utilized. Although bilateral superficial cervical plexus blockade is permissible, bilateral deep cervical plexus blockade should be avoided due to the risk of bilateral diaphragm paralysis.

Nerve Injury   Injury to the components of the cervical plexus is uncommon, although tumor invasion of the neck may result in pain or dysesthesias in the distribution of the branches of the plexus.

OCCIPITAL NERVES

Anatomy   The greater and lesser occipital nerves provide sensory innervation to the posterior two-thirds of the scalp. They are derived from the fibers of the cervical plexus. (The lesser occipital nerve was described previously.) The greater occipital nerve passes over the superior nuchal line in conjunction with the occipital artery, the pulsation of which is easily palpable. The lesser occipital nerve is located lateral to the greater occipital nerve. It, too, passes over the superior nuchal line, about one-third of the distance from the mastoid process to the greater occipital protuberance (Fig. 20–23).

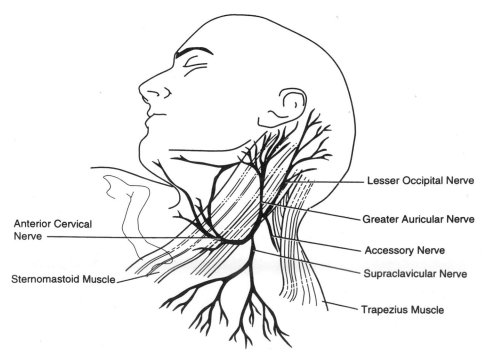

Figure 20–22 The nerves of the superficial cervical plexus as they emerge from the lateral border of the sternocleidomastoid muscle.

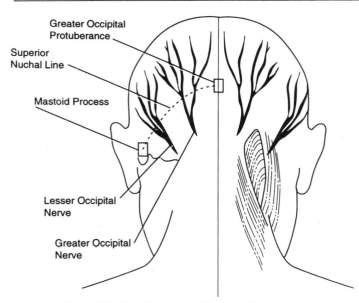

Figure 20-23 Anatomy of the occipital nerves.

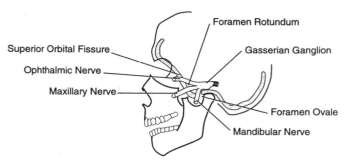

Figure 20-24 Anatomy of the trigeminal nerve and gasserian ganglion.

Neural Blockade Blockade of the occipital nerves is used as part of a series of nerve blocks to render the scalp anesthetic for minor surgical procedures. It is also used in the treatment of some headache syndromes.

Nerve Injury Occipital nerve injury may result from whiplash injury and, rarely, prolonged compression of the occiput.

TRIGEMINAL NERVE: OPHTHALMIC, MAXILLARY, AND MANDIBULAR DIVISIONS

Anatomy The trigeminal nerve (also known as the fifth cranial nerve) provides sensorimotor function to the face. The roots of this nerve emerge from the pons and supply sensory fibers to the gasserian ganglion (Fig. 20-24). The gasserian ganglion lies at the intersection of the middle and posterior cranial fossa; it sits at the top of the petrous bone, inside the skull, and just above the foramen ovale. It is bounded medially by the cavernous sinus (containing the carotid artery and cranial nerves III, IV, and VI), superiorly by the inferior surface of the temporal lobe of the brain, and posteriorly by the brainstem. About two-thirds of the ganglion posteriorly is contained in a cerebrospinal fluid (CSF)-bathed dural sleeve.

Distal to the gasserian ganglion, the trigeminal nerve divides into three major branches. The uppermost branch, the ophthalmic division (V_1), passes through the skull, into the superior orbital fissure, and enters the orbit. Now referred to as the frontal nerve, it divides into supraorbital and supratrochlear branches just above the orbit. The supraorbital nerve is found at the supraorbital notch; the supratrochlear nerve is located at the medial border of the orbit (Fig. 20-25). These two branches supply sensation to the ipsilateral forehead, eyebrows, upper eyelids, and nose (Fig. 20-26).

The middle branch of the trigeminal nerve, the maxillary division (V_2), contains only sensory fibers (as does V_1). It emerges from the gasserian ganglion and exits the cranial cavity via the foramen rotundum (Fig. 20-24). It then traverses the pterygopalatine fossa (bounded anteriorly by the maxilla, medially by the palatine bone, and posteriorly by the pterygoid process of the sphenoid). The maxillary nerve enters the floor of the orbit at the inferior orbital fissure. Sphenopalatine and posterior dental branches arise from the maxillary nerve within the aforementioned pterygopalatine

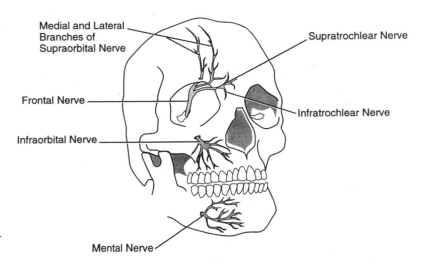

Figure 20-25 Anatomy of the ophthalmic (V_1) division of the trigeminal nerve in the orbit.

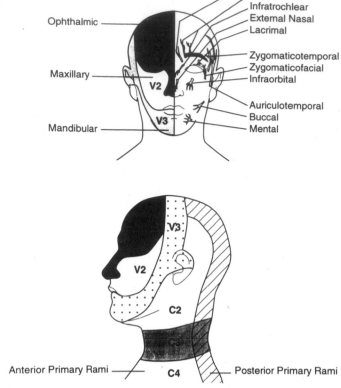

Figure 20–26 Innervation of the face by the divisions of the trigeminal nerve.

fibers. It emerges from the gasserian ganglion and exits the skull through the foramen ovale (Fig. 20–24). Situated just posterior to the lateral pterygoid plate of the sphenoid, the nerve lies in the infratemporal fossa (Fig. 20–27). This fossa is bounded anteriorly by the posterior maxilla wall, posteriorly by the carotid sheath and styloid apparatus, laterally by the coronoid process and ramus of the mandible, and medially by the lateral pterygoid plate. In this fossa, the mandibular nerve gives off its terminal branches, including the mental nerve (which exits through the mental foramen near the midline at the anteriormost aspect of the mandible), the buccal nerves, and the auriculotemporal nerve. The mandibular nerve and its branches provide sensation to the lower jaw, the tongue, the lower teeth, the buccal cheek surface, the skin overlying the lower jaw (mental), the temporal area, and much of the external surface of the ear (auriculotemporal); (Fig. 20–26). They also supply motor innervation to the masticatory muscles.

Neural Blockade   Regional anesthesia techniques requiring blockade of the trigeminal nerve are practiced rarely, primarily due to concerns about airway control and complications arising from proximity of the nerves to other structures (e.g., eye, carotid, brain, CSF, etc.). Peripheral blockade of the V_1 branch can be used for limited scalp or forehead surgeries, such as laceration repair. The peripheral branches of the maxillary and mandibular divisions (V_2 and V_3) are commonly blocked for disabling trigeminal neuralgia. This can be done with a local anesthetic, with a neurolytic agent, or by radiofrequency ablation. Unfortunately, gasserian ganglion blockade can be difficult to perform and has the potential for catastrophic side effects due to its proximity to the CSF.

Nerve Injury   Injuries to the trigeminal nerve resulting from positioning during anesthesia and surgery are rare. Trigeminal neuralgia (tic douloureux) is the major nerve lesion of the trigeminal nerve. In some cases, it is caused by pressure on the nerve from the superior cerebellar artery, tumors, aneurysms, or arteriovenous malformations.

fossa. At the infraorbital canal, anterior dental nerves give off from the main nerve trunk. Finally, the infraorbital nerve emerges from the infraorbital foramen just below the eye and lateral to the nose. Terminal palpebral, nasal, and labial nerves arise from the infraorbital nerve. The maxillary nerve provides sensation to the upper jaw, lateral nasal wall, nasal septum, and the hard palate. The distal infraorbital nerve innervates the skin of the middle third of the face (Fig. 20–26).

The lowermost branch of the trigeminal nerve, the mandibular division (V_3), contains both motor and sensory

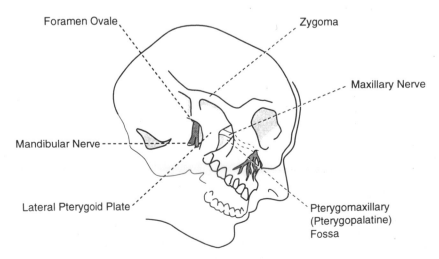

Figure 20–27 Anatomy of the mandibular nerve (V_3) in the infratemporal fossa (the mandible has been removed to expose the fossa and nerve).

The author and editors would like to thank illustrator Diane Raeke-Heilig for her excellent drawings and Paul Bockhoj for his expertise and influence.

BIBLIOGRAPHY

Clemente CD: *Anatomy: A Regional Atlas of the Human Body*, 2d ed. Baltimore, Urban and Schwarzenberg, 1981.

Cousins MJ, Bridenbaugh PO: *Neural Blockade in Clinical Anesthesia and Management of Pain*, 2d ed. Philadelphia, Lippincott, 1988.

Gray H: *Anatomy: Descriptive and Surgical*, 5th ed. Philadelphia, Henry C. Lea, 1870.

21

Central Neuroanatomy: An Operative Approach

Mark E. Shaffrey,
Christopher I. Shaffrey,
Andrew G. Chenelle,
and David J. Stone

Successful management of the neurosurgical patient is dependent upon effectual interactions between the neurosurgeon and the neuroanesthetist. One of the prerequisites for effective communication is a basic understanding of neuroanatomy. However, an isolated knowledge of neuroanatomy may not be sufficient if its application is unclear. Thus, our purpose is to describe and illustrate neuroanatomic terminology in its applied context, an operative approach.

☐ CALVARIAL ANATOMY: EVACUATION OF TRAUMATIC HEMORRHAGES

The cranium is composed of the cranial vault (or calvarium) and the cranial base. Simplistically, the calvarium is formed anteriorly by the frontal bone, superiorly by the parietal bones, posteriorly by the occipital bone, and inferiolaterally by the sphenoid and temporal bones (Fig. 21–1A).* The anterior cranial base is composed of the frontal bone, the ethmoid bone, and the sphenoid bone. The middle cranial base is bound anteriorly by the posterior border of the sphenoid bone, laterally by the squamous portion of the temporal bone, and posteriorly by the petrous portion of the temporal bone. The posterior cranial base is formed anteriorly by the petrous portion of the temporal bone, laterally by the squama of the occipital bone, and posteriorly by the anterior lip of the foramen magnum. The clivus is positioned medially within the posterior cranial base (Fig. 21–1B).

The calvarium is covered with periosteum on both its inner and outer surfaces. The inner periosteum is fused to the dura, forming the outer dural layer (Fig. 21–1C). The periosteum of the skull is markedly deficient in its osteogenic capacity compared with the periosteum of long bones. Relatively little bony regeneration would take place if a flap of bone were removed and not replaced (i.e., craniectomy). Thus, it is usually planned to replace any flaps of bone that are removed in neurosurgical procedures (i.e., craniotomy) unless conditions require that the bone flap cannot be replaced, as in states of severe cerebral edema, destruction of bone flap by underlying tumors, or infection.

One of the procedures that highlights the formation of a craniotomy flap is the evacuation of an acute traumatic subdural or epidural hematoma. During blunt closed head injuries that involve acceleration, deceleration, and/or rotational forces, the brain may undergo deformation, particularly in the frontal, temporal, and midline regions. This leads to the high incidence of frontal and temporal contusion as well as tearing of midline bridging veins (which connect the cortical veins to the sagittal sinus; Fig. 21–1C). Tearing the bridging veins is the mechanism most classically associated with acute subdural hematoma (Fig. 21–1D). Operative exposure must allow access to the frontal and temporal lobes and the anterior and middle cranial fossae and permit venous drainage of the frontal and temporal lobes.

Generally a large "question mark" skin incision is performed; this extends from the base of the zygoma to the anterior midline of the scalp (Fig. 21–1E). The crucial openings for a craniotomy flap are in the temporal bone at the base of the zygomatic arch (on the floor of the middle cranial fossa) and anteriorly in the region of the pterion (the anterolateral portion of the skull where the frontal, temporal, and sphenoid bones are adjoined; Fig. 21–1A). Prior to the craniotomy, an emergent subtemporal decompression is performed, using the temporal burr hole (Fig. 21–1F). The medial portion of the bone flap should be approximately 2 cm from the midline to allow visualization of bleeding from the sagittal sinus. Once the bone flap is removed, the blood clot can be gently

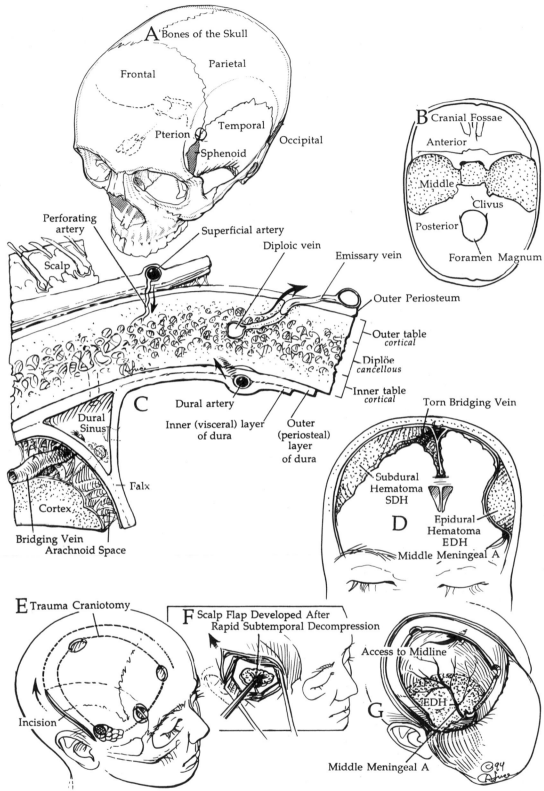

Figure 21–1   (*A*) The cranial vault, demonstrating the frontal, temporal, parietal, and sphenoid bones. (*B*) Skull base, demonstrating the anterior, middle, and posterior cranial fossae. (*C*) Cross section of the calvarium, demonstrating cortical and cancellous bone as well as emissary veins and dural layers. (*D*) Coronal section, demonstrating epidural and subdural hemorrhages. (*E*) Traditional scalp flap and craniotomy for acute subdural or epidural hemorrhage. (*F*) Emergent subtemporal decompression for immediate pressure relief prior to craniotomy. (*G*) Completed craniotomy, showing the middle meningeal artery, which will need to be coagulated, and the epidural hemorrhage.

evacuated from the cortical surface using a combination of irrigation, suctioning, and cup forceps. Large clot fragments should be removed; however, small clot fragments that lie beyond the craniotomy margin or near the venous sinuses should not be aggressively pursued due to a high potential for bleeding, which could be difficult to control.

An injury to the temporal area of the skull, with or without an associated temporal bone fracture, can produce an epidural (i.e., between the dura and the inner table of the skull) hematoma (Fig. 21–1D). This is because of the proximity of the middle meningeal artery associated with the dura directly beneath the temporal bone. Relatively minor trauma or fractures may lacerate the middle meningeal artery and produce bleeding between the inner table of the skull and the outer dural layer. Not all epidural hematomas are associated with laceration of the middle meningeal artery; however, this is a common presentation (Fig. 21–1G). Surgical treatment of the epidural hematoma is essentially the same as that for the subdural hematoma, through a large, standard craniotomy flap. This exposure allows decompression of the epidural hematoma, primarily by suction and irrigation. It is necessary to open the dura only if a contributory subdural or intra-parenchymal hemorrhage is suspected. It is very important to locate and coagulate the primary source of bleeding in both subdural and epidural hematomas.

☐ DURAL ANATOMY: DECOMPRESSIVE CRANIOTOMIES

The dura mater is the outer layer of the meninges, a dense, inelastic membrane composed of two layers that surround the convexity of the brain (Fig. 21–1C). As previously mentioned, the outer layer of dura is actually the inner periosteal layer of the skull. The inner dural layer is the meningeal portion, which folds into four double-layer partitions that compartmentalize the cranial vault (Fig. 21–2A, B). The falx cerebri is the fold of dura in the midline between the cerebral hemispheres; its free edge lies just above the corpus callosum. The falx cerebelli is a similar midline partition that separates the two cerebellar hemispheres. The tentorium cerebelli is the transversely oriented layer that separates the cerebral hemispheres (supratentorial compartment) from the cerebellum (infratentorial compartment). Finally, the diaphragma sellae forms the roof of the sella turcica and is perforated by the pituitary stalk.

This rigid compartmentalization of the cranial vault is clinically significant when intracranial pressure is elevated. Discrete intracerebral mass lesions or generalized cerebral edema that occurs in the supratentorial compartment can force the uncus of the temporal lobe through the notch in the tentorium, resulting in uncal (or transtentorial) herniation (Fig. 21–2C). The uncal pressure may then be translated to the brainstem, the oculomotor nerve, and/or the posterior cerebral artery. Pressure on the brainstem can affect the reticular formation and result in rapid, deep coma. Compression of the oculomotor nerve leads to the familiar dilation of the

pupil, or "blown pupil," frequently associated with this syndrome. Entrapment of the posterior cerebral artery can eventually lead to an infarction in this vascular territory if the patient survives the initial insult of brainstem compression.

Mass lesions in the mid- to upper portions of the frontal and parietal lobes can result in herniation of portions of these lobes, generally the cingulate gyrus, beneath the midline falx cerebri (Fig. 21–2D). This is termed *subfalcine herniation*. Subfalcine herniation may occur alone or in conjunction with uncal herniation. Although the effect on the results of the patient's neurologic examination is not usually so immediate or dramatic, compression of the branches of the anterior cerebral artery may result in corresponding vascular distribution infarction. Posterior fossa mass lesions may result in herniation of the cerebellar tonsils through the foramen magnum and cause compression of the brainstem, medulla, and upper cervical spinal cord (Fig. 21–2E). This tonsillar herniation may result in dramatic neurologic deterioration and eventually death if the pressure within the infratentorial compartment is not relieved.

When there is no focal mass lesion (e.g., intracerebral hemorrhage or tumors) and there is generalized edema, some neurosurgeons might consider a decompressive craniectomy to treat intractable intracranial hypertension. This involves the removal of a large portion of the calvarial bone on one side of the skull (hemicraniectomy) or both frontal bones in a single plate (bifrontal craniectomy, or Kjellberg procedure). These techniques have never been rigorously proven to improve the outcomes of patients with generalized cerebral edema.

☐ VENTRICULAR ANATOMY: CEREBROSPINAL FLUID DIVERSION

Knowledge of ventricular anatomy and cerebrospinal fluid (CSF) flow are crucial to the performance of one of the most basic neurosurgical procedures: the diversion of CSF. The ventricular system is a series of four communicating cavities lined by ependymal cells. The CSF is derived from blood and elaborated by the choroid plexus contained within the ventricular system. The components of the ventricular system include a pair of lateral ventricles: the third ventricle and the fourth ventricle (Fig. 21–3A, B).

The two lateral ventricles are contained within the cerebral hemispheres, and each is connected to the third ventricle through separate intraventricular foramina of Monro. Each lateral ventricle has four distinct parts. The anterior horn is the portion anterior to the intraventricular foramen and is located within the frontal lobe. Its anterior wall and roof are formed by the corpus callosum. The medial portions of the lateral ventricles are separated by a thin membrane known as the septum pellucidum (Fig. 21–3D). The body of each lateral ventricle lies posterior to the foramen of Monro and is located in the parietal lobe. Its roof is also formed by the corpus callosum. The choroid plexus of the lateral ventricle is found on the floor of the body. The posterior, or occipital, horn is located within the occipital lobe. The inferior, or tem-

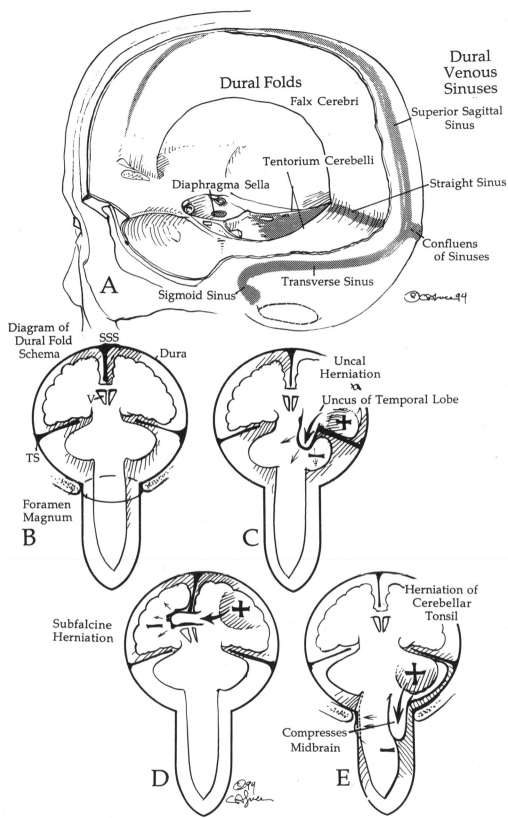

Figure 21–2 (*A*) Cutaway section of the skull with the brain removed, demonstrating the primary dural partitions and principal venous sinuses. Simplified coronal brain sections demonstrate a normal brain and the three common herniation syndromes: (*B*) normal, (*C*) uncal, (*D*) subfalcine, (*E*) tonsillar.

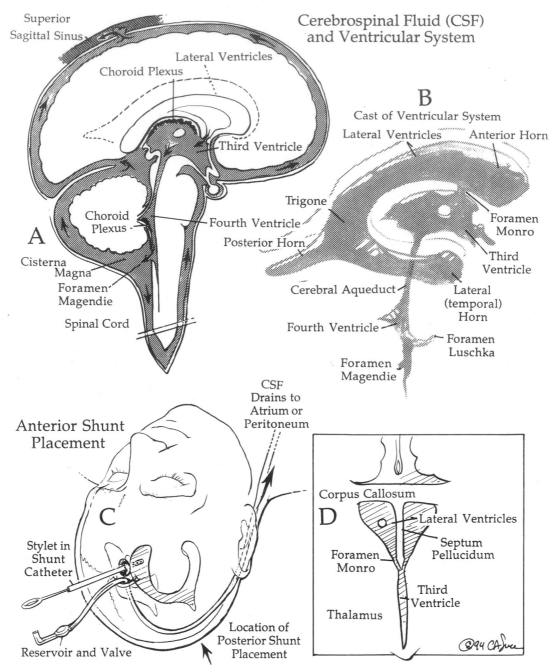

Figure 21–3 (*A*) Diagram of CSF flow from its production in the choroid plexus of the lateral and fourth ventricles out of the foramina of Luschka and Magendie into the subarachnoid space to ultimate absorption by the arachnoid granulations of the superior sagittal sinus. (*B*) Cast of the ventricular system demonstrating the anterior, posterior, and temporal horns of the lateral ventricles in addition to the foramen of Monro, the aqueduct of Sylvius (cerebral aqueduct), the third ventricle, the fourth ventricle, and the foramina of Luschka and Magendie. (*C*) Typical ventricular catheter placement. The burr hole is 2 cm anterior to the coronal suture at the midpupillary line. The catheter enters the ipsilateral frontal horn anterior to the foramen of Monro. (*D*) Simplified coronal cross section demonstrating the relationships of the lateral ventricles to the corpus callosum, foramen of Monro, septum pellucidum, and third ventricle. A shunt catheter is represented in the lateral ventricle.

poral, horn is contained within the temporal lobe. The trigone, or atrium of the lateral ventricle, is the cavity at the junction of the body, posterior horn, and inferior horn.

The CSF formed within the lateral ventricles passes through the paired intraventricular foramina of Monro to reach the third ventricle (Fig. 21–3*A*). The third ventricle is a thin, vertical chamber located in the midline between the paired lateral ventricles. Its roof is formed by a thin layer of

ependyma; its lateral walls are formed primarily by each thalamus. The CSF that exits the third ventricle flows caudally through the aqueduct of Sylvius, which communicates with the fourth ventricle. The fourth ventricle is a rhomboidshaped cavity that lies between the brainstem anteriorly and the cerebellum dorsally. This ventricle communicates with the subarachnoid space between two lateral foramina of Luschka and the midline foramen of Magendie. The CSF flows out of the fourth ventricle through the foramina of Luschka and Magendie. The CSF that exits these foramina flows in several directions: superiorly into the subarachnoid space surrounding the cerebellar hemispheres, caudally into the spinal subarachnoid space, and cephalad into the cisterns surrounding the brainstem (Fig. 21–3A).

The CSF is returned to the venous system through small membranous villi, called arachnoid granulations, that are located primarily in the superior sagittal sinus. The flow of CSF is generally unidirectional because of the pressure gradient that exists between its source of arterial blood within the choroid plexus and venous blood where it is eventually reabsorbed.

There are usually three major sources of accumulation of CSF within the brain (i.e., hydrocephalus). First, there can be communicating hydrocephalus, in which there is a failure to reabsorb CSF via normal pathways. This may happen, for example, in patients with meningitis or subarachnoid hemorrhage. Second, noncommunicating or obstructive hydrocephalus can occur, for example, when an intraventricular hemorrhage causes a blood clot to occlude normal CSF flow. Also, tumors may occlude many sites along the normal path of CSF flow. Finally, hydrocephalus can occur through overproduction of CSF; the most common example of this is a tumor of the choroid plexus known as a choroid plexus papilloma.

Catheters placed within the ventricular system can be either left to drain externally or internalized to any of several sites, such as the peritoneal cavity, the pleural cavity, or the atrium of the heart. The ventriculostomy catheter is generally placed either in a frontal location or in a parieto-occipital location (Fig. 21–3C). The ideal frontal ventriculostomy catheter is placed through a burr hole approximately 1 to 2 cm anterior to the coronal suture in the midpupillary line. The catheter is generally guided to the hypothetical junction point of the sagittal midline and a coronal line just anterior to the external auditory canal. This places the catheter tip just anterior to the foramina of Monro, in the frontal horn of the lateral ventricle, which is devoid of choroid plexus. Many proximal ventricular catheter malfunctions can occur because of obstruction of the catheter by choroid plexus.

The ideal placement of the parieto-occipital burr hole is less well-defined. However, most surgeons use landmarks several centimeters superior to the transverse sinus and several centimeters lateral to the sagittal sinus. In some series, parieto-occipital placement of ventricular catheters results in a lower frequency of epilepsy.

☐ LOCALIZATION OF CORTICAL FUNCTION: CEREBRAL LOBECTOMIES

Functional areas of the cerebral cortex that have been most well-defined include the primary motor area, the primary somatosensory area, the primary visual cortex, and language areas (Fig. 21–4A). The localization of cortical function is necessary in most cerebral lobectomies for either tumors or removal of epileptogenic foci.

The primary motor areas are located bilaterally along the anterior wall of the central sulcus (precentral gyrus). This layer of cortex is unusually thick and contains the giant pyramidal cells (of Betz). The corticospinal tracts arise in part from these areas and provide motor function to the opposite side of the body, especially skilled voluntary movements of the facial musculature, and flexion of the extremities. The location of cortical centers for specific movements of voluntary musculature varies somewhat in each individual; however, the sequence of these centers remains relatively constant. This sequence is described in the somatotopically organized motor homunculus, with lower extremity function lying most medially, upper extremity function lying lateral to that, and facial musculature and the swallowing apparatus lying most inferiorly (Fig. 21–4B).

The primary somatosensory areas recognize the source, quality (pain, temperature, pressure, light touch, proprioception, and kinesthesia), and quantification of sensory stimuli. The primary sensory cortices are located in each postcentral gyrus and receive somatosensory input relayed from the contralateral half of the body through the thalamus (Fig. 21–4C). Somatotopic organization of somatosensory input is similar to that of the motor cortex (somatosensory homunculus).

The primary visual cortex surrounds the calcarine fissure. It receives visual input from the ipsilateral nasal visual field and the contralateral temporal visual field via both the optic nerves and the ipsilateral optic tract, optic radiation, and geniculocalcarine tract. Destruction of visual pathways that lie in close proximity to or include the primary visual cortex cause homonymous visual field deficits (i.e., the ipsilateral nasal field and the contralateral temporal field will be affected relatively equally).

Language is grossly separable into two components: expression and reception. The region in the inferior aspect of the frontal lobe near the motor cortex, Broca's area, is involved in the articulation of speech (Fig. 21–4A). Lesions that affect Broca's area result in expressive (or nonfluent) aphasia, and these patients are unable to perform the coordinated movements necessary for language, despite understanding what they want to verbalize. The area in the temporoparietal region that is involved with language interpretation is known as Wernicke's area (Fig. 21–4A). Lesions involving Wernicke's area result in the inability to understand language, but, if Broca's area is intact, words may be produced without regard to meaning (fluent aphasia). Language is localized to the left hemisphere in approximately 96% of the population.

When performing a frontal lobectomy, specific attention must be given both to the primary motor areas and Broca's area if operating on the language-dominant hemisphere. Exposure to the frontal lobe may be carried through a modified transcoronal skin incision that begins at the zygoma on the ipsilateral side and extends to the contralateral superior temporal line. The bone flap should be approximately 1 cm from the midline and should extend close to the floor of the ante-

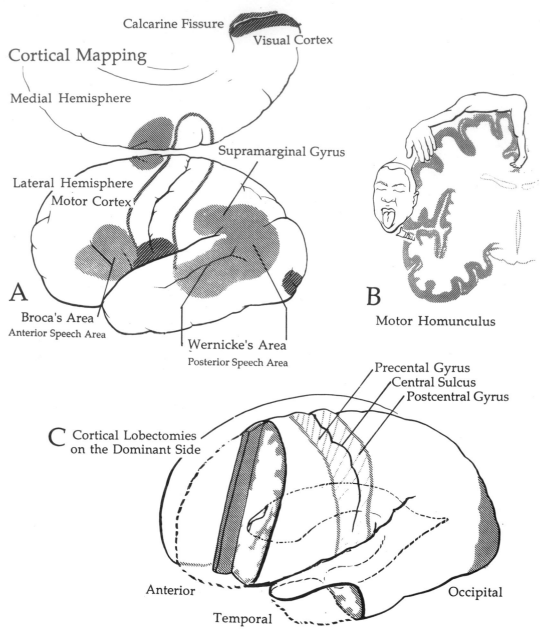

Figure 21–4 (*A*) Cortical localization of speech, motor, and sensory areas. (*B*) The motor homunculus, with the lower extremity medial in the interhemispheric fissure and the upper extremity and face more lateral. (*C*) Common lobectomies—frontal, temporal, and occipital—in the dominant hemisphere. Note the avoidance of speech areas.

rior cranial base. The frontal lobe may be resected up to 7 cm in the nondominant hemisphere, sparing the primary motor area. However, in the dominant hemisphere, this resection must be foreshortened to 5 cm, particularly in the inferior frontal gyrus, where the potential for injury to Broca's area is the greatest.

A temporal lobectomy is usually performed with the head in the lateral position. A small "question mark" skin incision may be extended from the ipsilateral zygoma. The size of the bone flap may be greatly reduced when exposure of only the temporal lobe is necessary. In the nondominant hemisphere, the temporal lobe can be resected to approximately 6 cm from the temporal tip, primarily risking a small quadrant visual field defect if the resection line includes any of the

geniculocalcarine visual fibers. Conventional wisdom contends that the resection of temporal lobe be reduced to less than 5 cm in the dominant hemisphere to avoid language deficits. Speech arrest has been elicited even as close as 2.5 cm from the dominant temporal tip.

An occipital lobectomy may be performed with the patient in a variety of positions from semisitting to prone. Often, a triangular or U-shaped skin incision is used, extending from beneath the level of the transverse sinus to the level of the ear. In the nondominant hemisphere, the cortical incision can be safely placed 6 cm anterior to the occipital pole. However, in the dominant hemisphere, the anterior extent of the resection is more conservative, limited to approximately 4 cm, to avoid receptive language dysfunction and dyscalculia. The probability of neurologic deficits in any of the cerebral lobectomy procedures can be greatly reduced through the use of cortical mapping.

☐ PARASELLAR ANATOMY: TRANSSPHENOIDAL HYPOPHYSECTOMY

The sella turcica sits at the base of the skull bordered anteriorly and posteriorly by the anterior and posterior clinoid processes (Fig. 21–5A). Macroadenomas of the pituitary gland may erode the clinoids. The sella turcica is bordered laterally by the cavernous sinuses. Superiorly, the sella is covered by the diaphragma sellae, a thin membrane that separates the sella from the rest of the cranial cavity. Running through the diaphragma sellae is the infundibulum, or pituitary stalk (Fig. 21–5B).

The cavernous sinuses, lateral to the sella turcica, run from the superior orbital fissure anteriorly to the petrous portion of the temporal bone posteriorly. These sinuses drain the ophthalmic veins and the sphenoparietal sinus. The cavernous sinuses drain into the superior and inferior petrosal sinuses.

Many important structures run in the cavernous sinus (Fig. 21–5B). The lateral wall of the cavernous sinus contains the oculomotor (III) nerve. This nerve contains both somatic motor fibers that innervate the levator palpebrae and most intrinsic eye muscles (other than the superior oblique and lateral rectus) and visceral motor fibers that provide the parasympathetic tone to the constrictor pupillae and ciliary muscles via the ciliary ganglion. The lateral wall of the cavernous sinus also contains the trochlear nerve (IV), whose somatic motor fibers innervate the superior oblique muscle, and the ophthalmic (V_I) and maxillary (V_{II}) branches of the trigeminal (V) nerve. These branches of the trigeminal nerve are generally somatic afferents that receive sensory input from the face, scalp, and dura. Running through the cavernous sinus are the carotid artery and the abducens nerve (VI), whose somatic motor fibers innervate the lateral rectus muscle of the eye.

The pituitary gland lies within the sella (Fig. 21–5C). The anterior pituitary gland (or adenohypophysis) makes ACTH, GH, LH, FSH, and prolactin (see Chapter 13); it is the site from which adenomas arise. The posterior pituitary gland (or neurohypophysis) is the site of release of oxytocin and vasopressin (ADH). The pituitary gland is connected to the hypothalamus by the infundibulum, or pituitary stalk, through which its portal venous system delivers releasing hormones to the pituitary.

A thin membrane, the diaphragma sellae, separates the sella from the CSF spaces of the anterior cranial fossa. Above this lie the optic (II) nerves, whose special sensory function conveys visual information from the retina. Above the optic nerves is the hypothalamus, which serves as an autoregulatory center for the body.

The transsphenoidal approach to the sella turcica was used frequently by Harvey Cushing (Fig. 21–5C, D, E). However,

with the advent of the operating microscope, the procedure was further refined and popularized by Jules Hardy. To start the operation, a transverse incision is made in the upper gingival mucosa or an inferior incision in the nasal mucosa carried on to the septum. A subperichondral separation of the nasal mucosa from the nasal septum is performed, usually on the left side, and carried back to the nasal spine. The nasal septum is then fractured at the base and displaced to the side. At the posterior end of the cartilaginous septum, a small bony septum is encountered that originates from the superior portion of the vomer and inferior portion of the perpendicular plate of the ethmoid. This bony septum, along with the perpendicular plate of the ethmoid, is then fractured and often removed, enabling the surgeon to visualize the anterior wall of the sphenoid sinus, which looks like a boat keel (Fig. 21–5D). The anterior wall of the sphenoid sinus is then removed, and the mucosa of the sphenoid sinus is stripped. It is important to note that the carotid arteries and their anterior loops are closely associated with the sphenoid sinus (Fig. 21–5B). The sella floor is easily visualized once the mucosa has been removed and a lateral x-ray film is taken to delineate the anterior and posterior extents of the sella. An opening is then made in the anterior wall of the sella (Fig. 21–5E). The cavernous sinuses are closely adherent to the lateral walls of the sella, and, in removing the sella floor, it is not uncommon to cause bleeding from the cavernous sinus.

Once the sella floor is exposed, the dura (Fig. 21–5E) is opened sharply with a knife. Dural opening that extends too far superiorly can enter the suprasellar recess and cause a CSF leak; opening the dura too far laterally can open the cavernous sinus and cause profuse bleeding.

Once the dura is opened, the tumor may be removed (Fig. 21–5E). In the cases of macroadenoma, a flattened pituitary gland can almost always be identified and spared. It is usually displaced posteriorly and superiorly. Preoperative localization by magnetic resonance imaging (MRI) and/or petrosal venous sampling can aid in gland exploration. Small incisions in the gland in the side of the localization usually enable the surgeon to find the microadenoma with minimal trauma to the normal gland. When microadenomas are debulked, the diaphragma sellae usually falls into the sella turcica. The infundibulum is often visualized as it pierces the diaphragma sellae. Care must be taken in resecting tumors with suprasellar extension not to damage the overlying optic nerves.

If a large suprasellar tumor is removed during the transsphenoidal route, a lumbar drainage catheter can be helpful. The tumor can then be outlined on the lateral skull radiograph with the insertion of 5 to 10 mL of air through the lumbar drain catheter. In addition, the insertion of a small amount of air through the lumbar drainage catheter can often push suprasellar tumor extension down into the sella, making it easier and safer to remove.

If a CSF leak is encountered, the sella is packed with fat harvested from a small incision on the patient's abdomen or thigh. Finally, the sella is packed with a small amount of gel foam and/or fat, and the bony nasal septum is fashioned to fit

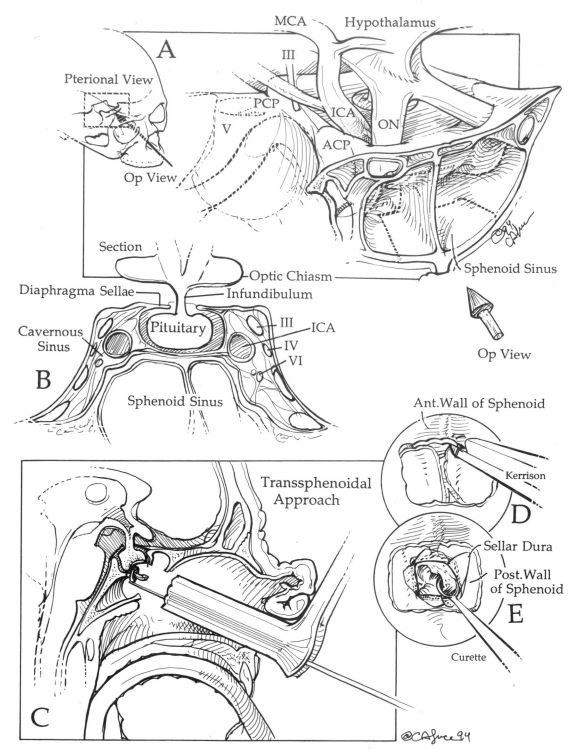

Figure 21–5 (*A*) Pterional view of the parasellar region. The pituitary gland lies beneath the optic chiasm. MCA = middle cerebral artery; ICA = internal carotid artery; ON = optic nerve; ACP = anterior clinoid process; PCP = posterior clinoid process. (*B*) Coronal section of the sella showing the surrounding cavernous sinuses with intercavernous structures. III = oculomotor nerve; IV = trochlear nerve; VI = abducens nerve. Transsphenoidal removal of a pituitary adenoma: (*C*) Sagittal view of the completed approach. The tumor is being removed with the use of a ring curette. (*D*) The anterior wall of the sphenoid sinus is removed with a Kerrison rongeur. (*E*) The posterior wall of the sphenoid (floor of the sella) is removed. The dura is opened, and the tumor is being removed.

under the dura, thus reconstructing the sella floor. The nasal septum is then brought back into place, the mucosa is brought against the nasal septum, and the sublabial and/or nasal incisions are closed with chromic suture and the nose is packed.

☐ THE CIRCLE OF WILLIS: BASILAR ARTERY ANEURYSM

The circle of Willis is formed by the anterior and posterior communicating arteries and the proximal portions of the anterior, middle, and posterior cerebral arteries (Fig. 21–6A). This arterial network surrounds the optic chiasm, the pituitary stalk, and the mamillary bodies. The circle of Willis is subject to frequent anatomic variation, and a "normal" circle is found in only slightly greater than 50% of the population. The most common variations include posterior cerebral arteries that arise directly from the internal carotid arteries and abnormalities of the anterior communicating arteries. The circle of Willis can provide an alternative supply of blood to regions affected by arterial occlusions.

The basilar artery is formed by the confluence of the two vertebral arteries. Its principal branches are the anterior inferior cerebellar arteries, the superior cerebellar arteries, and numerous penetrating and short circumferential branches, especially to the pons (Fig. 21–6A). The basilar artery terminates distally in the paired posterior cerebral arteries. They provide the major blood supply to the midbrain and supply the posterior half of the thalamus and the medial and lateral geniculate bodies. The posterior cerebral arteries also supply the occipital lobe, the visual cortex, and the inferior surface of the temporal lobes. Aneurysms of the distal basilar artery at either the apex of the basilar artery or at the origin of the superior cerebellar artery represent approximately half of all posterior circulation aneurysms. Important neural and vascular structures are very close to these aneurysms (Fig. 21–6A). The height of the basilar bifurcation helps determine the approach to aneurysms in this area. Most commonly, the bifurcation is at or just above the dorsum sellae. A pterional exposure will give adequate exposure of the neck of a basilar bifurcation aneurysm that originates between the middle of the sella turcica to a height 1 cm above the posterior clinoid process (Fig. 21–6B, C). Aneurysms below the middle of the sella are best approached by a subtemporal or subtemporal/transtentorial route.

The pterional approach is used for exposure of most anterior circulation aneurysms. The distance between the carotid artery and the basilar bifurcation is less than 2 cm. Following positioning with a skull fixation device, a pterional craniotomy with an anterior decompressive temporal craniectomy is performed (Fig. 21–6B). The sphenoid ridge is removed with a high-speed burr or bone rongeurs to allow maximal exposure. Following the opening of the dura, the Sylvian fissure is opened to increase exposure and limit the force of retraction on the frontal and temporal lobes (Fig. 21–6D). The posterior communicating artery is followed until it pierces a thickened arachnoid band called the membrane of Lilliequist. Opening of this membrane gains entrance into the interpeduncular cistern. The segment of the posterior cerebral artery from its origin at the basilar artery to the junction point with the posterior communicating artery is called the P1 segment (Fig. 21–6A). This segment crosses the oculomotor nerve before passing around the cerebral peduncle. Many small important thalamoperforating branches arise from the P1 segment. These perforators supply the anterior and posterior thalamus, the hypothalamus, and the posterior internal capsule. Occlusion of these branches can result in profound neurologic deficits, including hemiplegia, altered consciousness, and ocular motility difficulties. Subsequent segments of the posterior cerebral artery supply the remaining portions of its distribution.

Identification of the P1 segment and the contralateral superior cerebellar artery and P1 segments is the key to a successful aneurysm clipping. Temporary clipping of the basilar artery and P1 segments is possible at this point prior to definitive aneurysm clipping. The oculomotor nerve passes between the posterior cerebral artery and the superior cerebellar artery before piercing the dura and entering the cavernous sinus (Fig. 21–6A). The proximity of the oculomotor nerve to the posterior cerebral artery makes it vulnerable to direct injury or indirect injury due to retraction. The trochlear nerve is the only cranial nerve to exit from the dorsal aspect of the brainstem. It exits at the junction of the mesencephalon and pons and then passes around the lateral surface of the midbrain between the posterior cerebral artery and the superior cerebellar artery before penetrating the dura at the anterior attaching fold of the tentorium. The trochlear nerve is a fine structure, easily disrupted at its entry into the tentorium, especially with subtemporal and subtemporal/transtentorial approaches. Because of the large number of perforating vessels in the region of the basilar tip, clear definition of the entire aneurysm neck is needed to reduce postoperative deficits.

Aneurysms arising below the middle of the sella usually require a subtemporal approach with or without division of the tentorium to obtain adequate exposure. This approach requires elevation of the temporal lobe and can compromise the inferior anastomotic vein (of Labbé) as it traverses from the posterior/inferior temporal lobe to the junction of the transverse and sigmoid sinuses. Venous compromise can cause edema or hemorrhagic infarction. A curvilinear incision is frequently used for the subtemporal approach. This begins at the zygoma and travels to the postauricular region. A craniotomy is performed, centered above the external auditory canal. Brain relaxation is a key feature, and CSF drainage, osmotic agents, and hyperventilation are often used to allow gentle elevation of the temporal lobe. With elevation of the uncus, the oculomotor nerve becomes visible due to arachnoid attachments in this region. The trochlear nerve is identified as it enters the tentorium and protected if a tentorial retraction suture is placed or the tentorium is divided. The superior cerebellar artery is often identified where it passes around the cerebral peduncle to enter the cisterna ambiens and is followed from this point to its origin at the basilar artery. The ipsilateral P1 segment and the contralateral P1

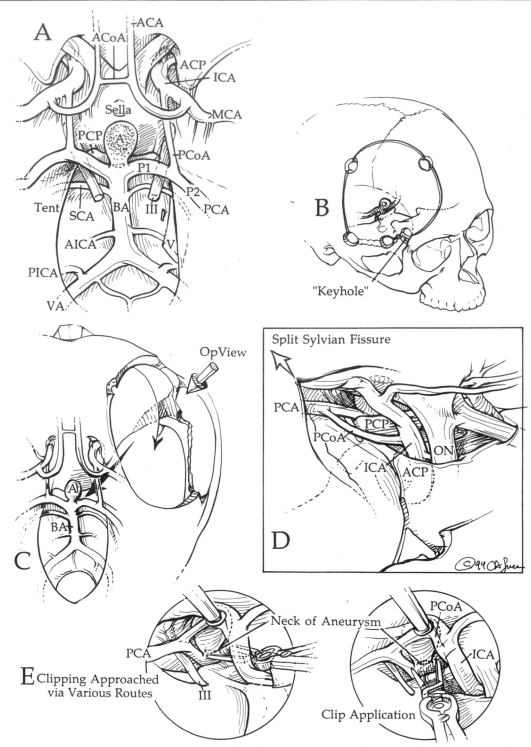

Figure 21–6 (*A*) The circle of Willis viewed from above. A basilar tip aneurysm (A) is present. Note nerve III passing between the SCA and the P1 segment. ACA = anterior cerebral artery; ACP = anterior clinoid process; ACoA = anterior communicating artery; ICA = internal carotid artery; MCA = middle cerebral artery; P1 = first segment of the posterior cerebral artery; P2 = second segment of the posterior cerebral artery; PCA = posterior cerebral artery; BA = basilar artery; SCA = superior cerebellar artery; AICA = anterior inferior cerebellar artery; PICA = posterior inferior cerebellar artery; VA = vertebral artery. (*B*) Standard pterional craniotomy for aneurysm, demonstrating the "keyhole" burr hole in the pterion. (*C*) Cutaway drawing showing the vascular anatomy and the operative view afforded the surgeon. A = aneurysm; BA = basilar artery. (*D*) Typical view of the vascular anatomy after pterional craniotomy and the splitting of Sylvian fissure. ON = optic nerve; ICA = internal carotid artery; PCoA = posterior communicating artery; ACP = anterior clinoid process; PCP = posterior clinoid process. (*E*) Clipping of a basilar tip aneurysm both medial (A) and lateral (B) to the internal carotid artery. PCA = posterior cerebral artery; PCoA = posterior communicating artery.

and superior cerebellar artery are then identified. For low-lying basilar tip aneurysms, the tentorium is frequently divided and retracted to improve exposure and to gain proximal control of the aneurysm. From this point, clipping proceeds as described above, with great attention given to prevent occlusion of the contralateral P1 segment, perforation of vessels, or impingement on the opposite oculomotor nerve.

POSTERIOR FOSSA ANATOMY: MICROVASCULAR DECOMPRESSION AND ACOUSTIC NEUROMA

The trigeminal nerve (V) has special visceral efferent fibers that innervate the muscles of mastication and general somatic afferent fibers that convey sensory information from the scalp, face, teeth, and dura. The trigeminal nerve originates on the lateral surface of the pons. The sensory ganglion lies in a depression in the floor of the middle cranial fossa called Meckel's cave. From the ganglion there are three major

branches of the trigeminal nerve. The ophthalmic (V_I) branch exits the skull through the superior orbital fissure. The maxillary (V_{II}) branch exits the skull through the foramen rotundum. The mandibular (V_{III}) branch exits through the foramen ovale. The motor root runs with the mandibular division.

The vascular anatomy around the trigeminal nerve is quite complex. The superior cerebellar arteries arise from the rostral basilar artery. They course laterally to supply the superior surface of the cerebellum and often have a significant inferior loop in their lateral course. The anterior inferior cerebellar arteries arise from the caudal basilar artery and loop superiorly and laterally to supply the caudal pons and inferior cerebellum. Both of these vessels can be close to the trigeminal nerve anteriorly. The petrosal vein drains the anterior brainstem and superior cerebellum and then runs into the superior petrosal sinus. It courses posteriorly to the trigeminal nerve (Fig. 21-7B).

The transverse and sigmoid sinuses are important anatomic structures in the approach to the trigeminal nerve. The paired transverse sinuses arise at the confluence of sinuses, run laterally in an indentation in the occipital bone to

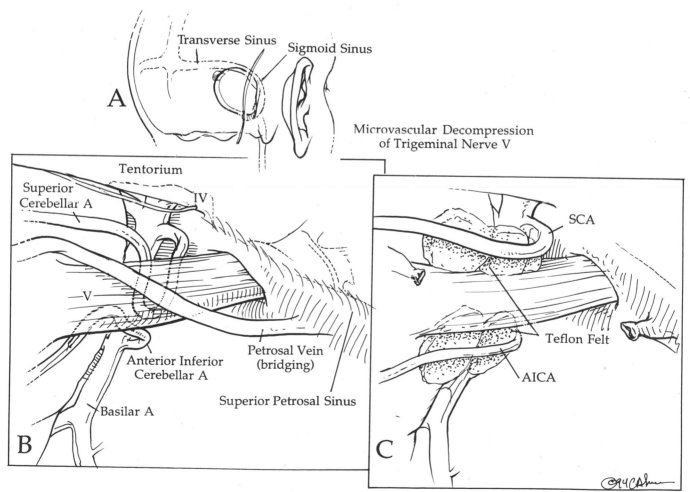

Figure 21-7   (A) Surgeon's view from the posterior of the typical craniotomy for microvascular decompression. Both the transverse and sigmoid sinuses are exposed. (B) Loops of the anterior inferior cerebellar artery or the superior cerebellar artery may compress the Vth nerve anteriorly. The overlying petrosal vein may need to be divided in the approach to the nerve. (C) Postprocedure separation of the vessels from the Vth nerve and padding with Teflon felt. In most cases, only one vessel compresses the nerve; however, in this drawing, both vessels are shown for the sake of simplicity.

the occipitopetrosal junction, and then curve inferiorly and posteriorly to form the sigmoid sinuses, which drain into the internal jugular veins.

MICROVASCULAR DECOMPRESSION

The first observation that vascular compression of the trigeminal nerve in the cerebellopontine (CP) angle could cause trigeminal neuralgia was made by Walter Dandy in 1925. The operative technique for microvascular decompression of the trigeminal nerve was advanced in the 1970s by Peter Jannetta. Cadaveric anatomic studies confirm that the superior cerebellar artery often makes contact with the trigeminal nerve at its origin from the brainstem. It is hypothesized that the etiology of trigeminal neuralgia is vascular compression of the trigeminal nerve at the brainstem, most often by the superior cerebellar artery; however, it is not unusual to find other vascular structures compressing the trigeminal nerve, such as the anterior inferior cerebellar artery (AICA) or the petrosal vein (Fig. 21–7B). It is thought that the vascular pulsations of these vessels cause the typical lancinating pain of trigeminal neuralgia.

Microvascular decompression is usually performed in the lateral position or with the patient supine and the head turned to the contralateral side. The surgical technique involves a vertical linear skin incision placed a finger-breadth behind the mastoid eminence. A half-dollar-sized retromastoid craniectomy is then performed, exposing the sigmoid and lateral sinuses (Fig. 21–7A). It is important to expose the junction of the sigmoid and lateral sinuses, since this is the angle at which the trigeminal nerve can be visualized with minimal cerebellar retraction. Occasionally, in performing this craniectomy, the mastoid air cells are entered. In this case, they must be packed with muscle and bone wax in order to prevent postoperative CSF leak.

Once the craniectomy is performed and the bone edges are waxed, the dura is opened, with careful attention to avoid entering the sigmoid and lateral sinuses. The arachnoid of the cerebellum is carefully opened, and a retractor blade is placed caudally just underneath the tentorium and used to locate the junction of the tentorium and the petrous dura. By following these two planes of dura, the trigeminal nerve can be found deeply anterior and caudal to the tentorium. When the patient is in the lateral position, gravity forms most of the cerebellar retraction.

Once the cerebellum is retracted, the petrosal vein is the first structure to be visualized. This is usually in an inverted Y or V shape. At this point, one must decide whether to sacrifice the vein in order to adequately visualize the trigeminal nerve. Occasionally, the petrosal vein causes vascular compression. During the retraction of the cerebellum, care must be taken not to injure the VIIth and VIIIth cranial nerves, which are anterior and caudal to the trigeminal nerve. Monitoring brainstem auditory evoked potentials is very helpful in this regard. When the trigeminal nerve is exposed, it is inspected for vascular compression. If the superior cerebellar artery is the cause of the compression, it occurs because a loop of the superior cerebellar artery comes from above, running anterior to the nerve. In the rare cases where the anterior inferior cerebellar artery is the cause of the vascular compression, the AICA makes a superior loop that again runs anterior to the trigeminal nerve.

Once the cause of trigeminal compression is identified, the artery or vein is carefully separated from the nerve and a small piece of gel foam, muscle, or Teflon pad is placed between the vessel and the nerve (Fig. 21–7C). Prior to closure, the cisterns are filled with saline solution. The dura is then closed in a watertight fashion, and the rest of the wound is closed in layers.

ACOUSTIC NEUROMAS

Three traditional approaches are utilized in removing acoustic neuromas: the suboccipital approach, the translabyrinthine approach, and the middle fossa approach. Surgical morbidity, including cranial nerve dysfunction, remained high until the development of microsurgical techniques. Acoustic neuromas arise from the vestibular nerves; the facial and cochlear nerves are displaced by the tumor but are almost never the source of the neoplasm. With improvements in operative technique and intraoperative monitoring, facial nerve preservation is routine, and preservation of useful hearing is possible in certain cases.

The suboccipital approach is performed by many surgeons when tumors are large (> 2.5 cm) or when hearing preservation is a consideration. The patient is supine with the head turned away from the side of the tumor or placed in a lateral "park bench" position. The use of the sitting position has largely been abandoned except for very large tumors because of the risk of air emboli. The patient is monitored intraoperatively with brainstem auditory evoked potentials and facial nerve electromyograms. Most frequently, a curvilinear incision posterior to the ear is performed, followed by a suboccipital craniectomy, which partially exposes the transverse sinus superiorly and the sigmoid sinus laterally (Fig. 21–8A). The dura is opened and the junction between the petrous bone and the tentorium identified. The cerebellar hemisphere is gently retracted, and the cerebellopontine cistern is exposed. This cistern contains the superior and anterior inferior cerebellar arteries, the superior petrosal vein, and cranial nerves V, VI, VII, and VIII (Fig. 21–8C).

The AICA usually arises from the basilar artery and rarely from the vertebral artery. The main trunk of AICA crosses the cranial nerve VII-VIII complex and can occasionally pass between the facial and vestibulocochlear components of the complex (Fig. 21–8C). The labyrinthine artery, which is most often a branch of AICA, enters the internal auditory canal. Damage to this branch can cause loss of hearing due to cochlear infarction despite preservation of the cochlear nerve. The petrosal vein drains the brainstem and empties into the superior petrosal sinus. If the petrosal vein is inadvertently torn, bleeding can be profuse. Sacrifice of the petrosal vein does not produce clinical sequelae.

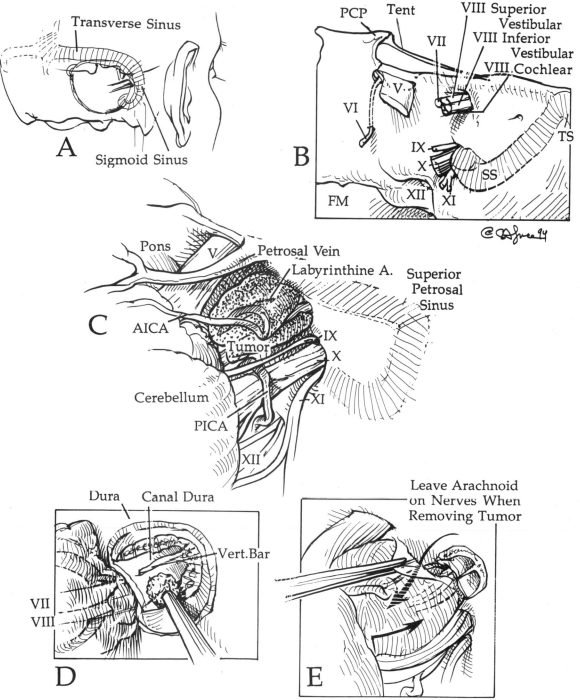

Figure 21–8   (*A*) Typical posterior fossa craniectomy for removal of an acoustic neuroma. (*B*) Region of the internal auditory meatus with the brainstem cut away. Note the four nerves entering the internal acoustic meatus, with the VIIth nerve anterior and superior, the cochlear nerve anterior and inferior, and the superior and inferior vestibular nerves posterior. FM = foramen magnum; TS = transverse sinus; SS = sigmoid sinus; PCP = posterior clinoid process. (*C*) Surgeon's view of an acoustic neuroma. Note the anterior inferior cerebellar artery (AICA) closely associated with the tumor. The VIIth nerve is pushed anteriorly by the tumor. (*D*) Drilling of the internal acoustic meatus. (*E*) Separation of the tumor from the arachnoid plane after internal debulking.

The facial and vestibulocochlear nerves emerge from the brainstem in the region of the pontomedullary sulcus. The facial nerve arises approximately 2 mm anterior to the point where the vestibulocochlear nerve arises. The nerves then travel laterally and superiorly to enter the internal auditory meatus. The internal auditory meatus is divided into four portions by bony septae known as the transverse and vertical crests. The cochlear portion of the VIIIth nerve is anterior and inferior; the facial nerve is anterior and superior. The inferior vestibular nerve is posterior and inferior, and the superior vestibular nerve is posterior and superior in location. The glossopharyngeal (IX), vagus (X), and spinal accessory nerves (XI) arise from the medulla along the margin of the inferior olive. These nerves travel superiorly and laterally to enter the jugular foramen (Fig. 21–8B).

In most patients, the facial nerve is displaced either anteriorly or inferiorly by the acoustic neuroma. Intraoperative electrical stimulation is utilized to locate the nerve. With large tumors, the trigeminal nerve may be displaced along the superior surface, and the glossopharyngeal, vagus, and accessory nerves may be displaced along the inferior surface. The tumor is separated from these nerves by arachnoid, and identification of this arachnoid plane is an important aspect of the tumor resection (Fig. 21–8D). In general, the tumor is initially internally decompressed, and then the cranial nerve VII-VIII complex is identified at the exit from the brainstem and followed from medial to lateral as the tumor is removed. Other surgeons prefer to identify individual nerves at the internal auditory canal and follow the facial nerve from lateral to medial. Often the dura overlying the internal auditory canal is opened, and the underlying bone is removed with a high-speed burr to fully remove the tumor and to assist in identifying the nervous structures (Fig. 21–8D). Following tumor removal, hemostasis is checked, and any mastoid air cells opened during bony dissection are sealed to prevent leakage of CSF.

The translabyrinthine approach for removal of acoustic neuromas is preferred by many surgeons, particularly with small to moderate-sized tumors when useful hearing has already been lost on that side. Potential advantages of this approach include avoidance of cerebellar retraction and identification of the facial nerve during the bony dissection for this approach. A small postauricular incision is made, and a mastoidectomy is performed using a high-speed burr. Mastoid air cells are removed to the mastoid antrum, and the semicircular canals are identified. As removal of the semicircular canals proceeds, the facial nerve is gradually identified under a thin covering of bone from the external genu to the stylomastoid foramen. The bone is subsequently removed in the area of the internal auditory canal. The dura is opened between the internal auditory meatus and the sigmoid sinus. The tumor is internally decompressed, and then dissection around the capsule is performed as the tumor is infolded into the resection cavity. Following tumor removal, the mastoid cavity is filled with a fat or muscle graft to reduce the possibility of CSF leakage.

The middle fossa approach is limited to small acoustic neuromas. It is used most often with intracanalicular tumors with preservable hearing. The patient is supine with the head turned so the appropriate ear faces upward. A vertical incision is made from the zygoma to the superior temporal line. The temporalis muscle is divided, and a craniotomy exposes the middle cranial fossa. The middle meningeal artery and its exit from the foramen spinosum are identified. The foramen ovale (where cranial nerve V_{III} exits) and the greater superficial petrosal nerve (a branch of cranial nerve VII, which supplies the lacrimal, nasal, and palatine glands) are next identified. The greater superficial petrosal nerve is followed back to where it joins the geniculate ganglion by removing a thin covering of bone. The labyrinthine portion of the facial nerve is then followed from the geniculate ganglion to the internal auditory canal, with additional bone removal in this region. At this point, the tumor can be removed, with preservation of facial nerve function and cochlear nerve function in some cases.

*All figures in this chapter are reproduced with permission from: Stone DJ, Sperry RJ, Johnson JO, Speikerman BF: Yemen. *Handbook of Neuroanesthesia*. Mosby, 1996.

BIBLIOGRAPHY

Carpenter MB, Sutin J: *Human Neuroanatomy*, 8th ed. Baltimore, Williams & Wilkins, 1983.

Dan NG, Wade MJ: The incidence of epilepsy after ventricular shunting procedures. *J Neurosurg* 65:19–21, 1988.

Dandy WE: Section of the sensory root of the trigeminal nerve at the pons: Preliminary report of operative procedure. *Johns Hopkins Med J* 36:105, 1925.

Hardy DG, Rhoton AL: Microsurgical relationships of the superior cerebellar artery and trigeminal nerve. *J Neurosurg* 49:669–678, 1978.

Hardy J: Transsphenoidal hypophysectomy. *J Neurosurg* 34:582–594, 1971.

Jannetta PJ: Arterial compression of the trigeminal nerve at the pons in patients with trigeminal neuralgia. *J Neurosurg* 26:159–162, 1967.

Ojemann GA: Individual variability in cortical localization of language. *J Neurosurg* 50:164–169, 1979.

Schmidek HS, Sweet WH: *Operative Neurosurgical Techniques*, 2d ed. Orlando, Grune & Stratton, 1988.

22

Cardiac Anatomy

Maria A. de Castro

An understanding of the anatomic relationships of cardiac structures is important in anesthetizing patients for cardiac surgery. Intraoperative transesophageal echocardiography (TEE) builds upon a knowledge of the anatomy of the heart and great vessels. The purpose of this chapter is to review those aspects of cardiac anatomy of particular importance to the anesthesiologist. In this chapter, correlations are made to horizontal and longitudinal echocardiographic images in order to enhance the reader's understanding of the anatomic relationships of the various cardiac structures. Several references at the end of the chapter provide extensive review of TEE imaging, including specific discussions of the technology and technique involved in performing the TEE examination.

☐ THE PERICARDIUM

The heart is enclosed within the pericardium, which is composed of two layers. The inner, visceral pericardium is a serous membrane. The outer, parietal pericardium is a fibrinous sac that extends onto the great vessels and attaches to the diaphragm and sternum. The two layers are joined at the level of the great vessels superiorly and at the central tendon of the diaphragm inferiorly. The space between the visceral and parietal pericardial layers normally contains up to 50 mL of fluid, which is an ultrafiltrate of plasma.

The pericardium folds back on itself to form four recesses: the superior sinus, the transverse sinus, the postcaval recess, and the oblique sinus. Two of these can be important echocardiographic landmarks. The transverse sinus is formed by the pericardial reflection behind the ascending aorta and pulmonary artery to the right of the superior vena cava and superior to the right and left pulmonary veins. The oblique

sinus is formed by the reflections of pericardium around the pulmonary veins. Pericardial effusions or cysts can enlarge these sinuses (Fig. 22–1).

Branches of the vagus nerve, left recurrent laryngeal nerve, and esophageal plexus innervate the pericardium. The stellate ganglion, first dorsal ganglion, and other sympathetic ganglia provide its sympathetic innervation. The phrenic nerves course laterally, encapsulated in the pericardial sac. This anatomic relationship explains how the phrenic nerves can be injured during surgical resection of the pericardium.

☐ CARDIAC CHAMBERS

RIGHT ATRIUM

The right atrium forms the right heart border. It lies to the right and behind the right ventricle. Its medial wall abuts the ascending aorta, with the right atrial appendage wrapping around the aortic root. The inner surfaces of the free wall of the right atrium and atrial appendage are composed of the pectinate muscles, while the posterior and septal walls are smooth.

The right atrium receives venous inflow posteriorly and medially from the superior vena cava and inferior vena cava (Figs. 22–2 and 22–3). A muscle ridge, the crista terminalis, extends between the superior and inferior venae cavae (Fig. 22–2). The entrance of the superior vena cava usually has no valve. The entrance of the inferior vena cava, however, is covered by a rudimentary valve, the eustachian valve, which is the inferior extension of the crista terminalis (Fig. 22–3).

Between the entrance of the inferior vena cava and the tricuspid valve lies the entrance of the coronary sinus with its valve, the Thebesian valve. The fossa ovalis of the interatrial

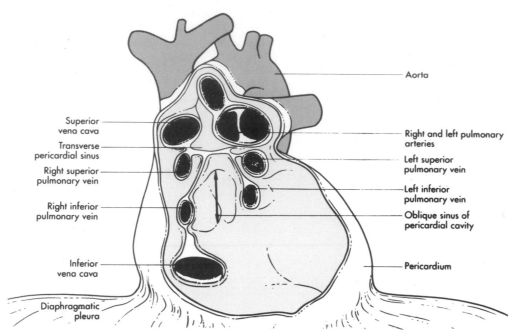

Figure 22–1 Dorsal view of the pericardial cavity demonstrating the pericardial reflection. (Reproduced with permission from Cheitlin and Finkbeiner, 1991.)

septum lies superior to the entrance of the inferior vena cava (Fig. 22–2). It is the remnant of the foramen ovale, which is closed by the septum secundum. Its superior rim has a prominent fold, the limbus of the fossa ovalis, which is an important landmark in echocardiography and angiography (Fig. 22–4).

RIGHT VENTRICLE

The right ventricle forms most of the anterior surface of the heart. It is triangular in shape. In cross section, as in the TEE transgastric short-axis view, it is crescent-shaped (Fig.

22–5). In contrast to the thicker left ventricle, the right ventricular walls are thin. The inner surfaces of the lateral and anterior walls of the right ventricle are heavily trabeculated muscle, the trabeculae carnae. The moderator band is a distinct muscle band connecting the septum to the anterior papillary muscle. The trabeculated anterior and inferior walls and the tricuspid valve form the right ventricular inflow tract. The superior portion of the right ventricle is the smooth-walled right ventricular outflow tract, also termed the infundibulum or conus. The inflow and outflow tracts are divided by a muscle band, the crista supraventricularis. In congenital heart disease, recognition of these characteristic

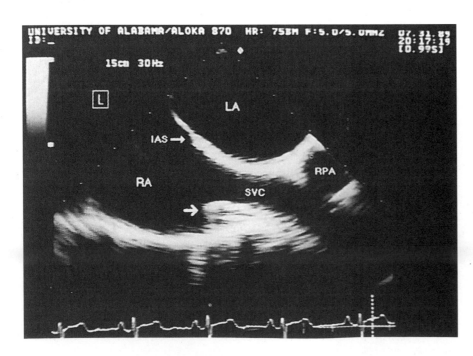

Figure 22–2 Transesophageal echocardiographic (TEE) view of the superior vena cava (SVC) entering the right atrium (RA). IAS, interatrial septum; LA, left atrium; RPA, right pulmonary artery; the arrow points to the crista terminalis. (Reproduced with permission from Maurer G: *Transesophageal Echocardiography.* New York: McGraw-Hill, 1994.)

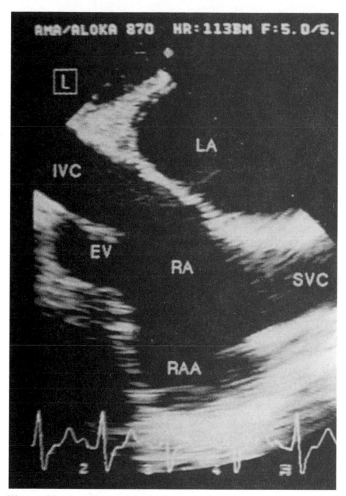

Figure 22-3   TEE view of inferior vena cava (IVC) entering RA. EV, eustachian valve; RAA, right atrial appendage. (Reproduced with permission from Maurer G: *Transesophageal Echocardiography.* New York: McGraw-Hill, 1994.)

features is important in identifying the morphologic right ventricle.

LEFT ATRIUM

The left atrium forms the superior posterior surface of the heart. The aortic root is anterior to the left atrium. The right atrium is anterior and to the right of the left atrium. The left atrial appendage curves laterally around the pulmonary artery. Immediately posterior to the left atrium is the esophagus. This relationship allows excellent imaging of the left atrium with TEE (Figs. 22-6, 22-7, and 22-8). The inner surface of the left atrium is smooth. Pectinate muscles are present only in the left atrial appendage. The four pulmonary veins drain into the left atrium posteriorly. The right superior and inferior pulmonary veins drain near the atrial septum. The left superior (Fig. 22-8) and inferior pulmonary veins drain laterally, posterior to the left atrial appendage.

LEFT VENTRICLE

The left ventricle forms the left heart border. It is roughly oval-shaped. In cross section, it is circular, with the muscular interventricular septum acting as the medial portion of the left ventricle (Fig. 22-5). The left ventricle is two to three times as thick as the right ventricle, and its trabeculae carnae are somewhat smoother and flatter than in the right ventricle. The mitral valve annulus, both leaflets of the mitral valve, and their chordae tendinae form the inflow tract of the left ventricle. The inferior surface of the anterior leaflet of the mitral valve, the superior portion of the muscular ventricular septum, the superior membranous ventricular septum, and a portion of the anterior left ventricular free wall form the left

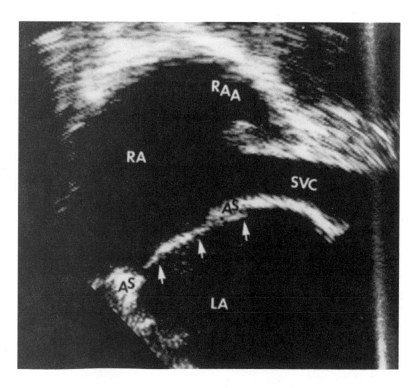

Figure 22-4   Biplane view of the limbus of the atrial septum (AS). (Reproduced with permission from Seward, et al., 1990.)

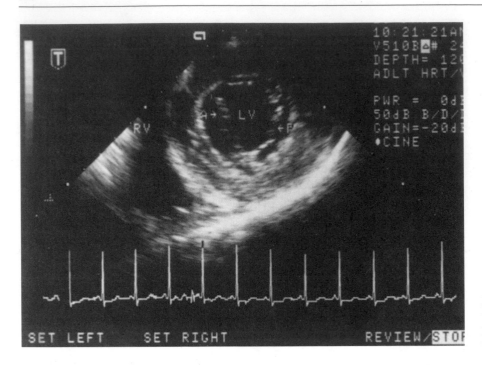

Figure 22–5 Short-axis view of the right ventricle (RV) and left ventricle (LV). (Reproduced with permission from Konstandt S, et al., 1993.)

ventricular outflow tract. The anterior leaflet of the mitral valve divides the inflow and outflow tracts.

☐ CARDIAC VALVES

TRICUSPID VALVE

The tricuspid valve attaches more apically than the mitral valve, such that the two atrioventricular (AV) valves do not lie in the same plane. The tricuspid valve has a nearly circular fibrous annulus. It is composed of three leaflets: anterior, posterior, and septal. The anterior leaflet is the largest. The septal leaflet, which is formed in part from the embryologic

endocardial cushion, attaches medially to the membranous portion of the interventricular septum (Figs. 22–6 and 22–9). Chordae tendinae attach the valve leaflets to the anterior, posterior, and septal papillary muscles.

PULMONIC VALVE

The pulmonic valve lies superior to the level of the aortic valve. It has no discrete annulus. Like the aortic valve, it is composed of three cusps: right, left, and anterior. The valve cusps also have fibrous thickening at their points of coaptation, although these areas are less prominent than in the aortic valve. Unlike the aortic valve, however, the pulmonic valve is

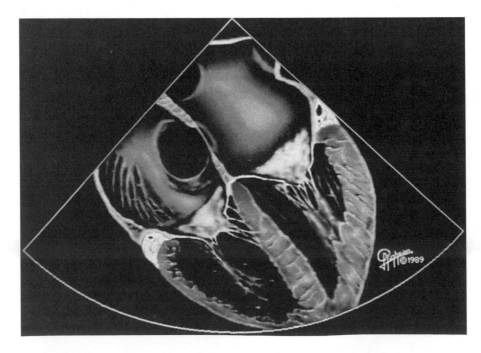

Figure 22–6 Artist's representation of TEE transverse plane four chamber view of the heart. (Reproduced with permission from Maurer G: *Transesophageal Echocardiography*. New York: McGraw-Hill, 1994.)

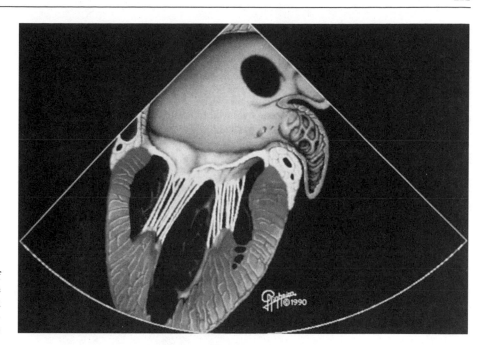

Figure 22–7 Artist's representation of TEE longitudinal two chamber view of the LA and LV. (Reproduced with permission from Maurer G: *Transesophageal Echocardiography*. New York: McGraw-Hill, 1994.)

separated from its AV (tricuspid) valve by the right ventricular outflow tract (Fig. 22–10). In contrast, the mitral and aortic valves are attached to each other at the ventricular septum.

MITRAL VALVE

The mitral valve is composed of an anterior and a posterior leaflet. The posterior leaflet has a true fibrous annulus, while the anterior leaflet attaches to the ventricular septum and to the left and noncoronary cusps of the aortic valve (Figs. 22–6, 22–7, and 22–11). Chordae tendinae attach the two mitral valve leaflets to the anterolateral and posteromedial papillary muscles.

AORTIC VALVE

The aortic valve is composed of three cusps: left, right, and noncoronary, also termed posterior (Figs. 22–12 and 22–13). The sinuses of Valsalva are the outpouchings in the aortic vessel wall behind each aortic cusp. The left and right coronary arteries originate in the sinus of Valsalva of the left and right cusps, respectively. The right and noncoronary sinuses are in contact with the right atrium and right ventricular outflow tract. The left sinus is adjacent to the left atrium and the superior portion of the interventricular septum. The points of contact of the aortic leaflets are marked by nodular fibrous thickenings, the noduli Arantii.

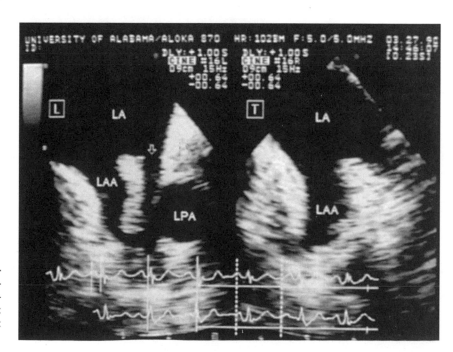

Figure 22–8 TEE view of the LA; left atrial appendage (LAA); LPA, left pulmonary artery. Arrow points to the left upper pulmonary vein. (Reproduced with permission from Maurer G: *Transesophageal Echocardiography*. New York: McGraw-Hill, 1994.)

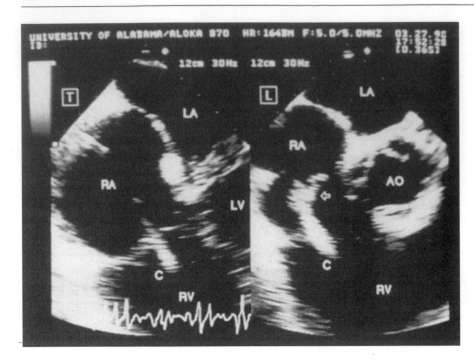

Figure 22–9 TEE image of tricuspid valve (TV) between RA and RV; C, catheter passing through TV. (Reproduced with permission from Maurer G: *Transesophageal Echocardiography.* New York: McGraw-Hill, 1994.)

☐ CONDUCTION SYSTEM

Although the landmarks of the cardiac conduction system are not grossly visible, familiarity with the location and arterial supply of the major portions of the cardiac conduction system is important for the anesthesiologist. In most hearts, the sinus node is located subepicardially lateral to the junction of the superior vena cava and the right atrium (Fig. 22–14). The blood supply to the sinus node is from the sinus node artery. In 55 to 60% of cases, the sinus node artery arises from the right coronary artery. In 40 to 45%, this vessel arises from the left circumflex artery. In approximately 10%, there is a dual blood supply.

The AV node is also located subepicardially within a triangle bounded by the orifice of the coronary sinus, the septal leaflet of the tricuspid valve, and the orifice of the inferior vena cava (Fig. 22–14). The AV nodal artery supplies the AV node. It arises from the right coronary artery (RCA) in 90% of cases and from the circumflex coronary artery in 10% of cases.

The distal portion of the AV node continues as the His bundle, which traverses the membranous interventricular septum. At the junction of the membranous and muscular portions of the interventricular septum, the His bundle divides to form the left and right bundle branches. The left bundle then further divides into anterior and posterior fasci-

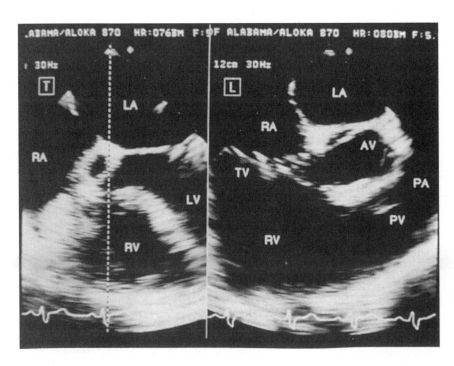

Figure 22–10 TEE view of RV outflow tract separating TV and pulmonic valve (PV). (Reproduced with permission from Maurer G: *Transesophageal Echocardiography.* New York: McGraw-Hill, 1994.)

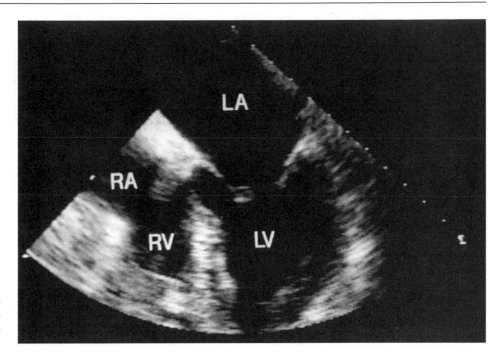

Figure 22–11 TEE longitudinal plane view of mitral valve (MV). (Reproduced with permission from Oh, Seward, and Tajik, 1994.)

cles. Branches of the left anterior and posterior descending coronary arteries supply the His bundle and the left and right bundle branches.

☐ CORONARY ARTERIES

The right and left coronary arteries (RCA and LCA, respectively) arise from the coronary ostia in the right and left sinuses of Valsalva. The RCA emerges behind the main pul-monary artery and passes underneath the right atrial appendage and into the AV sulcus. Its first branch is the conus artery, which can emerge separately from its own coronary ostium. The sinus node artery may arise as a branch of the RCA. The RCA then gives rise to several atrial and ventricular branches, including the large acute marginal branch, which supplies the anterior wall of the right ventricle. The RCA further contributes to the blood supply of the conduction system by giving off branches to the AV node and to the proximal bundle branches. In most cases, the posterior descending artery, which travels in the posterior interventricular

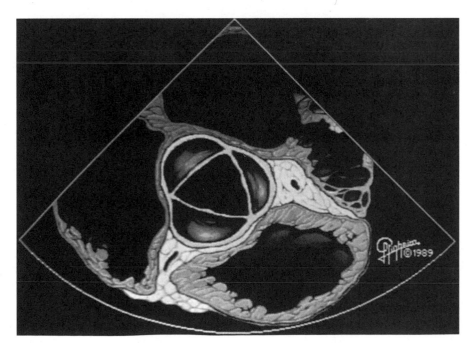

Figure 22–12 Artist's representation of short-axis view of the aortic valve (AV). (Reproduced with permission from Maurer G: *Transesophageal Echocardiography.* New York: McGraw-Hill, 1994.)

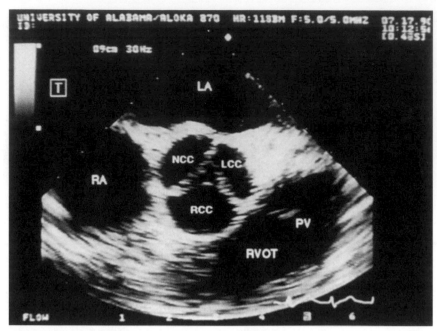

Figure 22–13   TEE short-axis view of AV. RCC, right coronary cusp; LCC, left coronary cusp; NCC, noncoronary cusp. (Reproduced with permission from Maurer G: *Transesophageal Echocardiography.* New York: McGraw-Hill, 1994.)

septum, is a branch of the RCA. This type of coronary anatomy is termed right dominant. The posterior descending coronary artery supplies the inferior, or diaphragmatic, walls of the left and right ventricles. Its branches, the septal perforators, supply the posterior septum. The terminal branches of the RCA supply the posterior aspect of the left atrium and ventricle.

The left main coronary artery emerges from behind the pulmonary artery and in front of the left atrium. It is variable in its length before dividing into the left anterior descending

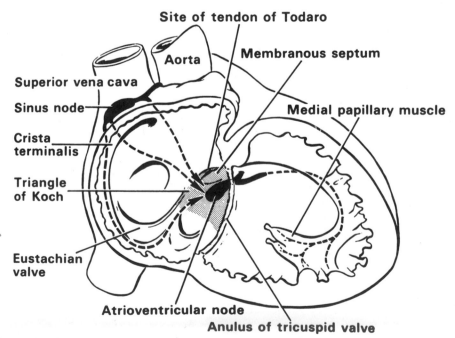

Figure 22–14   Location of sinus node at the entrance of the SVC into the RA. (Reproduced with permission from Waller and Schlant, 1994.)

(LAD) and left circumflex (LC) branches. The LAD branch lies in the interventricular sulcus. Its first branch, the first diagonal, supplies the lateral free wall of the left ventricle. Its second branch, the first septal perforator, supplies the interventricular septum. The LAD branch may or may not give rise to a right ventricular branch before giving off other septal perforators and other diagonal branches.

The LC branch travels in the left AV sulcus. Its branches include several anterior, lateral, and posterior branches to the left atrium. Its largest branch, the obtuse marginal (anterolateral marginal), supplies the lateral wall of the left ventricle. It also gives off a number of posterolateral marginals before terminating as the distal circumflex. In a minority (15%) of cases, the posterior descending coronary artery originates from the LC branch. This type of anatomy is termed left-dominant.

The transgastric short-axis view of the left ventricle at the midpapillary muscle level is used most commonly for intraoperative monitoring for ischemia. At this level, all three coronary arteries perfuse the left ventricle (Fig. 22–15).

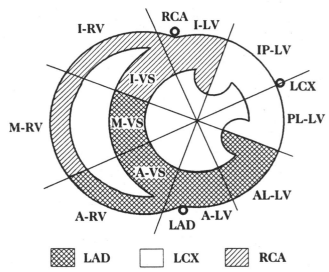

Figure 22–15   Artist's representation of blood supply of the left and right ventricles on TEE short-axis view. (Reproduced with permission from Maurer G: *Transesophageal Echocardiography.* New York: McGraw-Hill, 1994.)

BIBLIOGRAPHY

Cheitlin MD, Finkbeiner WE: Cardiac Anatomy, in Chaterjee K, Parmley WW (eds): *Cardiology: An Illustrated Text/Reference.* New York, Gower Medical, pp 1.2–1.18, 1991.

Choe YH, Im J-G, Park JH, et al: The anatomy of the pericardial space: a study in cadavers and patients. *Am J Radiol* 149: 693–697, 1987.

Konstandt S, Reich DL, Thys DM, Aronson S: Transesophageal Echocardiography, in Kaplan JA (ed): *Cardiac Anesthesia,* 3d ed. Philadelphia, Saunders, pp 342–385, 1993.

Nanda NC, Pinheiro L, Sanyal RS, et al: Transesophageal Biplane Echocardiographic Imaging: Technique and Image Planes, in Maurer G (ed): *Transesophageal Echocardiography.* New York, McGraw-Hill, pp 41–65, 1994.

Oh JK, Seward JB, Tajik AJ: *The Echo Manual.* Boston, Little, Brown, 1994.

Oliver WC, de Castro MA, Strickland RA: Uncommon Diseases and Cardiac Anesthesia, in Kaplan JA (ed): *Cardiac Anesthesia,* 3d ed. Philadelphia, Saunders, pp 819–864, 1993.

Seward JB, Khanderia BK, Edwards WD, et al: Transesophageal echocardiography: Technique, anatomic correlations, implementation, and clinical applications. *Mayo Clin Proc* 63:649–680, 1988.

Seward JB, Khanderia BK, Edwards WD, et al: Biplanar transesophageal echocardiography: Anatomic correlations, image orientation, and clinical applications. *Mayo Clin Proc* 65: 1193–1213, 1990.

Waller BF, Gering LE, Branyas NA, Slack JD: Anatomy, histology, and pathology of the cardiac conduction system: Part 1. *Clin Cardiol* 16(3):249–252, 1993.

Waller BF, Gering LE, Branyas NA, Slack JD: Anatomy, histology, and pathology of the cardiac conduction system: Part 2. *Clin Cardiol* 16(4):347–352, 1993.

Waller BF, Schlant RC: Anatomy of the Heart, in Schlant RC, Alexander RW (eds): *Hurst's the Heart: Arteries and Veins,* 8th ed. New York, McGraw-Hill, pp 59–111, 1994.

Watanabe H, Panopoulos J, Oka Y: TEE Assessment of Left Ventricular Function for Intraoperative Monitoring, in Maurer G (ed): *Transesophageal Echocardiography.* New York, McGraw-Hill, pp 257–276, 1994.

CHAPTER
23

Airway Anatomy, Innervation, and Embryology

Benjamin Gruber

☐ BASIC ANATOMY OF THE AIRWAY

OVERVIEW

It is easy to focus on the larynx and trachea when dealing with airway anatomy, but consideration of the nasal and oral air passages is also important (Fig. 23–1). The anesthesiologist should remember that structures are functionally interrelated, and obstruction of one component can significantly influence the overall management of the airway. For example, significant nasal obstruction will usually require the use of an oral airway during anesthetic induction. The surrounding structures, as well, are important. They provide structural support to the airway, and an abnormality in these areas can significantly alter the anatomy (e.g., compression of the oropharynx by a large carotid body tumor, or tracheal deviation from a substernal goiter). An otherwise normal larynx may appear unusual due to rotation and anterior displacement from an adjacent neck mass.

NASAL CAVITY, NASOPHARYNX, AND OROPHARYNX

Skeletal Considerations   The nasal cavity extends from the opening of the nostrils to the nasopharynx, a distance of roughly 8 cm in adults. The right and left nasal cavities are separated by the nasal septum, a rigid structure made of bone and cartilage. The septum may be very crooked, creating a tortuous passage. The lateral walls of each passage have bony protruberances covered with vasomotor tissue, known as turbinates. Only the inferior turbinate affects the nasal airway. The middle and superior turbinates are involved with the structure and function of the sinuses. It is important to re-

member that the nasal cavity is rigid and irregular and that there is a limit to the amount of space that can be obtained by topical decongestion. Significant damage to the intranasal structures can occur with forceful introduction of a nasogastric tube, a nasopharyngeal airway, or a nasotracheal tube. The size of a person's nostrils is not related to the critical dimensions within the nose itself.

The influence of the mandible on the airway should not be underestimated. The dimensions of the arch of the mandible are highly variable, even among individuals of the same age and sex. Although the distance from the teeth to the tip of the endotracheal tube is measured on the endotracheal tube, one should be cautious about accepting "normal" values or formulas for calculating this distance. Neither precludes selective mainstem intubation or accidental extubation during the surgical procedure.

Soft Tissue Considerations   The mucosa of the nasal cavity is vasomotor and responds to environmental or hormonal stimuli by vascular engorgement, causing a variable degree of nasal obstruction. Some individuals abuse over-the-counter topical decongestants, which may complicate the intraoperative management of hypertension. Nasal polyps are benign growths of the nasal mucosa that cause sinus and nasal airway obstruction. This condition is frequently associated with asthma, and the presence of nasal polyps should alert the anesthesiologist to potential for pulmonary problems. These patients are often remarkably free of obstructive symptoms, possibly because of the longstanding obstruction. Introduction of tubes and probes into the nose in these individuals may shear the polyps and cause bleeding or airway obstruction.

The pharyngeal airway is subject to obstruction by enlargement of the adenoids or tonsils and retrodisplacement of

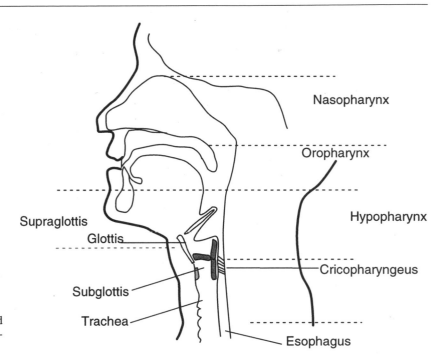

Figure 23–1 Sagittal section of adult head and neck showing major subdivisions of the upper airway.

a large tongue. The tissues of the hypopharynx have a tendancy to collapse without constant muscle tone of the pharyngeal musculature. Some individuals develop obstruction during sleep (sleep apnea), and these patients require special attention to the airway during anesthesia.

Innervation The sensory innervation of the nasal cavity and the nasopharynx is via the trigeminal nerve. Intense stimulation of the nasopharynx, such as with a posterior nasal pack or aggressive placement of a nasogastric or nasotracheal tube, can cause reflex hypopnea or bradycardia—the so-called nasopulmonary reflex. Sensory innervation of the oro- and hypopharynx involves cranial nerves V, VII, IX, and X. Coordinated control of the pharyngeal musculature by cranial nerves V, IX, X, XII, and XI indirectly maintains the patency of the pharyngeal airway during wakefulness and sleep.

LARYNX

Cartilage and Bony Skeleton The cartilage skeleton of the larynx provides a framework that prevents collapse of the airway and sites for attachment of the intrinsic and extrinsic musculature (Fig. 23–2). Some of the cartilage framework is especially flexible in infancy and later in life becomes ossified.

The largest and most prominent of the laryngeal cartilages is the shield-shaped thyroid cartilage, which is suspended from the hyoid bone by the thyrohoid membrane and ligaments. The hyoid bone itself is suspended from the skull base and mandible by the stylohoid ligaments and the digastric and mylohyoid muscles. Inferiorly, the hyoid bone and thyroid cartilage are attached to the sternum and clavicles by the strap muscles.

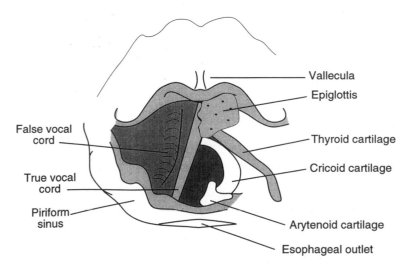

Figure 23–2 Half-cut section, viewed from above the glottis, showing the cartilagenous skeleton of the larynx.

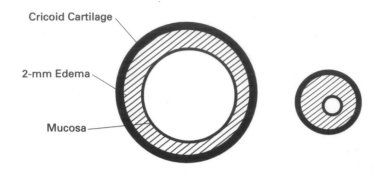

Cricoid Cartilage

2-mm Edema

Mucosa

| | Adult | | Infant | |
	Baseline	Postinjury	Baseline	Postinjury
Diameter (mm)	18	14	6	2
Percent decrease in airflow	—	53	—	96

Figure 23–3 Effect of 2 mm of postintubation edema on subglottic airway (level of cricoid) in an adult and an infant. These calculations are based on Poiseuille's equation and assume a constant driving pressure (respiratory effort or ventilating pressure), tracheal length, and gas viscosity as well as laminar flow conditions. When airflow is turbulent, the importance of the radius is even greater, since in the analogous equation it is raised to the fifth power.

The cricoid cartilage is the only structural element of the airway that forms a complete ring. The ring is signet-shaped, with the expanded lamina located posteriorly, fitting into the shield of the thyroid cartilage. Laterally, a true joint is formed where the cricoid cartilage meets the lateral alae of the thyroid cartilage.

Because the cricoid is the only complete ring of the larynx and tracheobronchial tree, it represents the limiting dimension of the airway. This has important clinical implications. Placement of too-large an endotracheal tube can cause injury to the subglottic mucosa where it is compressed against the unforgiving cricoid cartilage. This is especially true in very small children, where the internal diameter of the cricoid ring may be only 6 mm. The development of acquired subglottic stenosis following intubation in the neonate may be more

likely to occur in those children with a congenitally small cricoid ring.

In an airway of small dimensions, even a small amount of tissue injury and edema result in a significant change in airflow. For a given driving pressure, laminar airflow in a tube such as the trachea is proportional to the tube's radius raised to the fourth power (Fig. 23–3). For this reason, laryngotracheobronchitis ("croup") is rarely seen in children over the age of 5 years.

Perched superiorly on the posterior lamina of the cricoid cartilage are the paired arytenoid cartilages (Fig. 23–4). Movement of these cartilages in relationship to the thyroid and cricoid cartilages open and close and tense the vocal cords. Schematically, each arytenoid cartilage can be viewed as a pyramid with a triangular base. The vocal cord is at-

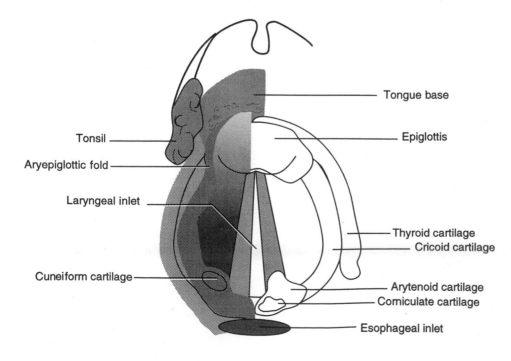

Figure 23–4 Half-cut section, viewed from a point superior and posterior to the glottis, revealing a "spine's eye view" of the airway, the major cartilaginous articulations of the larynx, and the attachments of the vocal cords.

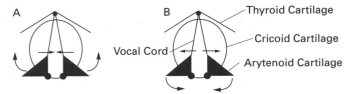

Figure 23–5 Action of cricoarytenoid muscles. (*A*) The lateral cricoarytenoid muscle causes anterior displacement of the muscular process of the arytenoid cartilage, adducting (closing) the vocal cords. (*B*) Contraction of the posterior cricoarytenoid muscle results in posterior displacement of the muscular process, abducting (opening) the vocal cords.

tached to the anterior corner of the triangle (vocal process), and the lateral and posterior cricoarytenoid (CA) muscles insert into the lateral corner (muscular process). The cartilage can then rotate on a vertical axis (Fig. 23–5). The CA joint is subject to fixation from trauma and can also be a site of rheumatic joint disease, especially in juvenile rheumatoid arthritis. Fixation of the CA joint can cause dysphonia, hoarseness, aspiration, and/or airway obstruction.

Two pairs of minor cartilages are also present in the supraglottic larynx. The corniculate cartilage sits atop the arytenoid cartilage, and the cuneiform cartilage is located floating within the aryepiglottic fold. These small cartilages are clinically important only when they are disproportionately large and contribute to the supraglottic collapse in congenital laryngeal stridor (laryngomalacia).

Vocal Cords The vocal cords are formed by the vocal ligaments, the vocal processes of the arytenoid cartilages, and their covering epithelium. The constant trauma of the vocal folds slamming and vibrating against each other during the respiratory cycle and vocalizations is tolerated because this stratified squamous epithelium continuously replaces its cells. The vocal ligaments are the thickened, superior-free edges of the conus elasticus, a well-developed layer of elastic tissue that arises from the upper border of the cricoid cartilage. Anteriorly, in the midline, the two edges of the conus elasticus come together to attach to the inner surface of the thyroid cartilage, forming the anterior commissure. Posteriorly, the ligaments are attached to the mobile arytenoid cartilages. The fibers of the vocalis muscle run parallel and just lateral to the vocal ligaments and also insert into the vocal process of the arytenoid cartilage.

Musculature The dynamic action of the vocal cords allows the larynx to serve two antagonistic functions. Adequate airflow through the larynx requires the vocal cords (glottis) to be open (abduction). Protection against aspiration and vocalization both require a closed glottis (adduction). In humans, the use of the larynx for speech is possible due to the high degree of specialized development of the laryngeal musculature. However, even the lowest amphibian uses its larynx for vocalization.

Four paired groups of muscles and one unpaired muscle act to close the vocal cords, while only one paired muscle

group opens the glottis. The adductor group includes the cricothyroid, lateral cricoarytenoid, interarytenoid, and the vocalis muscles. The interarytenoid muscle is unique among all the muscles of the body in that it receives bilateral innervation. Only the posterior cricoarytenoid muscles abduct the vocal cords (Fig. 23–5). Those muscles that act on the vocal cords by changing the relationship and orientation of the laryngeal cartilages are referred to as intrinsic laryngeal muscles. Extrinsic muscles attach the laryngeal cartilages to the surrounding structures, such as the esophagus, hyoid bone, mandible, skull base, and clavicles, and move the larynx as a unit. The cricopharyngeus, inferior constrictor, digastric, mylohyoid, styohyoid, and strap muscles are all extrinsic laryngeal muscles.

Innervation
Sensory
Sensation to the larynx is carried by cranial nerves IX and X. The tongue base and lingual surface of the epiglottis are innervated by branches of the glossopharyngeal nerve. Some of these nerve fibers carry the special sense of taste as well. The majority of the supraglottic structures and the laryngeal inlet are innervated by the superior laryngeal nerve (SLN), while the interior of the larynx and upper trachea are innervated by the recurrent laryngeal nerve (RLN). The SLN leaves the main trunk of the vagus high in the neck and divides into internal and external branches. The internal laryngeal nerve is only sensory, while the external branch has primarily motor fibers. Damage to the SLN from thyroid or other neck surgery can result in chronic aspiration and/or a change in pitch and strength of the voice (see "Motor").

Motor
The extrinsic muscles of the larynx receive their motor nerve supply from cranial nerves V, VII, IX, X, and XI. The intrinsic laryngeal muscles are all supplied by branches of the vagus nerve. The superior laryngeal nerve supplies the cricothyroid muscle, the primary function of which is to alter the tension in the vocal cords, thereby changing the pitch of the voice. This muscle also acts as an adductor in synergism with the other adducting muscles. All other intrinsic muscles of the larynx are supplied by the RLN. The major motor innervation of the larynx arises from a branch of the vagus nerve that is related to the sixth aortic arch in early embryogenesis. As the heart "descends" into the thoracic cavity, the laryngeal nerve is "pulled" with it. A portion of the sixth arch on the right disappears, resulting in looping of the recurrent nerve around the fourth arch, which later develops into the right subclavian artery. On the left, the sixth arch persists as the ductus arteriosis and later as the ligamentum arteriosum. It is possible, although rare, for either or both nerves to be nonrecurrent. The RLN divides into a posterior abductor branch, supplying primarily the posterior cricoarytenoid muscle, and an anterior adductor branch. Vocal cord paralysis due to injury to the RLN is common and results in hoarseness and/or aspiration or airway obstruction (see next page).

TRACHEA AND BRONCHIAL TREE

A complete discussion of bronchial anatomy is beyond the scope of this chapter. However, a brief description of the tracheobronchial anatomy will aid in understanding the structure of the airway.

The framework of the trachea and major bronchi is made up of C-shaped cartilagenous "rings" connected by fibroelastic tissue. Smooth muscle fibers, oriented transversely, are located between the rings. In small children, these muscles can cause tracheospasm, a reactive airway condition analogous to asthma, causing intermittent stridor.

The rings are roughly the same size until the trachea branches into the right and left mainstem bronchi at the carina. There are generally 15 to 20 rings in the trachea, which measures roughly 11 cm from the cricoid cartilage to the carina (in the adult male), which occurs at about the level of the sternal angle. The trachea deviates to the right side of the vertebral column just before it divides; hence, the left mainstem bronchus is longer than the right by approximately the width of a vertebral body. The right mainstem bronchus tends to be more in line with the trachea, while the left mainstem bronchus comes off at a more oblique angle. Thus, an endotracheal tube or an inhaled foreign body is more likely to go into the right mainstem than the left. In small children, however, the difference in angle is not so great, and foreign bodies are as likely to be found in the left as in the right bronchus.

The mainstem bronchi each divide into lobar bronchi. On the right, there is an upper, a middle, and a lower lobe bronchus, while on the left side there is only an upper and lower lobe bronchus. They, in turn, subdivide into the bronchopulmonary segments, the basic functional unit of the lung, each having its own bronchus and branch of the pulmonary artery. On the right side, there are generally 10 bronchopulmonary segments, and the left usually has 8 segments.

The sensory innervation of the tracheobronchial tree is entirely via the vagus nerve. Sensory receptors are primarily of the irritant receptor type. Motor innervation to the bronchial smooth muscle is via the vagus and sympathetic nerves.

☐ EMBRYOLOGY OF THE AIRWAY

NASAL CAVITY, NASOPHARYNX, AND OROPHARYNX

The oral cavity begins as a depression in the head of the embryo, the stomodeum. The nasal cavity develops separately as an invagination of the nasal placode (primitive olfactory organ). The embryogenesis of each of these cavities is intimately related to that of the other and to the development of the face. By the fifth week of gestation, the major primodia of these structures are all formed.

LARYNX

Organogenesis of the larynx occurs during a period of rapid embryonic development from 4 to 8 weeks of gestation. During this time, the embryo grows from only a few millimeters in length to approximately 3 cm. By the end of the embryonic period (8 weeks), the larynx is a well-developed organ, with identifiable cartilagenous and muscular structures.

The developing larynx and trachea are first seen as a midline ventral groove in the embryonic foregut as early as 20 days' gestation, when the embryo is less than 3 mm in length. Once the respiratory primordium begins to descend, forming the lung buds, the digestive and respiratory passages develop along independent courses. Swellings on the floor of the pharynx, which will later form the arytenoid cartilages, and a laryngeal inlet are identifiable at approximately 32 days' gestation (5 to 7 mm). Between the arytenoid swellings, a platelike collection of epithelial cells develops (epithelial lamina). A triangular condensation of undifferentiated mesenchyma forming the laryngeal primordium can be seen surrounding the respiratory diverticulum at roughly 33 days' gestation (7 to 9 mm). At approximately 37 days' gestation, the primordia of the superior and recurrent laryngeal nerves are evident, and the pharyngotracheal canal becomes patent within the epithelial lamina. By 40 days' gestation (11 to 14 mm), the larynx is clearly identifiable, and cellular differentiation of the cartilaginous and muscular structures begins. The cricoid cartilage begins as a ventral condensation. The cricoid ring is complete at around 44 days' gestation, at which time the concave shape of the epiglottis is also defined. Over the next 2 weeks of gestation, further cellular rearrangement, cavitation, and sculpting occur, with delineation of the major laryngeal cartilages and muscle groups.

The physiologic development of the laryngeal muscles depends more on the swallowing reflex than on respiratory movements. The reciprocation of glottic closure and cricopharyngeal opening during swallowing and glottic opening with cricopharyngeal closure during respiration is the key in developing the dynamic function of the larynx. The cricoid cartilage acts as the common fulcrum for both musculature valves.

During the third month of gestation, there is a ventral fusion of the lamina of the thyroid cartilages, and further cartilaginous development of the arytenoid and cricoid cartilages. The laryngeal ventricle and saccule become clearly defined, and the lining differentiates into pseudostratified columnar epithelium with a definite basement membrane. Swallowing activity is first observed during this period. Further differentiation of the cartilage framework, along with development of glandular elements, takes places through the remainder of fetal development and continues into the first decade or more of postnatal life.

TRACHEA AND BRONCHIAL TREE

The respiratory diverticulum develops in a rostral-to-caudal sequence (i.e., the larynx develops before the pulmonary structures). The pulmonary primordium is first identifiable at about 22 days' gestation and divides into a right and left bud shortly thereafter. The lung buds begin to descend from the pharynx at approximately day 26. The trachea is evident as a separate luminal structure at about 28 days' gestation, and development of cartilage rings can be seen as early as day 40 of gestation. Tracheal mucous glands are evident by the end of the fourth month, and the main elements of the respiratory tree are formed by the sixth month of intrauterine development. Development of the tracheobronchial tree and lungs continues throughout the first 7 years of life.

☐ AIRWAY VARIATIONS

DIFFERENCES BETWEEN THE ADULT AND THE NEONATAL AND PEDIATRIC AIRWAY

Location of Larynx   In the infant, the larynx is located higher in the neck and can be elevated so that the epiglottis slides up behind the soft palate into the nasopharynx. The superior border of the larynx may be as high as the first cervical vertebra. When the edges of the soft palate seal against the lateral pharyngeal walls, the respiratory pathway becomes separate from the oral cavity and the digestive tract. This enables the infant to suckle and breathe simultaneously, and explains why newborn infants are obligate nose breathers. The ability to swallow liquids while breathing is progressively lost after 6 months of age. There is a gradual descent of the tongue base into the neck during the first 5 years of life, resulting in a lowering of the larynx. In the adult, the considerable separation between the larynx and the soft palate requires that the hypopharynx function both as an air passage and as a food conduit. This change in anatomic relationship allows food impaction to cause airway obstruction ("cafe coronary").

Differences in Laryngeal Anatomy   In addition to the difference in location, there are several important anatomic considerations in the larynx of the young child. The newborn larynx is roughly one-third the size of the adult larynx. Because the larynx is located high in the neck, the hyoid cartilage (bone) can be anterior, rather than superior, to the thyroid cartilage. The shape of the epiglottis is more tubular in the small child, assuming the configuration of the Greek letter omega (Ω). The lumen of the larynx is larger than the trachea in the infant, and the cricoid cartilage is the limiting dimension in this "funnel." The subglottic airway extends backward and downward in the infant, whereas it is nearly vertical in the adult. This is important to consider when intubating a small child, since the curve of the endotracheal tube is opposite to the natural configuration of this portion of the airway.

Differences in Tracheal Anatomy   When viewed endoscopically in the newborn child, the trachea is often ovoid in

Table 23–1 TRACHEAL DIMENSIONS (cm)

Dimension	Infant (1 year)	Child (10 years)	Adult Male	Adult Female
Diameter of trachea	0.6–0.7	0.8–1.1	1.5–2.2	1.3–1.8
Length of trachea (cricoid to carina)	4.7	7	8.5–15	10
Distance from upper incisors to carina	12	17	26	23

cross section, compressed in the anteroposterior dimension, whereas the anteroposterior dimension of the adult trachea is usually greater that the lateral dimension. The flexibility of the tracheal and bronchial cartilage in the infant allows for extrinsic compression by the vascular structures in the neck and mediastinum. In severe cases, this can cause airway obstruction and/or recurrent pneumonia. The cervical portion of the trachea in a small child is longer than the thoracic portion, since the carina is generally at the level of the third thoracic vertebra. In the adult, the thoracic portion of the trachea is longer, and the carina is approximately at the level of T5 (See Table 23–1).

CONGENITAL ANOMALIES

For a complete description of congenital anomalies of the airway, the reader is referred to textbooks on pediatric otolaryngology and/or craniofacial disorders. Only a few commonly encountered conditions are discussed here. Most congenital anomalies that cause airway compromise are clinically evident within hours of birth. Others present as chronic respiratory problems within the first few months of life.

Upper Airway Anamolies   Pierre Robin syndrome is felt to be due to lack of adequate development of the mandibular primordium prior to 9 weeks' gestation, causing the tongue to be located more posteriorly and thereby interfering with the closure of the palatal shelves. This results in varying degrees of mandibular hypoplasia and a rounded cleft palate. The degree of mandibular hypoplasia causes varying degrees of airway obstruction, making these children difficult, if not impossible, to intubate with a rigid laryngoscope. Many of these children require tracheostomy. If allowed to thrive, these patients will eventually outgrow their mandibular deficit.

Mandibulofacial dysostosis, or Treacher Collins syndrome, is an autosomal dominant disorder characterized by downward slanting eyes, malar hypoplasia, mandibular hypoplasia, external and middle ear anomalies, and cleft palate.

In these patients, as well, the relative underdevelopment of the mandible may narrow the airway to an extent where a temporary tracheostomy is required.

Other congenital conditions associated with hypoplasia of the mandible (facio-auriculo-vertebral spectrum) can result in airway anatomy that is sufficiently altered so that routine intubation is not possible.

The most common craniofacial anomaly, cleft lip with or without cleft and palate, does not cause airway obstruction when no additional anomalies are present. Other craniofacial syndromes may include varying degrees of nasal obstruction as part of the midface anomaly, but generally no intervention is necessary.

Failure of the oronasal membrane to disintegrate during embryogenesis results in choanal stenosis or atresia. Because newborns are obligate nose breathers, a child with this condition obstructs unless it is crying and breathing through its mouth. Unilateral stenosis or atresia is sometimes undiagnosed until the child is several years old. A unilateral atresia rarely causes airway problems, but the persistent nasal discharge eventually prompts a thorough evaluation.

Laryngeal Anomalies   A great variety of laryngeal anomalies have been described, most presenting as severe airway problems in the newborn. Minor abnormalities may not present until approximately 6 months. Congenital vocal cord paralysis presents as a hoarse, weak cry in the newborn. Airway compromise is usually not a problem, and the condition is frequently self-limited. Some cases of congenital vocal cord paralysis are associated with an intracranial pathologic condition involving the posterior fossa. Congenital cysts and webs present as stridor and may occur in any portion of the larynx. Subglottic hemangioma is a space-occupying lesion of the airway that will eventually regress, usually by age 2 years. However, serious airway compromise usually requires intervention (laser excision and/or tracheostomy).

Congenital Laryngeal Stridor   A fairly common condition in the very young child is laryngomalacia, or congenital laryngeal stridor. This presents as coarse inspiratory stridor, and infants frequently have more severe symptoms while supine than when they are prone. A variety of mechanisms contribute to the supraglottic collapse during inspiration in this condition, including immaturity of the laryngeal musculature, structural immaturity (malacia) of the epiglottis, and redundancy of the aryepiglottic folds and mucosa overlying the arytenoid cartilages. This disorder rarely persists beyond 12 weeks of age.

COMMONLY SEEN ANATOMIC VARIATIONS

Variants in the Epiglottis   In some individuals, the epiglottis retains its omega shape from childhood. This is a completely normal condition and is referred to as infantile epiglottis. In others, the epiglottis is unusually curled or extremely short, even apparently absent when performing routine laryngoscopy. If there is redundant pharyngeal mucosa in the

hypopharynx, the latter two conditions may make intubation difficult. Mucosal cysts of the epiglottis are occasionally encountered and are for the most part asymptomatic and require no treatment. These cysts, however, can become quite large and cause airway obstruction, especially in small children.

Benign and Malignant Lesions of the Vocal Cords   Vocal cords are normally white and glistening. Any change from this represents a pathologic condition, most of which fortunately are benign. Vocal cord polyps and nodules are common and usually symptomatic because of the resultant hoarseness. Polyps can completely obstruct the laryngoscopist's view of the vocal cords in a patient with surprisingly few symptoms of obstruction. Occasionally this mild or intermittent laryngeal obstruction caused by the vocal cord polyps is manifested by a wheeze, and the patient has been misdiagnosed as having asthma. Masses of granulation tissue (granulomas) can be seen in previously intubated patients (posttraumatic) or in individuals with severe gastroesophageal reflux. Callus-like lesions are generally the result of overuse of the voice. Laryngeal papillomas, a virally induced neoplasm related to venereal warts, are important to recognize because dislodging pieces of these lesions during intubation can result in implantation of the tumor fragments in the distal tracheobronchial tree. Malignant lesions of the vocal cords are generally exophytic and friable, and bleeding can result from the intubation process. The anesthesiologist has the opportunity to significantly affect the patient's care if a small lesion can be identified as an incidental finding during routine intubation for an unrelated elective procedure (Table 23–2).

COMMONLY ENCOUNTERED CLINICAL PROBLEMS

Hypognathia   In newborn infants, underdevelopment of the arch of the mandible, such as in the Pierre Robin syndrome, can cause airway obstruction by retrodisplacement of the tongue base. In adults, however, the tongue base is below the mandible, and the patient with a receding jaw has little if any airway problems, except under anesthesia. In addition to presenting extremely challenging intubation problems, maintenance of an adequate pharyngeal airway before intubation may be difficult in such patients. Awake fiberoptic intubation is often recommended in these instances.

Sleep Apnea Habitus   Many obese patients have sleep apnea, a condition manifested by upper airway obstruction during sleep. This disorder may be present without the individual's being aware of the problem or present to the anesthesiologist in preparation for elective nonairway surgery. While awake, these persons have no airway problems, and it is up to the anesthesiologist to anticipate airway problems before they develop. Some of these patients have enormous tonsils and/or adenoid tissue or an extremely large and thick tongue, which makes visualization of the posterior pharynx difficult. Most patients, however, have no obvious cause of

Table 23-2
COMMONLY ENCOUNTERED PATHOLOGIC CONDITIONS OF THE VOCAL CORDS

Pathologic Condition	Laryngoscopic Appearance	Location on Vocal Cord
Nodule	Small, submucosal bump	Junction of anterior and middle thirds
Polyp	Pale, grapelike, smooth, mucosa-covered	Anterior or entire cord
Granuloma	Red, friable, round, bleeding	Posterior
Leukoplakia	Flat, white, rough surface	Anterior
Papilloma	Pale red, irregular, may be multiple, bleeds easily, pedunculated, microcobblestone surface	Anywhere in larynx
Squamous carcinoma	Irregular; friable; red, white, or pale; alters structure of surrounding tissue	Anywhere in larynx, but primarily anterior third of cord (early)

their obstruction, which is said to be due to anatomic disproportion of the pharyngeal structures—slightly retrognathic, moderate tonsils, moderately enlarged tongue, thick soft palate—all of which add up to not having enough room to breathe. The anesthesiologist should also be aware of enlarged lingual tonsils. This diffuse lymphoid tissue of the tongue base can obscure the larynx during intubation, and edema in this tissue after a traumatic intubation can cause obstruction after extubation. Every massively obese patient and every patient with a history of sleep apnea should be treated as a difficult airway and approached cautiously, anticipating the possible use of fiberoptic intubation and/or nasopharyngeal airways after extubation. Some patients will require nasotracheal intubation or tracheostomy postoperatively.

Special mention should be made of adult and pediatric patients with trisomy 21 (Down's syndrome). These patients often have an extremely large tongue and relative hypognathia, and control of the oropharyngeal airway is difficult. Such individuals may or may not have diagnosed sleep apnea or cervical spine instability.

Obstructing Pharyngeal and Laryngeal Tumors As with obese patients, individuals with known tumors of the upper airway should be treated cautiously. Close cooperation between the anesthesiologist and the otolaryngologist is essential to avoid emergency situations in these patients. The otolaryngologist may say that there was no problem visualizing the larynx in the office, but this does not mean that intubation will be easy. Moreover, even if the intubation is uneventful, the trauma from the surgical procedure can frequently cause enough edema to result in airway obstruction postoperatively. The safest approach to these patients is tracheostomy under local anesthesia (sedated) before induction.

Vocal Cord Paralysis Injury to the RLN and vocal cord paralysis can occur from both iatrogenic and natural mechanisms. Natural causes include carcinoma of the lung, thyroid cancer, thoracic aortic aneurysm, traction neuropathy from violent coughing or vomiting, mediastinal inflammatory disease, and idiopathic neuropathy. Common iatrogenic causes of RLN injury are thyroidectomy, anterior cervical disk fusion, carotid artery surgery, and cardiac surgery (e.g., patent ductus ligation). Vocal cord paralysis is also occasionally seen following endotracheal intubation and upper gastrointestinal endoscopy, the mechanism of which is poorly understood.

Tracheal Compression This condition is most often encountered in patients with large thyroid masses, usually of the multinodular goiter type. The larynx and trachea can be displaced laterally to a surprising degree. Laryngeal anatomy is often distorted. Adequate visualization of the larynx can be extremely difficult with a rigid laryngoscope, and intubation may be problematic. In these situations, use of a flexible fiberoptic laryngoscope is recommended. The placement of the endotracheal tube must checked carefully to avoid obstruction of the tube in the tortuous trachea.

Laryngectomy Individuals who have had the larynx removed in the treatment of cancer have complete separation of the airway and the digestive tract. These patients breathe only through the hole in their neck and often, but not always, through a tracheostomy tube. The nasal and oral cavities and pharynx are no longer connected to the tracheobronchial tree. Delivery of oxygen via nasal cannula or face mask is therefore of no benefit. Delivery of respiratory gasses is directed to the tracheostoma.

BIBLIOGRAPHY

Crelin ES: Development of the upper respiratory system. *CIBA Clin Symp* 28(3), 1976.

Hollingshead WH: *Anatomy for Surgeons: The Head and Neck*, vol. 1, 3d ed. Philadelphia, Harper & Row, 1982.

CHAPTER
24

Basic Physics for Anesthesiologists

Robin Chorn

☐ THE GAS LAWS

MOLECULAR THEORY

All substances are composed of atoms or compounds of atoms, that is, molecules. In a solid, the atoms or molecules are regularly arranged in a lattice in which each molecule exerts a force upon its neighbor; in a liquid, these forces have broken down due to the application of heat energy, and the substance has melted. If more heat is added to the liquid, the molecules escape from the surface of the liquid and are able to move about freely in space; this is a gas, or vapor.

Avogadro's hypothesis states that equal volumes of gases at the same temperature and pressure contain the same number of molecules. Note that equal volumes of different gases at the same temperature and pressure have different masses but that the number of particles is the same.

THE GAS LAWS

The first gas law, or Boyle's law, states that at *constant temperature* the volume of a given mass of gas varies inversely with the absolute pressure. That is, if pressure is doubled, the volume will halve. Hence,

$$V = \frac{1}{P} \text{ and } P \times V = k \tag{1}$$

The second gas law, or Charles's law, states that at *constant pressure* the volume of a given mass of gas is directly proportional to its absolute temperature. That is, if the temperature is doubled, the volume of gas will double. Hence,

$$V \propto T \text{ and } \frac{V}{T} = k_2 \tag{2}$$

The third gas law states that at *constant volume* the absolute pressure of a given mass of gas varies directly with the absolute temperature. That is, if the temperature is doubled, the pressure will double. Hence,

$$P \propto T \text{ and } \frac{P}{T} = k_3 \tag{3}$$

The concept of the perfect gas laws can be combined with Avogadro's hypothesis and the mole as follows:

$$PV = k_1; \quad \frac{V}{T} = k_2; \quad \frac{P}{T} = k_3 \tag{4}$$

Therefore,

$$PV = nRT \tag{5}$$

where n = number of moles of gas
T = absolute temperature
R = universal gas constant, $8.3 \text{ J} \cdot \text{mol}^{-1} \cdot \text{K}^{-1}$

CRITICAL TEMPERATURE

When a liquid boils it becomes a vapor; if pressure is applied to the vapor, it can be liquefied even though the temperature of the liquid is above its boiling point. However, eventually a temperature will be reached at which no amount of pressure will liquefy the vapor. This temperature is the *critical temperature*, defined as the temperature above which a substance cannot be liquefied regardless of the amount of pressure applied.

The distinction between a vapor and a gas is thus: a vapor can be converted back to liquid if sufficient pressure is applied (because the temperature is below its critical temperature), while a gas can never be liquefied. By this definition, the volatile agents are vapors (they are obviously not gases, because they exist in liquid form at room temperature and are thus below their respective critical temperature), while oxygen is definitely a gas: no amount of pressure will convert it back to liquid at room temperature because its critical temperature is $-119°C$. Nitrous oxide (N_2O) may be both in the clinical situation: its critical temperature is $36.5°C$ and may therefore be a gas (in the tropics or if the air-conditioning fails) or a vapor. The *critical pressure* is that vapor pressure exerted by the substance at its critical temperature.

Entonox (50% O_2 and 50% N_2O) has no real critical temperature because the term applies to a single gas. However, there is a specific "critical temperature" at which Entonox may split into its two constituent gases; this is known as a pseudo-critical temperature and is *not* analogous to critical temperature as explained above. If the cylinder temperature falls below $-5.5°C$, Entonox may separate into N_2O and O_2. The initial gas delivered will be oxygen, followed by nitrous oxide as the tank empties, which will result in delivery of a hypoxic gas mixture.

☐ PRESSURE

DEFINITIONS

Pressure is defined as force applied per unit area. In the SI system, the unit of pressure is the pascal (Pa), and 1 Pa equals a force of 1 newton (N) acting over 1 m². Because 1 Pa is a very small pressure, the kilopascal (kPa) is used. A non-SI unit, the bar (which equals 100 kPa), is also in common usage and is approximately equal to atmospheric pressure at sea level (1 atm).

$$P = \frac{f}{a} \tag{6}$$

where P = pressure, Pa
f = force, N
a = area, m²

GAUGE AND ABSOLUTE PRESSURES

In most cases, we use gauge pressures when comparing pressures. When a cylinder is empty, the gauge reads 0, but there is still "ambient" pressure (1 atm) within the cylinder (unless a vacuum pump has been used to completely evacuate the cylinder). Hence, the absolute pressure within the cylinder equals 1 atm:

Absolute pressure = gauge pressure +

atmospheric pressure (7)

PRESSURE IN LIQUIDS

The pressure in a column of water (or other liquid) is independent of the cross-sectional area of the column and varies only with the height (and density) of the column of liquid. The reasoning is as follows:

$$f = m \cdot g \text{ (from Newton's second law)} \tag{8}$$

where f = force, N
m = mass, kg
g = acceleration, m/s²

From above,

$$P = \frac{f}{a} \tag{9}$$

Therefore, the pressure exerted by the column of liquid equals the force exerted by the liquid over the cross-sectional area of the column:

$$P = \frac{m \cdot g}{a} \tag{10}$$

Now, the mass of any fluid is a function of the density and volume of the fluid such that mass divided by volume equals density (ρ, rho) in kilograms per cubic meter as follows:

$$\rho = \frac{\text{mass}}{\text{volume}} \tag{11}$$

and therefore

$$m = \rho \cdot \text{volume} \tag{12}$$

Therefore, substituting Eq. 12 into Eq. 10, we get

$$P = \frac{\rho \cdot \text{volume} \cdot g}{a} \tag{13}$$

Now, the volume of a liquid in a cylinder equals the cross-sectional area times the height of the column, or

volume (m³) = area (m²) × height (m) (14)

Substituting Eq. 14 into Eq. 13 yields the following:

$$P = \frac{\rho \cdot \text{area} \cdot \text{height} \cdot g}{a} \tag{15}$$

Since the area measurements in the numerator and denominator cancel, we finally arrive at the relationship between pressure and the height of a column of liquid.

$$P = \rho \cdot h \cdot g \tag{16}$$

Since g (the acceleration due to gravity) is a constant, the only variables that determine the pressure of a column of liquid are the density of the liquid and the height of the column; the pressure of a column of liquid is not a function of the cross-sectional area of the column.

☐ FLUID FLOW

LAMINAR FLOW

Flow is the quantity of fluid (gas, blood, etc.) in liters or milliliters, passing a given point in unit time. The analogy with electric current is well-established, in which current strength (in amperes) is equivalent to fluid flow, because an ampere is a quantity of charge (electrons) per unit time. This leads to the common expression:

$$V = I \times R \qquad (17)$$

where V = voltage or potential difference (analogous to pressure difference)

I = current strength (analogous to fluid flow or cardiac output)

R = resistance (analogous to systemic vascular resistance)

For hemodynamics, the expression is

$$BP = CO \times SVR \qquad (18)$$

where BP = blood pressure, mmHg or torr

CO = cardiac output, L/min

SVR = systemic vascular resistance, dyn · s/cm^{-5} (unit derived from blood pressure divided by cardiac output)

In laminar flow, fluid moves steadily through the tube (e.g., blood vessel or bronchus) without turbulence or eddies. This normally occurs in smooth tubes at low rates of flow. The flow is greatest at the center of the tube, being about twice the mean flow, while at the walls of the tube, the flow may be so slow as to approach 0. Of note is that in laminar flow, flow is a function of the pressure difference across the ends of the tube (i.e., resistance is constant) and is equal to the ratio of the pressure to the flow. The Hagen-Poiseuille equation describes this relationship mathematically:

$$\Delta Q = \frac{\Delta P \pi r^4}{8 \eta l} \qquad (19)$$

where ΔQ = flow rate

ΔP = pressure difference across ends of tube

r = radius of tube

η = viscosity of the fluid, Pa · s, or poise

l = length of tube through which fluid flows

By substitution, resistance R (which equals pressure divided by flow) can be seen to be equal to the following:

$$R = \frac{8 \eta l}{\pi r^4} \qquad (20)$$

Thus, resistance is directly proportional to the viscosity of the fluid and the length of the tube and inversely proportional to the fourth power of the radius of the tube.

TURBULENT FLOW

In turbulent flow, fluid no longer flows in a smooth fashion but swirls and eddies, with higher resistance than for the same laminar flow. Turbulent flow is not directly proportional to pressure, and resistance is not constant for the system but varies with the flow. The mathematical relationships are as follows:

$$\Delta Q \propto \frac{\sqrt{P}}{\sqrt{\rho l}} \qquad (21)$$

where ΔQ = flow

P = pressure across ends of tube

l = length of tube

ρ = density of fluid (as opposed to viscosity in laminar flow)

From this, it can be seen that the property of the fluid important in turbulent flow is the density, which equals mass divided by volume (kg · m^{-3}).

An index known as the Reynolds number (Re) can be used to determine whether, in any given system, fluid flow will be predominantly laminar or turbulent. The Re is calculated as follows:

$$Re = \frac{v \rho d}{\eta} \qquad (22)$$

where v = linear velocity of fluid in tube

ρ = density of fluid

d = diameter of tube

η = viscosity of fluid

If Re exceeds about 2000, the flow is likely to be turbulent, whereas if Re is less than 2000, the flow is likely to be laminar. It can be seen that as the velocity and the density of the fluid increase and as the viscosity of the fluid decreases, the likelihood of turbulent flow increases. This is the rationale for the use of helium in respiratory disorders, because the density of the inhaled gases, and thereby the incidence of turbulent flow, is reduced. A lower resistance to breathing results because the transition from turbulent to laminar flow is associated with a marked decrease in resistance to flow through a tube.

☐ ELECTRICITY

AMPERES AND CURRENT MEASUREMENT

The ampere (A) is the unit of current in the SI system and is equal to a flow of 6.24×10^{18} electrons per second past a given point (i.e., 1 C/s). A coulomb (C) equal 6.24×10^{18} electrons.

When a current flows, heat and light are produced. A potential difference must be present across the ends of the wire (or other electrical device) in order for the electrons to flow through the device. This is analogous to the idea that a pressure difference must be present in order for fluid to flow through tubing. The unit of potential difference is the volt (V), defined as the potential difference required to produce a current of 1 amp when the rate of energy dissipation is 1 watt:

$$\text{Volts} = \frac{\text{power (watts)}}{\text{current (amperes)}} \qquad (23)$$

Because a current of 1 A is equal to 1 C/s and a power of 1 W equals a rate of energy expenditure of 1 joule per second (J/s), Eq. 23 can also be written as:

$$1\text{ V} = \frac{1\text{ J}}{1\text{ C}} \qquad (24)$$

From Eq. 24, it can be seen that the volt is a measure of the energy (joules) required to move an amount of electric charge (coulombs). Resistance, measured in ohms (Ω), is the ratio between the potential difference and the flow of current (i.e., what potential difference is required to produce a given flow of electrons):

$$\text{Resistance }(\Omega) = \frac{\text{volts}}{\text{amperes}} \qquad (25)$$

Again, the analogy with fluid dynamics is clear, in which systemic vascular resistance (SVR) is a measure of the blood pressure required to produce a given cardiac output.

ELECTRICAL SAFETY

When the flow of electric current through a person is excessive, there is the risk of electric shock and burns. In order to understand how this arises, consider how electricity is supplied to the hospital. If a person touches a live wire in the hospital, an electric current can be completed through that person's body, to the earth, and back to the supply station. The effect of the shock perceived depends on the size of the current that flows. From Eqs. 23 through 25:

$$\text{Current (amperes)} = \frac{\text{potential difference (volts)}}{\text{resistance }(\Omega)} \qquad (26)$$

where resistance implies the total impedance to current flow presented by the person, including the person's skin, footwear, and so on. If this is, for example, 240 kΩ, then the current flow will be small:

$$\text{Current} = \frac{120\text{ V}}{240{,}000\ \Omega} = 0.50\text{ mA} \qquad (27)$$

which is barely discernible to the person. However, skin impedance is not constant, and assuming the person is standing in a pool of conductive fluid (e.g., saline solution) holding faulty apparatus, he or she may be subject to a significant shock because the person's impedance to the current may be only 5000 Ω, resulting in a current of 24 mA (Table 24–1).

The risk of ventricular fibrillation is increased by additional factors, such as the timing of the arrival of the impulse at the heart. The risk is also much greater if the current

Table 24–1
EFFECTS OF A 60 Hz CURRENT ON AN AVERAGE HUMAN FOR A 1 s CONTACT

Current, mA	Effect
MACROSHOCK	
1	Threshold of perception
5	Maximum harmless current
10–20	"Let-go" current; above this, the person would not be able to let go due to sustained muscle contraction
50	Pain, injury, fainting; cardiorespiratory function continues
100–300	Ventricular fibrillation; respiratory center still intact
6000	Sustained myocardial contraction, then normal heart rhythm; temporary respiratory paralysis
MICROSHOCK	
0.1	Ventricular fibrillation
0.01	Maximum leakage current at 60 Hz

passes through the heart during the phase of repolarization of muscle cells (during the early T wave of the electrocardiogram). Another factor is the form of the electric pulse. Mains alternating current of 50 to 60 Hz is more dangerous than a very high-frequency current of 1000 Hz or more. Note from the table that very small currents are able to cause ventricular fibrillation if they pass directly through the heart, as may occur during cardiac catheterization or the placement of pacemaker leads, and so on (see Table 24-1, under "Microshock").

☐ VAPORIZERS

A vaporizer is a device for adding a clinically useful concentration of anesthetic vapor to a stream of carrier gas. Vaporizers are classified according to various specifications, including their ability to deliver constant concentrations of vapor in spite of fluctuating temperatures, their specificity for anesthetic agents, the method used for varying the concentration of vapor, the method of vaporization, and the position in the breathing circuit.

According to this classification, the Dräger vaporizer is a temperature-compensated, agent-specific, variable-bypass, flow-over, out-of-circuit vaporizer.

TEMPERATURE COMPENSATION

Temperature compensation is an important characteristic of vaporizers. Indeed, all modern vaporizers employ some method of compensating for changes in temperature. The need for temperature compensation is apparent when one realizes that, as an anesthetic agent is vaporized, it takes heat (the latent heat of vaporization) from the remaining fluid and from the surrounding vaporizer walls, resulting in a fall in temperature of the remaining fluid. A fall in temperature renders the anesthetic agent less volatile and thus reduces the amount of anesthetic vaporized, thereby rendering the concentration dialed on the vaporizer inaccurate.

Most vaporizers utilize a property of metal known as the coefficient of expansion. In the Fluotec vaporizers, a bimetallic strip (consisting of two metals with different coefficients of expansion bonded together) bends or straightens, depending on the temperature, thereby allowing more or less vapor to flow through the vaporizer and thus compensating for reduced vaporization at lower temperatures.

FLOW DEPENDENCE

Since the saturated vapor pressure of volatile anesthetic agents at room temperature is many times greater than that required for clinical anesthesia, vaporizers reduce their output by splitting the gas flowing into the vaporizer into two streams. One stream passes through a vaporizing chamber, while the other bypasses the vaporizing chamber and flows through the bypass channel. These two streams are then reunited in the appropriate ratio to produce a clinically useful concentration and delivered to the patient.

PRESSURE EFFECTS ON THE VAPORIZER

Gas is supplied to the vaporizer at a constant flow rate from the rotameters, but during intermittent positive-pressure ventilation there is intermittent back pressure from the ventilator, which can be transmitted to the vaporizer outlet. This intermittent back pressure can cause gas containing a volatile agent to flow into the bypass channel (which is usually free of anesthetic agent) and thereby increase the output concentration of the vaporizer. This is known as the pumping effect.

The pumping effect can be overcome by the use of a valve downstream of the vaporizer to prevent the transmission of back pressure from the ventilator to the vaporizer. Also, a long inlet channel to the vaporizing chamber can be provided so that retrograde flow from the vaporizing chamber does not reach the bypass channel.

USE AT HYPERBARIC PRESSURE

The depth of anesthesia is dependent on the partial pressure of anesthetic vapor rather than its percentage. Thus, at higher than normal ambient pressures, the vaporizer may deliver a reduced percentage of vapor but at the same partial pressure as before; hence, the depth of anesthesia should be unaltered. For example, if the ambient pressure is 100 kPa (1 atm) and the vaporizer delivers 1% halothane, the partial pressure of the halothane is 1 kPa (1% of 100 kPa).

If the ambient pressure is doubled to 200 kPa, the saturated vapor pressure of the halothane in the vaporizer is unchanged: vapor pressure is affected only by temperature. Hence, the vaporizer will still deliver 1 kPa halothane, although the percentage of halothane will be reduced, from 1 to 0.5% (i.e., from 1% of 100 kPa to 0.5% of 200 kPa).

VAPORIZER POSITION

The vaporizers should be positioned between the flowmeters and the fresh gas outflow, and the emergency O_2 flush should be between the patient's breathing circuit and the vaporizers, so that the O_2 flush cannot be delivered through the vaporizer. In addition, the order of vaporizers on the vaporizer manifold should be in increasing vapor pressure from flowmeters to patient (e.g., enflurane 175 mmHg, then isoflurane 239 mmHg, and then halothane 243 mmHg). This procedure ensures that the more volatile agents cannot contaminate the less volatile agents with traces of anesthetic vapor.

☐ NATURAL EXPONENTIAL FUNCTIONS

In an exponential process, the rate of change of a quantity at any given time is proportional to the quantity at that time. We commonly encounter three types of exponential functions in anesthesia and medicine: the wash-in, or buildup, curve; the washout curve; and the breakaway curve.

The wash-in curve describes the buildup of anesthetic agent in the alveoli at the commencement of anesthesia as the rate of rise of alveolar gas over inspired gas approaches unity, that is, as F_A/F_I approaches 1 (Fig. 24–1).

The washout curve describes the rate of decline of anesthetic gas in the alveoli at the termination of anesthesia, when the inspired concentration is reduced to 0 (Fig. 24–2).

The breakaway curve (or compound interest curve) is described by, for example, a colony of bacteria growing in the presence of excess substrate (Fig. 24–3).

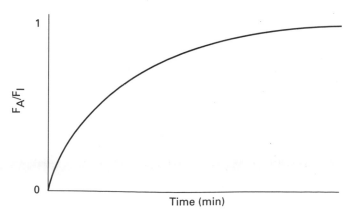

Figure 24–1 Depiction of how alveolar concentration (F_A) approaches inspired concentration (F_I) over time.

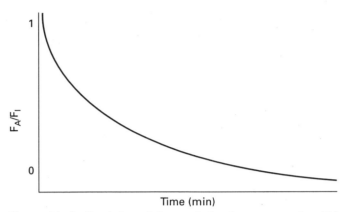

Figure 24-2 Depiction of decay of alveolar concentration (F_A) relative to inspired concentration (F_I) over time.

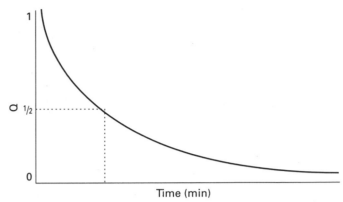

Figure 24-4 The half-life is the time taken for the quantity to fall to half its initial value.

HALF-LIFE AND TIME CONSTANT

In exponential processes in which the quantity is diminishing (Fig. 24-2), it never actually reaches 0. Consequently, the total length of time taken for the process is infinite, and the total time cannot be used to measure the process. Two alternative concepts are used: the half-life and the time constant. At one half-life (Fig. 24-4), the measured quantity (Q) decreases to half its initial value; at two half-lives, the quantity falls to one-quarter its initial value; at three half-lives, it falls to one-eighth its initial value, and so on.

As an alternative to the half-life, the rate of an exponential process can be measured by its time constant. The time constant is the time at which the process would have been complete had the initial rate of change continued unaltered. The time constant is symbolized by τ (tau), as shown in Fig. 24-5. Note that after one time constant, the quantity Q has fallen to 37% of its initial value. Therefore, the time constant is longer than the half-life. If lung expiration has a time constant of 0.3 s, then after 0.3 s, only 37% of the tidal volume is left to be exhaled; after 0.6 s, 13.7% is left (37% of 37%); and after three time constants (0.9 s), only 5% of the tidal volume is left. Therefore, expiration is 95% complete after three time constants.

☐ SOLUBILITY

If a liquid is placed in a closed container, an equilibrium is established between the vapor of the liquid and the liquid itself in which the partial pressure exerted by the vapor is known as the saturated vapor pressure. In this situation, the equilibrium occurs when dissolved gas molecules leave the liquid at the same rate as others enter the liquid.

In any given liquid-vapor equilibrium in a closed container, the amount of gas dissolved in the liquid is proportional to the pressure of the gas above the liquid, provided the temperature is kept constant. This principle is known as Henry's law, which states that at a particular temperature the amount of a given gas that is dissolved in a given liquid is directly proportional to the partial pressure of the gas in equilibrium with the liquid.

It is a general principle that as a liquid is warmed, less gas is dissolved in the liquid. This is observed when boiling water: as the water temperature increases, gas solubility decreases, and bubbles form in the water due to air coming out of solution. The liquid is also relevant when considering the solubility of gases. Different liquids have different capacities for a given gas at a given temperature. In summary, then, the solubility of a gas depends on the partial pressure, the temperature, and the gas and liquid concerned.

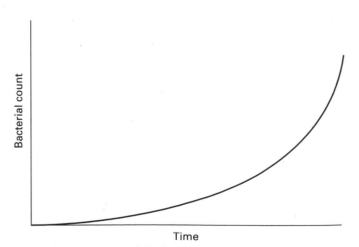

Figure 24-3 Exponentially increasing bacterial count in the presence of unlimited nutrient.

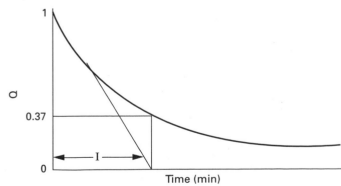

Figure 24-5 After one time constant (τ), the quantity Q has fallen to 37% of its initial value.

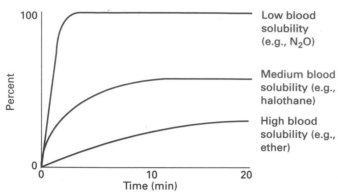

Figure 24–6 Alveolar concentration of anesthetic as a percentage of inspired concentration.

In anesthetic practice, the Ostwald solubility coefficient is used to describe the amount of gas dissolved in a given liquid. The Ostwald solubility coefficient is the volume of gas that dissolves in one unit volume of the given liquid at a given temperature. The Ostwald coefficient is independent of pressure. For example, water dissolves 16 mL nitrogen at 20°C, whereas blood dissolves 470 mL nitrous oxide at 37°C. These values demonstrate the wide variability of various gases to be dissolved in various liquids at various temperatures.

Solubility coefficients have clinical applications when considering anesthetic gas uptake and distribution. It is well known that ether is highly soluble in blood (12 L of ether per liter of blood), while halothane is moderately soluble (2.3 L/L of blood), and N_2O is insoluble (470 mL/L of blood). Because of its great solubility, ether is carried away from the lungs more rapidly than halothane or N_2O, and hence the concentration of ether in the alveolar air builds up more slowly than that of a less soluble anesthetic. Therefore, induction (and emergence) takes much longer with ether than with halothane or N_2O.

Figure 24–6 shows graphs of alveolar concentrations of anesthetic agents against time during the phase of rapid anesthetic uptake. It can be seen from Fig. 24–6 how the rate of rise of alveolar concentration of anesthetic agent will be delayed in the case of the soluble agents. With insoluble agents, there is a rapid rise of alveolar concentration and hence a rapid onset of anesthetic induction. Solubility of anesthetic agents in oil correlates closely with potency (the Meyer-Overton theory of anesthesia). An anesthetic with a high oil solubility is effective at low alveolar concentrations and has a high potency.

☐ DAMPING AND RESONANCE

Direct (invasive) pressure monitoring utilizes saline solution-filled tubing that transmits the force of the pressure pulse wave to a transducer that converts the beat-to-beat pressure changes into voltage changes. These voltage changes are then amplified, filtered, and displayed as the pressure tracing on the monitor. Analysis of the arterial pressure wave indicates that the frequencies present are between 1 and 30 Hz (cycles per second); most of the frequency components are below 10 Hz.

The fidelity of any fluid-coupled transducing system is constrained by two properties: damping (ζ, zeta) and the natural frequency (F_0) of the system. Zeta describes the tendency of the fluid in the measuring system to resist or extinguish motion. The F_0 describes the tendency of the measuring system to resonate, or vibrate.

Zeta and F_0 must be optimized to permit the to-and-fro movement of the coupling tubing and transducer to faithfully reproduce the range of frequencies contained in the pressure wave being measured. The bandwidth describes the range of frequencies from 0 Hz to the system's F_0 (the frequency at which resonance occurs). Conventional disposable transducers have bandwidths of approximately 20 to 30 Hz.

Optimally damped systems have a bandwidth of approximately two-thirds (0.68) of F_0; that is, the maximum measured frequencies are usually less than two-thirds of the resonating frequency. If the F_0 approaches the frequency found in the measured wave, estimates of the systolic pressure will increase because the fluid-filled system resonates. Ideally, the measured frequencies are well below the resonating frequency of the measuring system.

Studies have demonstrated that fidelity is optimized by stiff catheters and tubing when the mass of the fluid is small, the length of the tubing is short, and the number of stopcocks is limited. The resonant frequency of the system should be as high as possible. Air bubbles lower the natural frequency of the system.

In practice, underdamped systems overestimate systolic pressure by 15 to 30 torr. Excessive increases in ζ (overdamping) reduce fidelity and lead to underestimation of the pressure. Mean pressures are generally accurately monitored even when damping and resonance are not optimal. In practice, the typical clinical system has a damping coefficient $\zeta = 0.2$ to 0.3, even though the optimal damping coefficient is predicted at about 0.6 to 0.7 (see above).

BIBLIOGRAPHY

Barker SJ, Tremper KK: Physics Applied to Anesthesia. In Barash PG, Cullen BF, Stoelting RK (eds): *Clinical Anesthesia,* 2nd ed. JB Lippincott Company, 1992.

Litt L: Electrical Safety in the Operating Room. In Miller RD (ed): *Anesthesia,* 4th ed. Churchill Livingstone Inc, 1994.

Parbrook GD, Davis PD, Parbrook EO: *Basic Physics and Measurement in Anesthesia,* 2nd ed. New York, Appleton-Century-Crofts, 1986.

Index

ISBN 0-07-069134-7

90000>